Renal Handling
of Phosphate

Renal Handling of Phosphate

Edited by
Shaul G. Massry, M.D.

University of Southern California School of Medicine
Los Angeles, California

and
Herbert Fleisch, M.D.

University of Berne
Berne, Switzerland

Plenum Medical Book Company
New York and London

Library of Congress Cataloging in Publication Data

Main entry under title:

Renal handling of phosphate.

Includes index.
1. Kidneys. 2. Phosphorus metabolism. 3. Renal tubular transport. I. Massry, Shaul G. II. Fleisch, H.
QP249.R43   596'.01'49   79-18651

ISBN-13: 978-1-4615-9154-2   e-ISBN-13: 978-1-4615-9152-8
DOI: 10.1007/978-1-4615-9152-8

© 1980 Plenum Publishing Corporation
Softcover reprint of the hardcover 1st edition 1980
227 West 17th Street, New York, N.Y. 10011

Plenum Medical Book Company is an imprint of Plenum Publishing Corporation

To Our Wives

MEIRA MASSRY

MARIA PIA FLEISCH

.

Contributors

CLAUDE AMIEL, M.D. • Department of Physiology, Faculty of Medicine Xavier Bichat, Université Paris 7, Paris, France

LOUIS V. AVIOLI, M.D. • Department of Medicine, Division of Bone and Mineral Metabolism, Washington University School of Medicine and The Jewish Hospital of St. Louis, St. Louis, Missouri 63110

NORMAN BANK, M.D. • Department of Medicine, Albert Einstein College of Medicine, and Renal, Electrolyte, and Hypertension Division, Montefiore Hospital and Medical Center, Bronx, New York 10467

OLAV L. M. BIJVOET, M.D. • Clinical Investigation Unit, Department of Clinical Endocrinology and Metabolism, University Hospital, Leiden, The Netherlands

JÜRGEN BOMMER, M.D. • Sektion Nephrologie, Medizinische Universitätsklinik, D-6900 Heidelberg, Germany

JEAN-PHILIPPE BONJOUR, M.D. • Department of Pathophysiology, University of Berne, 3010 Berne, Switzerland

NACHMAN BRAUTBAR, M.D. • Division of Nephrology. Department of Medicine, University of Southern California School of Medicine, Los Angeles, California 90033

RUSSELL W. CHESNEY, M.D. • Pediatric Renal Disease Laboratory, Department of Pediatrics, The University of Wisconsin Center for the Health Sciences, Madison, Wisconsin 53792

JENNIFER W. CHILDERS, B.S., R.N. • Department of Physiology and Biophysics, University of Tennessee Center for the Health Sciences, Memphis, Tennessee 38163

THOMAS P. DOUSA, M.D., Ph.D. • Departments of Medicine and Physiology, Mayo Clinic and Foundation, Rochester, Minnesota 55901

GARABED EKNOYAN, M.D. • Department of Medicine, Baylor College of Medicine, and Medical Services, Harris County Hospital District, Texas Medical Center, Houston, Texas 77030

EDWARD M. FITZGERALD, B.S. • Department of Physiology and Biophysics, University of Tennessee Center for the Health Sciences, Memphis, Tennessee 38163

HERBERT FLEISCH, M.D. • Department of Pathophysiology, University of Berne, 3010 Berne, Switzerland

SARAH D. GLEASON, B.S. • Department of Physiology and Biophysics, University of Tennessee Center for the Health Sciences, Memphis, Tennessee 38163

MARTIN GOLDBERG, M.D. • Department of Medicine, University of Cincinnati College of Medicine, Cincinnati, Ohio 45267

STANLEY GOLDFARB, M.D. • Department of Medicine, Renal Electrolyte Section, University of Pennsylvania School of Medicine and Hospital of the University of Pennsylvania, Philadelphia, Pennsylvania 19104

ROBERT C. HANSON, Ph.D. • Department of Physiology and Biophysics, University of Tennessee Center for the Health Sciences, Memphis, Tennessee 38163

ANZELM HOPPE, M.D. • Department of Clinical Biochemistry, Medical Academy, 80-211 Gdansk, Poland

STEPHEN A. KEMPSON, Ph.D. • Department of Physiology and Biophysics, Mayo Clinic and Foundation, Rochester, Minnesota 55901

FRANKLYN G. KNOX., M.D., Ph.D. • Department of Physiology and Biophysics, Mayo Clinic and Foundation, Rochester, Minnesota 55901

WILHELM KREUSSER, M.D. • Sektion Nephrologie, Medizinische Universitätsklinik, D-6900 Heidelberg, Germany

KAI LAU, M.D. • Department of Medicine, Renal Division, University of Michigan School of Medicine, Ann Arbor, Michigan 48109

GERHARD MALNIC, M.D. • Department of Physiology, University of São Paulo, Institute of Biomedical Sciences, São Paulo, Brazil

MANUEL MARTINEZ-MALDONADO, M.D. • Department of Medicine and Physiology, University of Puerto Rico Medical School, and Medical Service, Veterans Administration Center, San Juan, Puerto Rico 00936

SHAUL G. MASSRY, M.D. • Division of Nephrology, Department of Medicine, University of Southern California School of Medicine, Los Angeles, California 90033

ROBERT A. PERAINO, M.D. • Department of Medicine, Baylor College of Medicine, Houston, Texas 77030

EBERHARD RITZ, M.D. • Sektion Nephrologie, Medizinische Universitätsklinik, D-6900 Heidelberg, Germany

EDWARD G. SCHNEIDER, M.D. • Department of Physiology and Biophysics, University of Tennessee Center for the Health Sciences, Memphis, Tennessee 38163

SUDHIR V. SHAH, M.D. • Department of Physiology and Biophysics, Mayo Clinic and Foundation, Rochester, Minnesota 55901

WADI N. SUKI, M.D. • Department of Medicine, Renal Section, Baylor College of Medicine and The Methodist Hospital, Houston, Texas 77030

Foreword

When Shaul Massry and Herbert Fleisch asked me to write a foreword for this book, I was honored and eagerly looked forward to reading the many chapters. As they came and I skimmed through them, my mind wandered back to the earliest classic contributions in this field in the late 1920s and early 1930s by Albright and his associates, Greenwald and Gross and Adolph, on the homeostatic regulation of inorganic phosphate and the central role of parathyroid hormone (PTH) in this regulation. They clearly showed the exquisite sensitivity of the renal handling of phosphate to varying dietary and parenteral loads and to changes in the level of PTH.

That two outstanding investigators in the field of divalent ion metabolism should choose to edit a book solely about the renal handling of inorganic phosphate shows how far we have progressed from these early classics to the recent almost exponential increase in the research and publications related to this subject. Despite this increase, I asked myself, is such a large new monograph, consisting of 13 chapters and 30 distinguished authors, warranted? My reading of these chapters and my learning so much from them convinced me that it is, and my pride was heightened in being asked to write the foreword for this book.

It is clear that the kidney has the most fundamental responsibility for the regulation of the concentration of inorganic phosphate in the body fluids and thereby, indirectly, for the cellular content of the organic phosphate compounds controlling all metabolism. Bijvoet, in his introductory chapter, most lucidly and incisively delineates the primacy of the renal tubular handling of phosphate in this regulation through his conclusive formulation of the concept of the renal threshold concentration, or Tm_{PO_4}/GFR. The subsequent chapters beautifully elucidate the intrarenal mechanisms for phosphate transport within various segments of the nephron and thus how the normal and diseased kidney fulfill this regulatory role.

Drs. Massry and Fleisch carefully chose those major known factors affecting the renal excretion of phosphate, and they then selected a group of authors, each of whose investigation has greatly contributed to our understanding of how a given factor influences the renal tubular transport of phosphate. Each author and his associates have written a critical in-depth analysis of their work and the relevant literature. Some chapters stress the systematic review of the literature, while others give a more synthesizing, integrative presentation with various conceptual models.

The net effect is that the reader can "whet his appetite" in every conceivable way. A "horn of plenty" is presented from which the reader can select the answer to almost every question or, at least, see the question discussed from almost every perspective.

The basic theme and objective of the editors was to leave nothing untold or unevaluated up to the time the authors submitted their chapters. They have fulfilled their goal.

Charles R. Kleeman, M.D.

Los Angeles

Preface

In recent years, we have witnessed a tremendous expansion in the knowledge related to the various processes involved in the regulation of phosphate metabolism. The central role of the kidney in the maintenance of phosphate homeostasis becomes quickly evident. Many laboratories all over the world have directed their efforts to delineate the renal and extrarenal processes, as well as the hormonal and nonhormonal factors involved in the control of the renal handling of phosphate. These investigations have furthered our understanding of the field and have provided a wealth of valuable information pertinent to the basic physiology and to the clinical pathophysiology of phosphate metabolism. It seems, therefore, that a book which presents the pertinent information on the renal handling of phosphate is both timely and useful.

In preparing this book, we attempted to have distinguished authorities contribute to this multiauthored monograph. We were most fortunate to have been able to achieve this goal. All of the chapters are written by scientists who contributed greatly to our understanding of phosphate homeostasis. Their investigations supplied, and continue to provide, new information to this ever-expanding field. We are most appreciative of their efforts.

We wish to give special thanks to Ms. Gracy Fick for her valuable assistance, which she performed with patience, dedication, and devotion.

Shaul G. Massry, M.D.
Herbert Fleisch, M.D.

Los Angeles and Berne

Contents

Chapter 1
INDICES FOR THE MEASUREMENT OF THE RENAL
HANDLING OF PHOSPHATE
Olav L. M. Bijvoet

1. Introduction 1
2. Glomerular Filtration and Tubular Transport 2
   2.1. The Composition of the Glomerular Filtrate 2
   2.2. The Direction of Tubular Transport 4
   2.3. The Concept of a Limit or Threshold Concentration ... 5
3. Threshold Concentration and Splay for Phosphate 9
   3.1. The Relation between Maximum Reabsorption and
        Glomerular Filtration 9
   3.2. Splay 11
4. Indices for the Measurement of the Renal Handling of
   Phosphate 17
   4.1. The Renal Threshold Concentration for Phosphate 17
   4.2. The Phosphate Clearance 19
   4.3. The Reabsorbed or Excreted Fraction of the Load 20
   4.4. The Excretion Rate of Phosphate 24
   4.5. The Plasma Phosphate Concentration 25
   4.6. The Choice between Indices 29
5. References 32

Chapter 2
SITES OF RENAL TUBULAR REABSORPTION
OF PHOSPHATE
Claude Amiel

1. Introduction 39
2. Phosphate Transport between the Glomerulus and the Late
   Accessible Proximal Convolution of the Superficial Nephron   39

2.1. Phosphate Reabsorption in the Intact Animal 39
2.2. Phosphate Reabsorption in the Absence of Parathyroid
     Hormone 42
2.3. Phosphate Secretion in the Proximal Tubule 43
3. Phosphate Transport in the Loop 45
   3.1. Evaluation by Micropuncture of the Late Accessible
        Proximal and Early Accessible Distal Convolutions
        Sampled at Random 45
   3.2. Evaluation by Micropuncture of the Late Accessible
        Proximal and Early Accessible Distal Convolutions of
        the Same Nephron 45
   3.3. Evaluation by Microinjection into the Late Accessible
        Proximal and Early Accessible Distal Convolutions 47
   3.4. Evaluation by *in Vivo* Microperfusion 47
   3.5. Evaluation by *in Vitro* Microperfusion 48
   3.6. Characteristics of Loop Phosphate Reabsorption 48
4. Phosphate Transport in the Terminal Nephron 50
   4.1. Evaluation by Micropuncture 50
   4.2. Evaluation by Distal Tubular Microperfusion and
        Microinjection 52
   4.3. Possible Sites of Phosphate Reabsorption in the
        Terminal Nephron 54
5. Conclusions 54
6. References 55

Chapter 3
IS PHOSPHATE SECRETED BY THE KIDNEY?

Edward G. Schneider, Robert C. Hanson, Jennifer W. Childers,
Edward M. Fitzgerald, and Sarah D. Gleason

1. Introduction 59
2. Phosphate Secretion by Kidneys of Lower Vertebrates 61
   2.1. Fishes 61
   2.2. Amphibians 62
   2.3. Reptiles 63
   2.4. Birds 65
   2.5. Summary of Phosphate Secretion by Nonmammalian
        Vertebrates 65
3. Is Phosphate Secreted by the Mammalian Kidney? 65
   3.1. Use of Clearance Techniques to Assess Phosphate
        Secretion by the Mammalian Kidney 65

    3.2. Evidence of a Peritubular-to-Luminal Flux of
         Phosphate in the Mammalian Kidney 69
 4. Conclusions 76
 5. References 76

Chapter 4
CELLULAR MECHANISMS OF PHOSPHATE TRANSPORT
Franklyn G. Knox, Anzelm Hoppe, Stephen A. Kempson,
Sudhir V. Shah, and Thomas P. Dousa

1. Introduction 79
 2. Transmembrane Movement of Phosphate 80
    2.1. Membrane Composition and Structure 80
    2.2. Phosphate–Membrane Interactions 83
    2.3. Enzymes of the Brush-Border Membrane 84
 3. Characteristics of Phosphate Transport 87
 4. Nonhormonal Factors 89
    4.1. Sodium Dependency of Phosphate Transport 89
    4.2. Glucose and Phosphate Transport 91
    4.3. Effect of Acid–Base Balance on Phosphate Transport . 93
 5. Hormonal Regulation of Phosphate at the Cellular Level ... 96
    5.1. Mechanism of Regulation by Cyclic Nucleotides 96
    5.2. Other Cellular Mechanisms in Regulation of Phosphate
         Transport 103
 6. References 104

Chapter 5
THE EFFECTS OF PARATHYROID HORMONE ON RENAL
PHOSPHATE HANDLING
Kai Lau, Stanley Goldfarb, and Martin Goldberg

1. Introduction 115
 2. Effects of PTH in Various Segments of the Nephron 116
    2.1. Proximal Convoluted Tubule 116
    2.2. Pars Recta—Loop of Henle 117
    2.3. Distal Convoluted Tubule and Terminal Nephron 118
 3. Mode of Action of PTH 120
 4. Mechanism of the Phosphaturic Effect of PTH 122
    4.1. Role of Adenyl Cyclase-cAMP System 123

    4.2. Role of Inhibition of Sodium Reabsorption—Sodium-
        Dependent Phosphate Transport Hypothesis 126
    4.3. Role of Tubular Fluid Alkalinization 128
  5. References 130

Chapter 6

EFFECTS OF HORMONES OTHER THAN PARATHYROID
HORMONE ON RENAL HANDLING OF PHOSPHATE

Eberhard Ritz, Wilhelm Kreusser, and Jürgen Bommer

1. Introduction 137
2. Growth Hormone (GH) 138
    2.1. Effects of GH on Serum Pi Levels 138
    2.2. Extrarenal Effects of GH on Pi Metabolism 139
    2.3. Effects of GH on Renal Handling of Pi 139
    2.4. Factors Related to the Effects of GH on Tubular
        Transport of Pi 141
3. Vasopressin (Antidiuretic Hormone; ADH) 142
    3.1. Effects of ADH on Serum Pi Levels 142
    3.2. Effects of ADH on Renal Handling of Pi 142
4. Thyroid Hormones (Thyroxine and Triiodothyroine) 145
    4.1. Effects of Thyroid Hormones on Serum Pi Levels 145
    4.2. Extrarenal Effects of Thyroid Hormones on Pi
        Metabolism 146
    4.3. Effects of Thyroid Hormones on Renal Handling of Pi   147
    4.4. Factors Related to the Effects of Thyroid Hormones
        on Renal Handling of Pi 148
5. Calcitonin (CT) 151
    5.1. Effects of CT on Serum Pi Levels 151
    5.2. Extrarenal Effects of CT on Pi Metabolism 152
    5.3. Renal Effects of CT 152
    5.4. Factors Related to the Effects of CT on Renal
        Handling of Pi 154
6. Glucagon 157
    6.1. Effects of Glucagon on Serum Pi Levels 157
    6.2. Effects of Glucagon on Renal Handling of Pi 157
    6.3. Factors Related to the Effects of Glucagon on Renal
        Handling of Pi 158
7. Insulin 159
    7.1. Effects of Insulin on Serum Pi Levels 159
    7.2. Effects of Insulin on Renal Handling of Pi 160

    7.3. Factors Related to the Effects of Insulin on Renal
           Handling of Pi 161
8.   Catecholamines 163
    8.1. Effects of Catecholamines on Serum Pi Levels 163
    8.2. Effects of Catecholamines on Renal Handling of Pi 163
9.   Glucocorticoids 167
    9.1. Effects of Glucocorticoids on Serum Pi Levels 167
    9.2. Extrarenal Effects of Glucocorticoids on Pi
           Metabolism 168
    9.3. Effects of Glucocorticoids on Renal Handling of Pi 168
    9.4. Factors Relating to the Effects of Glucocorticoids on
           Renal Handling of Pi 171
    9.5. Circadian Rhythm of Pi Excretion and Glucocorticoids 172
10.   Estrogens 173
    10.1. Effects of Estrogens on Serum Pi Levels................. 173
    10.2. Effects of Estrogens on Extrarenal Metabolism of Pi . 174
    10.3. Effects of Estrogens on Renal Handling of Pi 175
11.   Various Other Hormones 177
    11.1. Angiotensin II 177
    11.2. "Natriuretic Hormone" 178
    11.3. Prostaglandins (Bartter's Syndrome) 178
12.   Tumoral Hyperphosphaturia 178
13.   References 179

Chapter 7
EFFECTS OF VITAMIN D AND ITS METABOLITES ON
RENAL HANDLING OF PHOSPHATE
Louis V. Avioli

1. Studies in Humans 197
2. Studies in Animals 200
3. Summary 202
4. References 204

Chapter 8
EFFECT OF URINARY ALKALINIZATION ON RENAL
PHOSPHATE REABSORPTION
Norman Bank and Gerhard Malnic

1. Introduction 209
2. Clearance Studies 210

3. Micropuncture Studies 213
4. Microperfusion Studies 216
5. Studies of Luminal Membrane Vesicles 223
6. Theoretical Considerations 224
   6.1. Relation between H^+ and Phosphate Transport:
        Phosphate as a Buffer System 224
   6.2. Use of Phosphate in Renal Acidification Studies 227
   6.3. Physicochemical Properties of Anions 231
   6.4. Mechanism of Action of Acetazolamide and
        Bicarbonate 233
7. Clinical Implications 236
8. References 237

Chapter 9
TUBULAR ADAPTATION TO THE SUPPLY AND
REQUIREMENT OF PHOSPHATE
Jean-Philippe Bonjour and Herbert Fleisch

1. Introduction 243
2. Assessment of the Overall Tubular Capacity to
   Transport Pi 244
3. Tubular Adaptation to the Dietary Supply of Phosphate 245
4. Tubular Adaptation to the Phosphate Demand of the
   Organism 249
5. Role of $1,25(OH)_2D_3$ in the Tubular Adaptation in Pi
   Transport 252
6. Localization of the Tubular Adaptation in Pi Transport 254
   6.1. Influence of Phosphate Supply 254
   6.2. Influence of Phosphate Demand through EHDP
        Treatment 257
7. Tubular Adaptation and Acute Phosphaturic Response to
   PTH 257
   7.1. Influence of Dietary Phosphate 257
   7.2. Influence of EHDP 258
   7.3. Influence of $1,25(OH)_2D_3$ 259
8. Mechanism of Tubular Adaptation 259
9. Tubular Adaptation and Disorders of the Renal
   Pi Transport 260
10. Conclusions 261
11. References 261

Chapter 10
ROLE OF EXTRACELLULAR FLUID VOLUME EXPANSION
AND DIURETICS IN RENAL HANDLING OF PHOSPHATE
Manuel Martinez-Maldonado and Garabed Eknoyan

1. Introduction 265
2. Volume Expansion and Phosphate Excretion in the Rat and
   the Dog 266
3. Volume Expansion and Phosphate Excretion in Humans 270
4. Mechanism of Phosphaturia during Volume Expansion 270
5. Effects of Diuretics on Phosphate Excretion 271
   5.1. Osmotic Agents 272
   5.2. Mercurial Diuretics 273
   5.3. Carbonic Anhydrase Inhibitors 275
   5.4. Potassium-Sparing Diuretics 280
6. References 280

Chapter 11
INFLUENCE OF CALCIUM ON RENAL HANDLING OF
PHOSPHATE
Robert A. Peraino and Wadi N. Suki

1. Introduction 287
2. Physiologic Studies 287
   2.1. Effect of Calcium Infusion on the Serum Inorganic
        Phosphate Concentration and Its Filtration
        Characteristics 287
   2.2. Influence of Calcium on Renal Hemodynamics 290
   2.3. Effect of Calcium Infusion on the Absorption of
        Phosphate by the Renal Tubule 291
   2.4. Studies during Hypocalcemia 296
   2.5. Summary of Physiologic Studies 296
3. Pathologic Studies 296
   3.1. Introduction 296
   3.2. Renal Glomerular Insufficiency 298
   3.3. Primary Hyperparathyroidism 298
   3.4. Vitamin-D-Resistant Rickets with Hypophosphatemia .. 300
   3.5. Hypoparathyroidism 302
4. References 303

Chapter 12
RENAL HANDLING OF PHOSPHATE IN RENAL FAILURE
Shaul G. Massry and Nachman Brautbar

1. Introduction 307
2. Factors Affecting Renal Handling of Phosphate in Renal
   Failure 307
3. Role of Serum Phosphorus 313
4. Renal Handling of Phosphate after Renal Transplantation 316
5. References 317

Chapter 13
TUBULAR DEFECTS IN PHOSPHATE REABSORPTION
IN CLINICAL MEDICINE
Russell W. Chesney

1. Introduction 321
2. Diseases Manifested by a Tubular Phosphate Leak 323
   2.1. Primary Renal Tubular Phosphate Hyperexcretion 323
   2.2. Secondary Renal Tubular Phosphate Hyperexcretion ... 340
   2.3. Phosphate Loss as Part of a Complex Tubulopathy 345
3. Conditions Associated with Increased Renal Tubular
   Retention of Phosphate 349
   3.1. Pseudohypoparathyroidism (PHP) 349
   3.2. Other Conditions of Phosphate Retention 353
4. References 354

INDEX 367

Indices for the Measurement of the Renal Handling of Phosphate

OLAV L. M. BIJVOET

1. INTRODUCTION

Phosphorus is unique among the elements in its ability to harness energy for useful purposes. In biology, its most common forms are the derivatives of orthophosphoric acid, the phosphate (PO_4) tending to remain essentially an inorganic radical (Needham, 1965). Phosphate was first discovered in urine over three centuries ago, and urine—and, later, bones—were the main sources for isolation and purification for more than a century hence (Partington, 1961–1962).

Throughout the evolution of vertebrates, the kidney was the only organ through which the body could excrete phosphate (Bijvoet and Reitsma, 1977; Smith, 1930). Urinary phosphate ($U_{PO_4}V$) therefore reflected the excess that had to be removed from the vertebrate body in order to maintain a constant proportion of phosphate in its structural composition and a constant concentration of phosphate in the extracellular fluid. Environmental inorganic phosphate may have a role in the genesis and maintenance of phosphate cycling through living beings, but the only source of phosphate for the vertebrate organisms is the diet, especially the phosphate bound in food protein. The only excretory organ, and, therefore, the only organ that may regulate the phosphate content of the body, is the kidney. An intermediate mechanism for smoothing out or causing fluctuations in extracellular phosphate concentration is temporary exchange with phosphate stores of the body. A major store is the skeleton, where phosphate is deposited and released together with calcium. Thus, an inevitable link exists between the metabolism of calcium and phosphate. Interestingly, parathyroid hormone influences skeletal calcium and phosphate transport in the same direction but renal calcium and phosphate transport in opposite directions. This may have an evolutionary explanation, related to a role of hard tissue as a reservoir of base (Bijvoet, 1977), and is the cause of a reversal of the influence of parathyroid hormone on the plasma PO_4 when renal function fails (see Section 4.5.2). How the kidneys operate in equilibrating output with fortuitous changes in dietary input is what clinical indices for the measurement of renal handling of phosphate are meant to measure.

There are two essentially different ways to look at the renal handling of phosphate. One is the microanatomical and biochemical methods aimed at elucidation of the various steps in phosphate transport, how they operate and where they are localized. The micropuncture technique is an important tool for this approach. Such techniques have the advantage of direct observation of local changes in phosphate flux and concentration, yet they are beset by serious difficulties, such as inaccessibility of certain nephron segments that may have an important role in phosphate transport, functional heterogeneity between superficial and deep nephrons, and the problem of contamination of specimens. This type of study is essential for the understanding of the operation and disturbance of the mechanisms that together bring about the physiological functioning of the kidneys. The present chapter is not concerned with the techniques used in such studies.

Another approach is to evaluate and measure renal phosphate transport as a whole; it aims at understanding the role of the kidneys in phosphate homeostasis of the body and views renal phosphate transport in relation to net phosphate fluxes in other organs, such as the skeleton and the intestine. This type of assessment is important to the clinician because it may help to distinguish if, and to what extent, the kidneys contribute to or may be expected to withstand disturbances of homeostasis.

There are two main conditions that must be met in order for the indices of renal phosphate handling to be useful: They must be based on simple and clinically practicable measurements, but they should also allow interpretation in relation to other parameters of renal phosphate handling. These indices are, therefore, based on simple concentration measurements in samples of serum and urine and are preferably expressed in terms of glomerular filtration and tubular transport.

2. GLOMERULAR FILTRATION AND TUBULAR TRANSPORT

2.1. The Composition of the Glomerular Filtrate

In 1844, Ludwig held that in the renal capsule the proteins were filtered off from the remaining constituents of the plasma. However, it was not until 1924 that Wearn and Richards published their classical micropuncture studies of the frog, demonstrating that glomerular fluid is an ultrafiltrate of plasma. In 1928, Schmitt and White were the first to measure by a micropuncture technique the phosphate content of renal capsular fluid in *Necturus*; these measurements were repeated with an improved technique in 1932 (White, 1932). They found that the phosphate concentration was 94% of that of plasma, not very different from values found by Walker (1933) in necturi (94%) and in frogs (100%). The earliest micropuncture studies of phosphate excretion in rats were published by Strickler *et al.* (1964); however, no direct measurement of capsular phosphate concentration was possible. More recently, direct measurements of phosphate in glomerular filtrate became possible using a special strain of rats with glomeruli on the surface of the kidney (Brenner *et al.*, 1972). In such studies, glomerular filtrate was found to have a phosphate concentration of 93% of that of plasma water (Harris *et al.*, 1974). Since the water content of plasma is 930 g/liter, it is evident that the concentrations of PO_4 in total plasma and in the glomerular filtrate are the same.

It is very important to emphasize that measured concentrations of PO_4 in plasma and in glomerular filtrate or *in vitro* ultrafiltrates of plasma can only be the same when a significant portion of the plasma PO_4 is not ultrafilterable. This point has often caused confusion and has been extensively discussed by Walser (1961; Walser *et al.*, 1960). The assumption of nonfilterability of a portion of the plasma PO_4 is needed to offset two factors. The first is that in measuring plasma PO_4 concentrations, the volume occupied by proteins is not taken into account, and the second is that the presence of plasma proteins on only one side of an ultrafiltering membrane will, because of their charge, induce an electrochemical gradient across the membrane, resulting in an unequal distribution of ions along the two sides of the membrane (the Donnan equilibrium). Plasma water content is 930 g/liter, and the Donnan factor for plasma PO_4 is about 0.915 (Van Slyke *et al.*, 1923). If the plasma PO_4 were entirely ultrafilterable, the PO_4 concentration in the glomerular filtrate would have to be $1/(0.93 \times 0.915)$, and 1.175, times that of plasma. Walser (1961; Walser *et al.*, 1960) reviewed existing *in vitro* ultrafiltration studies of plasma PO_4 and found that many were unreliable because factors such as pH, pCO_2, or temperature had not been taken into account. However, the best available reported data and Walser's own studies of humans showed that whatever the absolute value of the plasma PO_4 concentration, ultrafiltrates of plasma have approximately the same PO_4 concentration as the plasma itself. On this basis, he reasoned that, on the average, 13% of the plasma PO_4 is protein bound and nonfilterable. Similar results have been obtained in studies of the distribution over plasma components after intravenous administration of radioactive phosphate (Fuchs and Fuchs, 1954a,b; Govaerts, 1947; Henry et al., 1953; Liljestrand and Swedin, 1952). Therefore, despite considerable protein binding, the PO_4 concentration in glomerular filtrate equals the plasma PO_4 concentration. The rate at which phosphate is filtered in the kidney (filtered load, L_{PO_4}; weight/time) can, therefore, be calculated as the product of plasma PO_4 concentration (weight/volume) and glomerular filtration rate (GFR; volume/time):

$$L_{PO_4} = [PO_4] \times GFR$$

2.2. The Direction of Tubular Transport

The phosphate content of the organism can only remain constant when the rate of phosphate excretion in the urine equals the rate at which phosphate is absorbed from the diet. One may postulate that the direction of renal tubular transport necessary to maintain the plasma PO_4 concentration around a certain value may depend on whether the phosphate filtered through the glomeruli is more or less than the phosphate absorbed by the gut. The rate of glomerular phosphate filtration (filtered load, L_{PO_4}) is equal to the product of GFR and plasma PO_4 concentration minus the phosphate reabsorbed from, or plus the phosphate secreted into, the tubular lumen by the tubular cells. To infer the general direction of tubular phosphate transport (secretion or reabsorption) necessary to maintain a constant extracellular phosphate concentration, one can compare available information about glomerular filtration, plasma PO_4 concentration, and phosphate absorbed from the diet.[*] In Table 1, these data are given

---

[*] References to this paragraph and more detailed information can be found in Bijvoet and Reitsma (1977), Smith (1961), and Marshall and Smith (1930).

Table 1. Phosphate Turnover in the Vertebrates[a]

Class	Input (μmol/kg/day)	GFR (ml/kg/day) ×	[PO₄] (μmol/ ml) =	Filtered (μmol/kg/ day)	S or R[b]
Cyclostomes	>1000	10 ×	<2 =	<20	S
Elasmobranchs	>1000	<100 ×	<3 =	<300	S
Teleosts					
Glomerular	>1000	<200 ×	<3 =	<600	S
Aglomerular	>1000	0 ×	<8 =	0	S
Amphibians		500 ×	≈1 =	500	R (S?)
Reptiles	≈1000	300 ×	<2 =	<600	R; S
Birds		300–2000 ×	<1 =	300–2000	R; S
Mammals	500	2000 ×	<2 =	<4000	R

[a] Bijvoet and Reitsma (1977).
[b] S, secretion; R, reabsorption.

for the various classes of the vertebrates (Bijvoet and Reitsma, 1977). It is evident that the filtration rate of phosphate in fish is lower than the rate at which they absorb phosphate. One has to deduce that fish maintain their plasma PO_4 concentration by tubular secretion. In the higher classes of animals, the situation has somewhat changed. The rate of phosphate filtration seems large enough to excrete more than the ingested phosphate, and, indeed, phosphate reabsorption has clearly been demonstrated in these animals. As pointed out, the development of a filtration–reabsorption system for water and salts was a major event in vertebrate evolution (Marshall and Smith, 1930). Observations in many mammals indicate that fluid and phosphate reabsorption in the proximal tubules may be proportional and that a threshold phosphate concentration of the glomerular filtrate exists below which most filtered phosphate is conserved and above which phosphate excretion is proportional to GFR. Because of the great proportion of extracellular fluid that is filtered through the glomerulus and returned through the proximal tubules per unit time, this threshold phosphate concentration, acting as a tubular phosphate sieve, largely determines the plasma phosphate concentration.

2.3. The Concept of a Limit or Threshold Concentration

The theory of glomerular filtration and selective tubular reabsorption to explain the operation of the kidney in mineral excretion was first for mulated by Ludwig in 1844 and later extended by Cushny (1917) to include Ambard's (Ambard and Weil, 1912) idea that there is a limit or threshold concentration below which excretion of some substances in the urine ceases. The term "threshold" originates with Claude Bernard (Ambard and Weil, 1912), who used it for glucose. Wigglesworth and Woodrow (1924), Adolph (1925), and Brain *et al.* (1928) raised the plasma PO_4 above this concentration and then found a linear relation between plasma PO_4 and $U_{PO_4}V$ with an intersection of the regression line with the plasma PO_4 axis, which they called the phosphate threshold (Fig. 1). The slope of the regression line was the same for a number of substances and, therefore, was called the proportionality constant; it was later found to measure GFR. The information in Fig. 1, which has been included for historical reasons, is somewhat imprecise. It is important to analyze more closely the pattern that emerges when the rate of phosphate excretion is compared with varying plasma PO_4 concentration, because the various elements emerging from an analysis of that pattern form the basis for understanding the nature and historical development of all clinical parameters for renal phosphate handling. Figure 2 shows such a pattern. It depicts the relationship between $U_{PO_4}V$ (mg/min) and plasma PO_4 (mg/100 ml) in a healthy person in the fasting state and during an infusion of phosphate. For com-

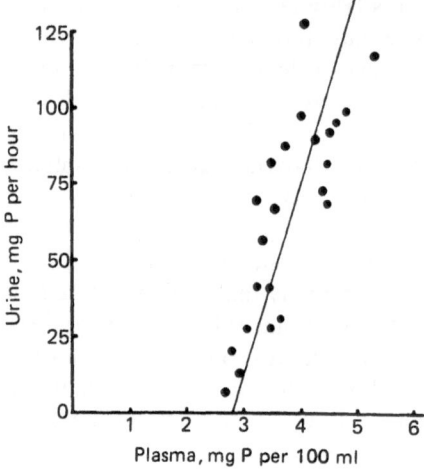

Fig. 1. The relationship between phosphate excretion rate and plasma phosphate concentration in six healthy persons after feeding with sodium glycerophosphate. (From Brain *et al.*, 1928.)

parison, the same relationship for inulin is also given. Because inulin is filtered entirely at the glomerulus and is neither reabsorbed nor secreted by the tubules, the rate at which inulin is excreted ($U_{in}V$; weight/time) is the same as the rate at which it is filtered in the glomerulus (plasma inulin; weight/time):

$$\text{Plasma inulin} \times \text{GFR} = U_{in}V$$

The line that relates ($U_{in}V$) to the plasma inulin concentration in Fig. 2 has, therefore, a slope that is equal to the GFR (volume/time):

$$\text{GFR} = U_{in}V/\text{Plasma inulin}$$

Note that the ratio of $U_{in}V$ to plasma inulin concentration, called the inulin clearance, just happens to be equal to GFR and is constant at all concentrations of inulin, because the regression line passes through the origin. The decision to use the word "clearance" for the ratio of excretion rate to concentration in the plasma, whether this is a constant (as with inulin) or not (as with phosphate in this figure), was an unhappy one that has been the cause of much confusion in interpretation, analysis, and communication. This is because the term that describes an effect on the plasma is used to designate a property of the kidney that can only be directly derived from the effect on the plasma in the case of inulin or creatinine. It makes perfect sense to talk about relative clearance of plasma PO_4 *through* kidney, but it is not appropriate to talk about the phosphate clearance *of* the kidney. If phosphate were not reabsorbed in the tubules, and if all of the filtered phosphate were excreted, then the same line that de-

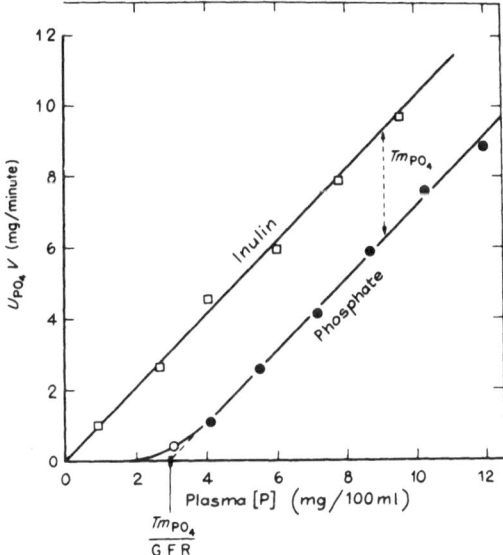

Fig. 2. The relationship between urinary excretion rate of phosphate ($U_{PO_4}V$; mg/min) and plasma phosphate [P] (mg/100 ml) in a healthy individual when fasting (open circle) and during an infusion of phosphate (closed circles). Note that [P] equals the phosphate concentration in the renal glomerular filtrate. The open squares show the relationship between urinary excretion rate and plasma concentration of inulin when inulin was infused simultaneously. (The inulin results are divided by 10.) The slope of the line through the infusion data for phosphate is the same as the slope of the line through the inulin data and is, therefore, the glomerular filtration rate (10^2 ml/min). The vertical distance between the two straight lines, or the negative intercept with the ordinate of the extrapolated straight line through the closed circles, is the maximum rate of tubular reabsorption of phosphate (Tm_{PO_4}; mg/min). The intercept with the abscissa of the line through the closed circles is the maximum tubular reabsorption of phosphate per 100 ml of glomerular filtrate (Tm_{PO_4}/GFR; mg/100 ml), which has also been called the "theoretical renal phosphate threshold." (From Bijvoet, 1969.)

scribes inulin would fit the relation between the excretion rate and the plasma concentration of phosphate. This is clearly not so. Actually, during the infusion of phosphate, whatever the concentration in the plasma, the rate of excretion is always less than the rate of filtration (represented by the inulin line) by a value that is indicated in the figure by the vertical dashed line with the symbol Tm_{PO_4}. The length of this line (Tm; weight/time) is the difference between two rates, the rate of filtration and the rate of excretion, and is, therefore, equal to the rate of reabsorption. Figure 2, therefore, shows that when the concentration of phosphate in the plasma is progressively raised above its value in the fasting state, indicated by an open circle, then the rate of reabsorption (Tm_{PO_4}; weight/

time) is the difference between two rates, the rate of filtration and the rate of excretion, and is, therefore, equal to the rate of reabsorption. When the concentration of phosphate in the plasma is progressively raised above its value in the fasting state, then Tm_{PO_4} gradually increases, but subsequently it ceases to rise and remains at a constant maximum rate. This constant maximum rate is generally called the maximum tubular reabsorption rate (Tm) for phosphate (Tm_{PO_4}; weight/time).

The slope of the regression line for the phosphate data is the same as the slope for the inulin data. This slope is, therefore, equal to the GFR. In a study of more than 60 patients, Arner (1964) demonstrated that GFR values calculated from this relationship of urinary PO_4 to plasma PO_4 are identical with inulin clearances over a wide range of GFRs.

When the straight line through the phosphate data in Fig. 2 is extrapolated downward, it cuts the abscissa at a certain plasma PO_4 concentration. The physiological meaning of this concentration is clear; it is a limit concentration. When the concentration of phosphate in the plasma or in the glomerular filtrate is lower than this, most of the filtered phosphate is reclaimed by the renal tubules and not much is excreted; however, when plasma PO_4 becomes higher than the threshold concentration, a substantial fraction of the filtered load is excreted. This threshold or limit concentration acts as a weir or sieve. It enables the kidney to maintain the concentration of phosphate in the plasma around that value.

Figure 2 also shows that, below the threshold concentration, phosphate reabsorption is not complete, and, as the concentration of phosphate in the plasma is raised, reabsorption reaches its maximum only gradually. This gradual transition, indicated by the curved part of the line, is called splay. If splay had not existed, phosphate reabsorption would just be maximal at the point where the concentration of phosphate in the plasma is equal to the threshold concentration. At this point, phosphate reabsorption would just have been equal to the filtered load. Thus:

$$[PO_4]_{thresh} \times GFR = Tm_{PO_4}$$

Therefore, the "phosphate threshold concentration" is numerically equal to maximum tubular reabsorption rate for phosphate per unit volume of glomerular filtrate:

$$[PO_4]_{thresh} = Tm_{PO_4}/GFR$$

The phosphate threshold concentration is often expressed as Tm_{PO_4}/GFR. An alternative name is the "theoretical phosphate threshold." The lowest concentration at which phosphate appears in the urine is called the "appearance threshold," and the concentration at which splay ends, the "saturation threshold" (Govaerts, 1950).

3. THRESHOLD CONCENTRATION AND SPLAY FOR PHOSPHATE

The analysis of renal phosphate handling that is contained in the previous section defined the terms "glomerular filtration rate" and "threshold concentration." But in this process arose the concept of Tm_{PO_4}, a maximum reabsorption rate, that is, the maximum rate of phosphate reabsorption when the plasma PO_4 is raised to abnormally high values by phosphate infusions. When renal phosphate handling is considered in the fasting person, the relation between $U_{PO_4}V$ and plasma PO_4 deviates from the regression line for infusion data; the deviation was referred to as splay by Pitts and Alexander (1944). These two concepts, Tm_{PO_4} and splay, will now be considered.

3.1. The Relation between Maximum Reabsorption and Glomerular Filtration

From the consideration in Section 2.3, it has become evident that the terms threshold concentration, glomerular filtration rate, and maximum tubular reabsorption rate for phosphate are related:

$$[PO_4]_{thresh} \times GFR = Tm_{PO_4}$$

or

$$[PO_4]_{thresh} = Tm_{PO_4}/GFR$$

At first sight, the threshold concentration might be considered as a maximum reabsorption rate, normalized for GFR. Because above splay the excretion rate is the difference between filtered load (plasma PO_4) and reabsorption (Tm_{PO_4}),

$$U_{PO_4}V = (Plasma\ PO_4 \times GFR) - Tm_{PO_4}$$

Normalization for GFR gives

$$U_{PO_4}V/GFR = Plasma\ PO_4 - (Tm_{PO_4}/GFR)$$

But there is more to this than normalization alone. It appears that the tubular reabsorption of phosphate, like that of other substances (glucose, bicarbonate, calcium, sodium, chloride), is proportional to GFR, not only when different persons are considered (that would justify normalization) but even within a single person and possibly within every single nephron. This phenomenon has been called "glomerulotubular balance" (Smith *et al.*, 1943; Wesson, 1964) and implies that variations of tubular reabsorption should be considered not in terms of rates (like Tm_{PO_4}) but in terms of concentrations (like threshold concentration). If this is so, the threshold concentration should not be defined in terms of Tm_{PO_4} and GFR, but rather the maximum reabsorption rate in terms of threshold concentration and GFR as $Tm_{PO_4} = [PO_4]_{thresh} \times GFR$.

The various elements that go into the argument stem from the physiology of glucose excretion (Smith *et al.*, 1943). Shannon and Fisher (1938) analyzed the relation between Tm, GFR, and threshold (Tm/GFR) for glucose and criticized Cushny's (1917) threshold theory (see Section 2.3), because a constant glucose threshold concentration would imply that there is no constant maximum rate of glucose reabsorption but rather that Tm for glucose should vary in proportion with GFR when the latter is experimentally reduced or increased. Considering Tm/GFR as a constant, they found, on the contrary, that Tm for glucose remained constant when GFR was varied by clamping the aorta. Theirs being the first study of this kind, their conclusion has decided terminology. But later, Smith and co-workers (1943) and Handley and Moyer (1955) demonstrated that between animals and even within the same animal, the Tm for glucose and GFR do vary together and that, therefore, the threshold concentration is the fundamental parameter for glucose reabsorption.

There was a long delay between the first classical studies of renal phosphate handling in humans by Adolph (1925) and the first experimental confirmation of a constant Tm_{PO_4} by Harrison and Harrison (1941) and Pitts and Alexander (1944) in dogs and by Schiess and co-workers (1948) again in humans. The finding has since been confirmed.* But because most of the authors examined Tm_{PO_4} at a constant GFR, the question of constancy of Tm_{PO_4} or rather of the threshold concentration remained untouched. It was noticed that Tm_{PO_4} might well be invariable within an individual, yet there were considerable variations when Tm_{PO_4} of different individuals, within a single study or reported by different authors, were compared (Thompson and Hiatt, 1957). Much of this variation could be accounted for by differences in GFR. This, as well as direct studies of the relation between Tm_{PO_4} and GFR, unequivocally demonstrated that Tm_{PO_4}/GFR rather than Tm_{PO_4} is the parameter of renal tubular phosphate handling that will distinguish variations in renal tubular phosphate transport that are not due to alterations of GFR or of filtered load (Fig. 3) (Anderson and Parsons, 1963; Bijvoet, 1969, 1976; Hellman *et al.*, 1964; Lewis and Ford, 1961). The Tm_{PO_4}/GFR may discriminate patients with different disease entities that alter renal tubular transport of phosphate

---

* Not all authors have found a constant Tm_{PO_4} or Tm_{PO_4}/GFR. More often than not, this was caused by technical errors. A more detailed discussion of this can be found in Bijvoet (1976).

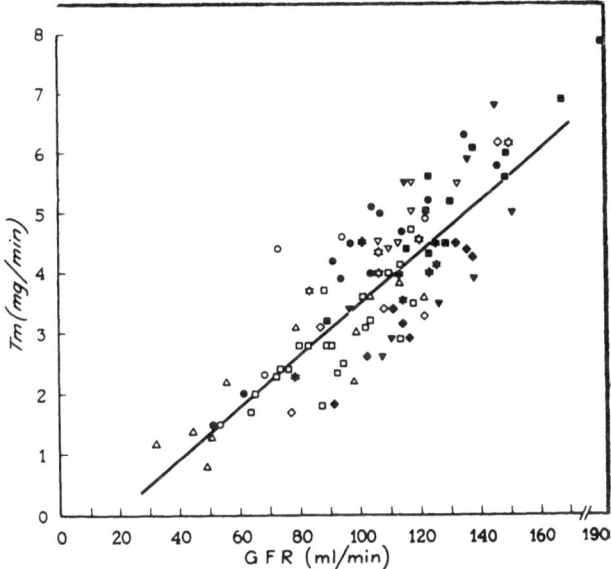

Fig. 3. The relationship between maximum rate of tubular reabsorption of phosphate (Tm; mg/min) and glomerular filtration rate (GFR; ml/min) in 101 persons collected from the literature. The equation of the regression line through the combined data is $y = 0.043x - 0.76$; $r = 0.86$. (From Bijvoet, 1969.)

(Bijvoet, 1969). For instance, it is possible to distinguish between groups of patients with hyper- or hypoparathyroidism or thyrotoxicosis by their Tm_{PO_4}/GFR, whereas Tm_{PO_4} alone is not helpful (Fig. 4). The role of Tm_{PO_4}/GFR in the setting of the plasma PO_4 concentration will be discussed later (Section 4.5.1).

3.2. Splay

I have already mentioned that the relation between $U_{PO_4}V$ and plasma PO_4 in the fasting person is determined by the splay (Fig. 2). Splay may be thought of as the deviation in units of plasma PO_4 of the points on the curve through low values of plasma PO_4 from the corresponding points on the extrapolated regression line for any given $U_{PO_4}V$. To derive Tm_{PO_4}/GFR for any measured pair of values of $U_{PO_4}V$ and plasma PO_4, splay should be exactly known. I will now proceed to an analysis of splay.

Figure 5 examines the relation between sets of values of $U_{PO_4}V$ and plasma PO_4 in persons in the fasting state and during infusions of phosphate. These are results of 100 studies of persons with a wide variation of Tm_{PO_4}/GFR from 1.1 to 6.9 mg/100 ml (Bijvoet, 1969; Bijvoet et al.,

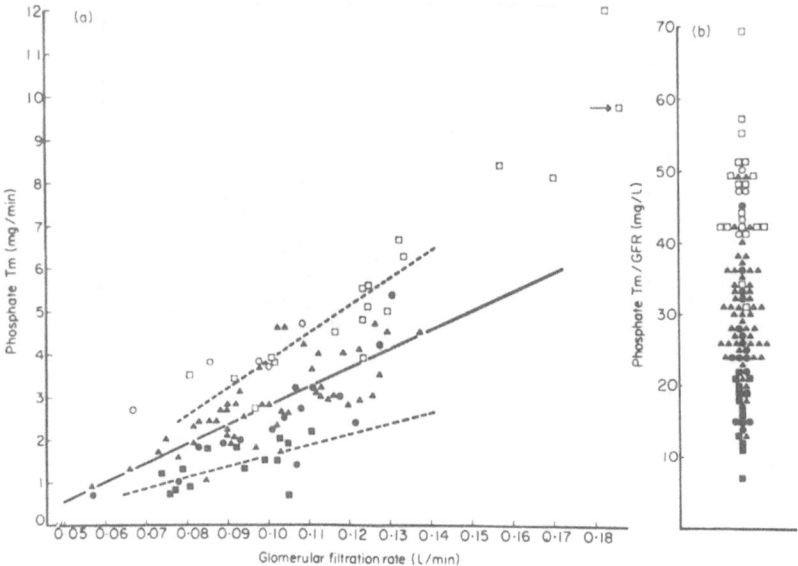

Fig. 4. (a) The relationship between maximum tubular reabsorption rate (Tm; mg/min) and glomerular filtration rate (GFR; liters/min) in 100 experiments. The dashed lines are regression lines calculated for the thyrotoxic (□) and hypoparathyroid groups (○) ($y = 65x - 2.0$; $r = 0.93$; $n = 23$) and for the hyperparathyroid patients (■) ($y = 25x - 0.6$; $r = 0.64$; $n = 14$). The solid line was calculated through the remaining data ($y = -4x - 1.2$; $r = 0.77$; $n = 63$). (b) Arrangement of the 100 experiments in (a) according to maximum reabsorption per liter of glomerular filtrate (Tm/GFR; mg/liter). The symbols refer to the diagnosis of the patient: □, thyrotoxicosis; ○, hypoparathyroidism; ●, kidney stones or nephrocalcinosis; ■, hyperparathyroidism; ▲, other diseases. (From Bijvoet, 1969.)

1969). Because of our interest in variation among persons due to variation in threshold concentration, the experiments have been ranged according to subsequent intervals of 1.0 mg/100 ml of Tm_{PO_4}/GFR. In order to keep the scale of the figure within reasonable limits, the highest values during infusion have been left out. Because the persons differed in GFR, which is responsible for the slope of the relation between $U_{PO_4}V$ and plasma PO_4, the values fan out at high values of plasma PO_4. The straight lines are the averages of regression lines through infusion data within each group. It should be realized that the range of Tm_{PO_4}/GFR within any single group is still 1 mg/100; this, and the variation of GFR, will contribute considerably to spread around the mean of splay. The figure shows that the data obtained during the fasting state deviate toward the left from the regression lines. This deviation, or splay, increases when the average Tm_{PO_4}/GFR is higher.

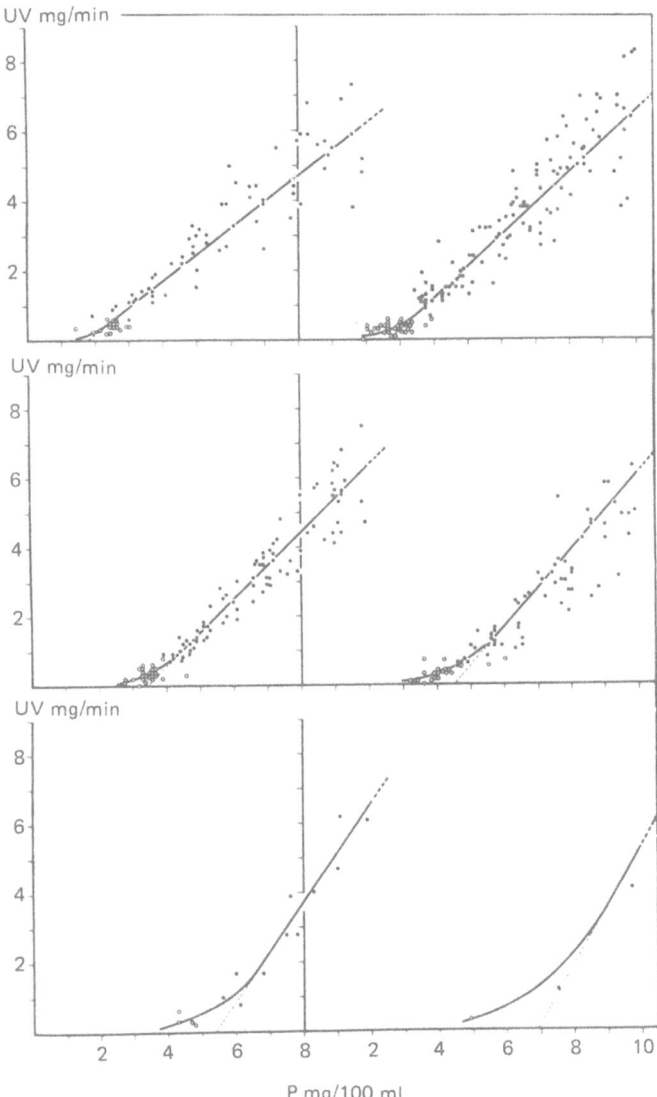

Fig. 5. The relationship between phosphate excretion rate (UV; mg/min) and plasma phosphate concentration (P; mg/100 ml) before (O) and during (●) infusions of phosphate. The results of 100 experiments were combined in six groups according to subsequent intervals of 1 mg/100 ml Tm/GFR. The average Tm/GFR values for the six groups were 1.6, 2.6, 3.4, 4.5, 5.4, and 6.9 mg/100 ml. The average GFR values were 75, 90, 96, 106, 139, and 174 ml/min. The straight lines were calculated from these averages from Fig. 6. (For clarity, the highest values of UV and P obtained during the infusions were not included in the figure.) (From Bijvoet, 1969.)

3.2.1. The Measurement of Splay

The realization that splay is proportional to Tm_{PO_4}/GFR is the basis for a quantitative analysis of splay and the possibility of estimating Tm_{PO_4}/GFR from a single pair of measurements of $U_{PO_4}V$ and plasma PO_4 and GFR (creatinine clearance) in the fasting person.

This is shown in Fig. 6a for measurements from four different persons. The variation among persons due to variations of GFR can be removed by plotting the relation between $U_{PO_4}V$/GFR (mg/100 ml) and the plasma PO_4 for each person (Fig. 6b). The slopes of all regression lines

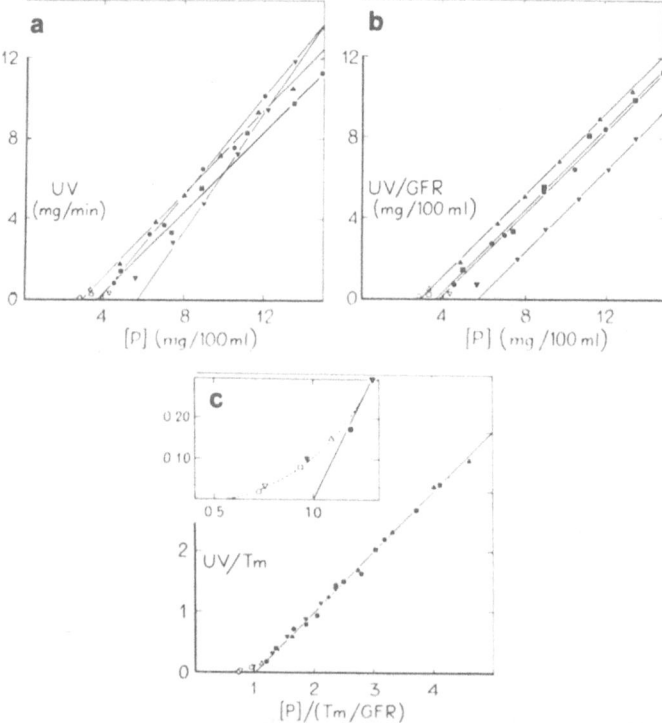

Fig. 6. (a) The relationship between rate of urinary excretion of phosphate (UV; mg/min) and plasma concentration of phosphate ([P]; mg/100 ml) in four persons. The open symbols represent the data obtained during fasting, and the closed symbols the data obtained during an infusion of phosphate. The regression lines through the data obtained during infusion differ in the slopes (GFR) and intercepts with the [P] axis (Tm/GFR). (b) The relationship between UV/GFR (mg/100 ml) and [P] in the same four persons as in (a). Variation between the studies due to variation in GFR has now been removed. The intercepts (Tm/GFR) still differ. (c) The relationship between UV/Tm = (UV/GFR) × (GFR/Tm) and [P]/(Tm/GFR) = (L/Tm) in the same four persons as in (a) and (b). The inset shows the lower values in more detail. (From Bijvoet et al., 1969.)

are now equal to unity, but the intercepts, which are still equal to Tm_{PO_4}/GFR, are, of course, still different. A general relation was obtained when this variation among persons due to Tm_{PO_4}/GFR was removed by expressing both $U_{PO_4}V/GFR$ and plasma PO_4 in terms of Tm_{PO_4}/GFR, that is $U_{PO_4}V/Tm_{PO_4}$ and plasma $PO_4/(Tm_{PO_4}/GFR)$ (Fig. 6c).

In Fig. 7, this general relation is shown for the results from 100 different infusion studies in healthy and diseased people. A smooth curve was drawn through the points which deviate from the regression line for data obtained during infusion. This curve represents the splay. The relation between $U_{PO_4}V/Tm_{PO_4}$ and Tm_{PO_4}/GFR defined by the splay in Fig. 7 was used to derive Tm_{PO_4}/GFR from GFR and the measurements of $U_{PO_4}V$ and plasma PO_4 made in the persons when fasting. In Fig. 8, this estimate was compared with the values of Tm_{PO_4}/GFR derived from the infusion values in the same studies. The figure shows that there is no systemic error in this estimate of Tm_{PO_4}/GFR, an observation which confirms that the splay has been adequately taken into account.

The general relation between $U_{PO_4}V/GFR$ and plasma PO_4 within splay has to be defined in terms of Tm_{PO_4}/GFR, the phosphate threshold concentration. Thus, the activity of phosphate reabsorption in the fasting persons varied in proportion to the threshold concentration, and it should be possible to predict the threshold concentration from measurements of $U_{PO_4}V$, GFR (or creatinine clearance), and plasma PO_4 in the fasting state.

3.2.2. The Cause of Splay

Smith and co-workers (1943) have suggested that splay is due to anatomical properties of the kidney. Every single nephron would reabsorb

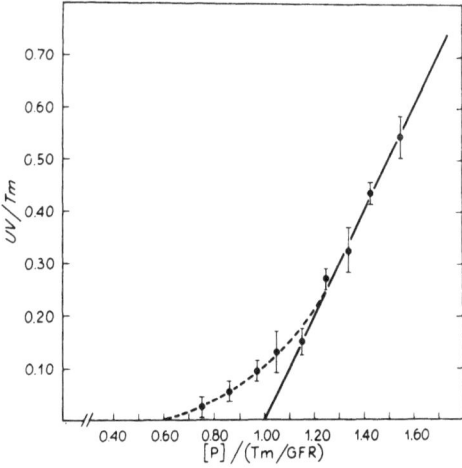

Fig. 7. The relationship between UV/Tm and [P]/(Tm/GFR) = (L/Tm) before and during an infusion of phosphate in 100 persons. The equation of the linear regression line through the data obtained during infusion is UV/Tm = (L/Tm) − 1. (From Bijvoet, 1969.)

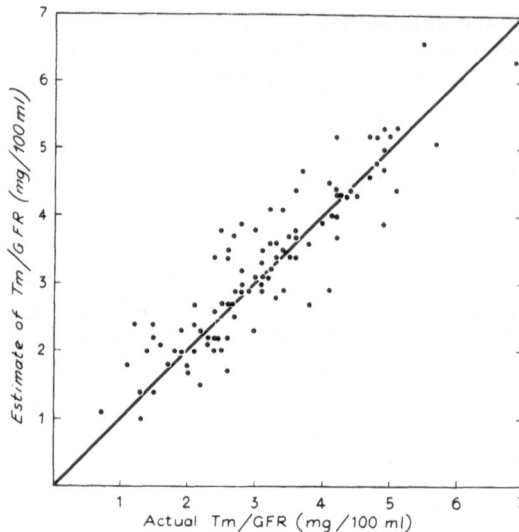

Fig. 8. The relationship in 100 experiments between the actual Tm/GFR, measured by the classical infusion technique (Fig. 1), and Tm/GFR estimated from $[PO_4]$, $U_{PO_4}V$, and GFR during fasting. The correlation coefficient between the 100 estimates and 100 measurements was 0.91; neither slope nore intercept was significantly different from the 45° line. Substituting creatinine clearance for GFR increased the SD by 0.1 mg/100 ml. (From Bijvoet, 1969.)

according to its own maximal capacity (tm_{PO_4}), and there would not be any splay within a single nephron. Because each nephron has a characteristic gfr, it also has a characteristic tm_{PO_4}/gfr. Because anatomical properties are never identical, Tm_{PO_4}/GFR values of the total nephron population will be distributed around the mean of all nephrons (corresponding to Tm_{PO_4}/GFR). Excretion starts when the concentration in the glomerular filtrate exceeds the lowest tm_{PO_4}/gfr, and the end of splay is reached when the reabsorptive capacity of all nephrons (Σtm = Tm) is saturated. The hypothesis does agree with proportionality of Tm_{PO_4}/GFR and splay.

Smith and co-workers calculated from their measurements of the splay in glucose reabsorption, which has the same configuration as the phosphate splay (Bijvoet, 1969), a hypothetical frequency distribution for anatomical properties. Oliver and McDowell (1961) actually compared glucose splay, measured in living dogs, with the distribution of the ratio of proximal tubular volume to glomerular surface, measured in anatomical preparations of the nephrons of the same dogs after sacrifice, and found that the distributions corresponded well.

Another approach compares the increase in tubular reabsorption rate to a maximum value, as the substrate (phosphate) concentration in the glomerular filtrate increases, with classical enzyme kinetics. Splay would be proportional to a Michaelis constant (K_m) and Tm to a maximal velocity (V_{max}). Reubi (1954) and Burgen (1956) tried, without definite success, to fit a kinetic model to glucose data. Their model does not agree with a proportionality of K_m and V_{max}. Marshall (1976) proposed a new kinetic model that does include this proportionality, but the latter model does not produce a sufficiently good fit with actual measurements. A fundamental property of models based on enzyme kinetics is that individual nephrons should show splay (unlike the anatomical model). It will not be long before actual measurements from micropuncture studies will give some indication about this, but the proposition of Smith *et al.* (1943) that the phosphate threshold will not be exactly similar throughout the kidney seems realistic enough to explain, at least in part, the origin of splay.

4. INDICES FOR THE MEASUREMENT OF THE RENAL HANDLING OF PHOSPHATE

4.1. The Renal Threshold Concentration for Phosphate

The most direct way to assess phosphate reabsorption would be to measure the renal phosphate threshold concentration (Tm_{PO_4}/GFR) by an intravenous infusion of phosphate. This is a complicated procedure involving an intravenous phosphate infusion at variable rates so that the plasma PO_4 rises linearly with time. The excretion rate is measured at short and precise intervals, and the threshold concentration can be obtained by extrapolation (Anderson and Parsons, 1963; Bijvoet, 1969; Stamp and Stacey, 1970).

The previous analysis showed that Tm_{PO_4}/GFR can be derived from measurements of excretion, plasma PO_4, and glomerular filtration in the steady state. It has been shown that the higher the actual plasma PO_4 concentration in relation to the phosphate threshold concentration (Tm_{PO_4}/GFR), the greater the fraction of the filtered load excreted. On the basis of the previous analysis of splay (Fig. 7), a quantitative description of the relation between the excreted fraction of the filtered load and the ratio of phosphate threshold concentration to actual plasma PO_4 concentration has become possible (Bijvoet *et al.*, 1969; Bijvoet and Morgan, 1971). The relation between the excreted fraction of the filtered load and the ratio of phosphate threshold to the plasma PO_4 can be derived from Fig. 7. Call the abscissa, plasma PO_4/(Tm_{PO_4}/GFR), x, and the ordinate, $U_{PO_4}V$/Tm_{PO_4}, y; then the excreted fraction of the load, $U_{PO_4}V$/(plasma $PO_4 \times$ GFR), equals y/x, and (Tm_{PO_4}/GFR)/plasma PO_4 equals $1/x$ (Fig. 9).

The ratio of phosphate clearance to creatinine clearance is C_{PO_4}/C_{cr}. This ratio is easily obtained from determinations of phosphate and creatine concentrations in plasma and urine:

$$C_{PO_4}/C_{cr} = (U_{PO_4}V \times \text{Plasma creatine})/(\text{Plasma } PO_4 \times U_{cr}V)$$

$$= (U_{PO_4} \times \text{Plasma creatine})/(U_{cr} \times \text{Plasma } PO_4)$$

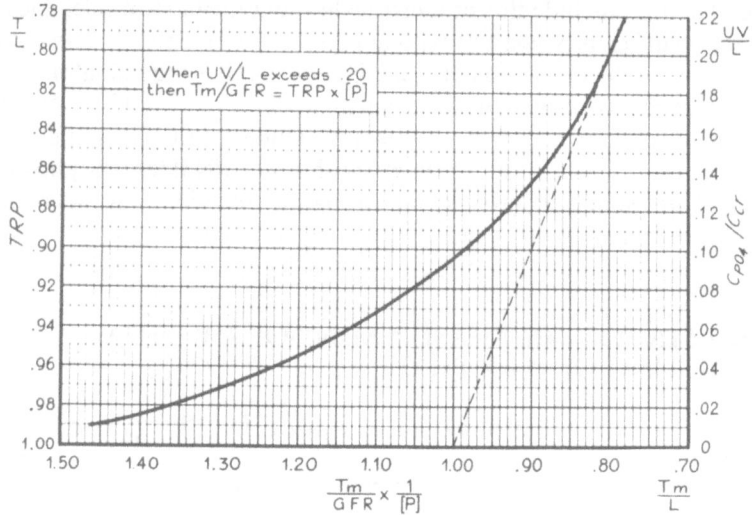

Fig. 9. A nomogram for the estimation of Tm/GFR from simultaneous measurements of the reabsorbed fraction of the filtered load (TRP; T/L) and [P]. TRP can be calculated from the concentrations of phosphate and creatinine in plasma ([P]) and ([Cr]) and in urine ([U_{PO4}] and [U_{cr}]). The rate of flow of urine (V) is not required. Thus: TRP = T/L = 1 − UV/L; UV/L = C_{PO4}/C_{cr} = [U_{PO4}] × V/[P] × [U_{cr}] × V/[Cr] = [U_{PO4}] × [Cr]/[P] × [U_{cr}]. When UV/L > 0.20 (TRP < 0.80), then Tm/GFR = TRP × [P]. When UV/L < 0.20 (TRP > 0.80), then the corresponding value of (Tm/GFR)/[P] can be obtained using the relationship shown by the continuous line in the figure. Tm/GFR is then this value multiplied by [P]. (From Bijvoet and Morgan, 1971.)

All that is needed is simultaneous collection of urine and plasma samples without taking the volume into account. Collections should preferably be made in the morning between 8 and 10 A.M. The patient should void at 8 A.M. The blood sample is taken at 9 A.M. and a urine sample at 10 A.M. Figure 9 can be used to derive Tm_{PO4}/GFR from C_{PO4}/C_{cr} and plasma PO_4 (Bijvoet, 1977; Bijvoet and Morgan, 1971). Find any value of C_{PO4}/C_{cr} or TRP, which is 1 − (C_{PO4}/C_{cr}), the corresponding value of (Tm_{PO4}/GFR)/ plasma PO_4 and multiply that value by plasma PO_4 to obtain Tm_{PO4}/GFR. Because the relation is linear at values of C_{PO4}/C_{cr} above 0.20 (reabsorption is above splay), Tm_{PO4}/GFR can then be directly calculated as follows:

$$Tm_{PO4}/GFR = TRP \times Plasma\ PO_4$$

Based on Fig. 9, a simpler device has been made to directly read Tm_{PO4}/GFR (Fig. 10) (Walton and Bijvoet, 1975). A straight line through the appropriate values of plasma PO_4 and TRP (or C_{PO4}/C_{cr}) passes through the corresponding values of Tm_{PO4}/GFR. The scales and units of the fig-

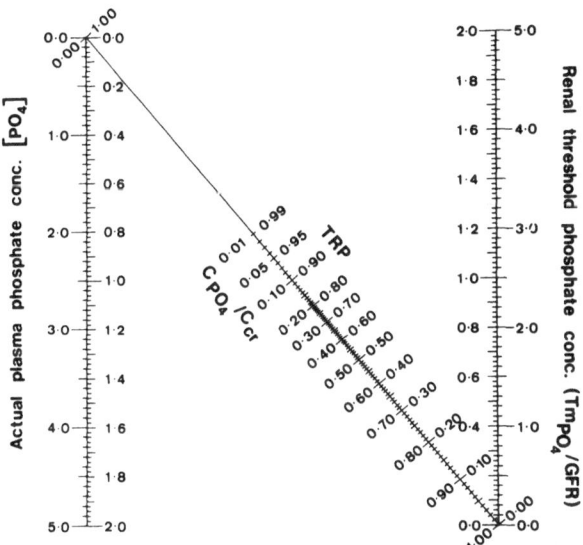

Fig. 10. Nomogram for the derivation of the renal threshold concentration for phosphate. (From Walton and Bijvoet, 1975.)

ures are arbitrary, provided consistent dimensions are used. Two scales have been chosen, one (0.0–2.0) close to values normally obtained in SI units, the other in mass units. If necessary, scales for plasma PO_4 and Tm_{PO_4}/GFR can be multiplied or divided by any number, provided the same number is used for both scales.*

4.2. The Phosphate Clearance

The phosphate clearance (C_{PO_4}) is the ratio of the phosphate excretion rate to the plasma PO_4 concentration. Figure 2 shows the relation between phosphate excretion and plasma PO_4 concentration at various values of the latter in a healthy person during an intravenous infusion of phosphate and at a fixed Tm_{PO_4}/GFR. C_{PO_4} is equal to the slope of a line linking any set of values ($U_{PO_4}V$ and plasma PO_4) with the origin. It is clear that C_{PO_4} rises as phosphate input (equal to excretion, $U_{PO_4}V$) rises until it reaches an asymptotic value equal to GFR. At any given constant $U_{PO_4}V$ and GFR, C_{PO_4} will vary inversely, but not in proportion, with

* The nomogram can be described by an empirical equation that can be solved with a moderately advanced programmable scientific calculator: When $C_{PO_4}/C_{cr} > 0.20$, then $Tm_{PO_4}/GFR = [(1 - (C_{PO_4}/C_{cr})] \times [PO_4]$; when $C_{PO_4}/C_{cr} < 0.20$, then $Tm_{PO_4}/GFR = [PO_4] \times e^p$, where $p = 10.318 (C_{PO_4}/C_{cr})^2 - 5.1848 (C_{PO_4}/C_{cr}) + 0.4022$.

Tm_{PO_4}/GFR. C_{PO_4} is, therefore, sensitive to variations in phosphate intake (equal to $U_{PO_4}V$ when in a steady state), GFR, and Tm_{PO_4}/GFR.

The absolute rate of excretion of phosphate in patients with hyperparathyroidism and a low phosphate threshold concentration is not different from normal (Chambers *et al.*, 1956), but the average plasma PO_4 of these patients as a group is lower than the normal average (Albright and Reifenstein, 1948; Chambers *et al.*, 1956). It is, therefore, not surprising that the average $U_{PO_4}V/plasma$ PO_4 or C_{PO_4} in such patients is higher than normal (Milne, 1951). However, the normal range is very wide, 2–33 ml/min or 8–38 ml/min when normalized for 1.73 m^2 body surface area (Dean and McCance, 1948). Other authors found a narrower, though still wide, range (4–16 ml/min), probably after better standardization of their conditions (Hodgkinson, 1961; Kyle *et al.*, 1958; Milne, 1951; Thomas *et al.*, 1958).

Administration of parathyroid hormone does cause an immediate increase of C_{PO_4} (Kleeman and Cooke, 1951; Kyle *et al.*, 1958), but such an observation pertains to transient changes of the steady state and gives only qualitative, not quantitative, information about the change of renal phosphate handling. A simple charting of the effect on excretion rate alone will give similar results.

Early authors (Kyle *et al.*, 1958; Milne, 1951) found a clear discrimination between healthy and hyperparathyroid persons on the basis of C_{PO_4}, the latter having a C_{PO_4} above 15 mol/min. This has not been confirmed by others (Hyde *et al.*, 1960; McGeown, 1961; Nordin and Smith, 1965; Pyrah *et al.*, 1966). GFR and phosphate intake do influence C_{PO_4} considerably. The sensitivity of C_{PO_4} to change in dietary phosphate input as distinct from changes in phosphate reabsorption was well illustrated by Pronovo and Bartter (1961), who pointed out that the main determinant of C_{PO_4} is the dietary phosphate content, not the renal phosphate handling.

4.3. The Reabsorbed or Excreted Fraction of the Load

The observation of Pitts (1933) that C_{PO_4} tends to approach GFR at very high values of plasma PO_4 prompted interest in the ratio of C_{PO_4} to GFR or C_{PO_4} to C_{cr}. The reabsorbed fraction of the filtered load (TRP) is, of course, equal to $1 - (C_{PO_4}/C_{cr})$. These notions were introduced by Smith *et al.* (1943), who, in contrast to most other authors, could not demonstrate a Tm_{PO_4} in dogs and suggested that the kidney reabsorbs a constant fraction of the filtered load. Their study consisted of measurements of phosphate reabsorption at rapidly decreasing plasma PO_4 concentration in four dogs. No allowance was made for the exponential nature of the decrease of plasma PO_4. Therefore, especially at high values of plasma PO_4, filtered load and reabsorption were probably overestimated and falsely suggested in three of the dogs an increase in reabsorption in proportion to filtered load.

The relation between C_{PO_4}/C_{cr} and Tm_{PO_4}/GFR can be seen in Figs. 6b and 11. In a chart relating $U_{PO_4}V/GFR$ to plasma PO_4, the clearance ratio is equal to the slope of a line, linking any set of values ($U_{PO_4}V/GFR$ and plasma PO_4) with the origin. It is clear that similar to C_{PO_4}, the ratio is sensitive not only to Tm_{PO_4}/GFR but also to changes of GFR and phosphate intake. Figure 11 shows that the index has some confusing properties: (1) The relation between C_{PO_4}/C_{cr} and plasma PO_4 is much steeper at a low value of Tm_{PO_4}/GFR than at a high value; a given increase of oral phosphate load, resulting in a given increase of $U_{PO_4}V$ (or of $U_{PO_4}V/GFR$), will cause a big rise of C_{PO_4}/C_{cr} and a small change of plasma PO_4 when Tm_{PO_4}/GFR is low, but will only cause a small change of C_{PO_4}/C_{cr} and a big change of plasma PO_4 when Tm_{PO_4}/GFR is high; and (2) a decrease in GFR will, at a fixed value of Tm_{PO_4}/GFR, have the same effect on C_{PO_4}/C_{cr} and on plasma PO_4 as a proportional increase of oral phosphate load, both resulting in an increase of $U_{PO_4}V/GFR$ in the same direction.

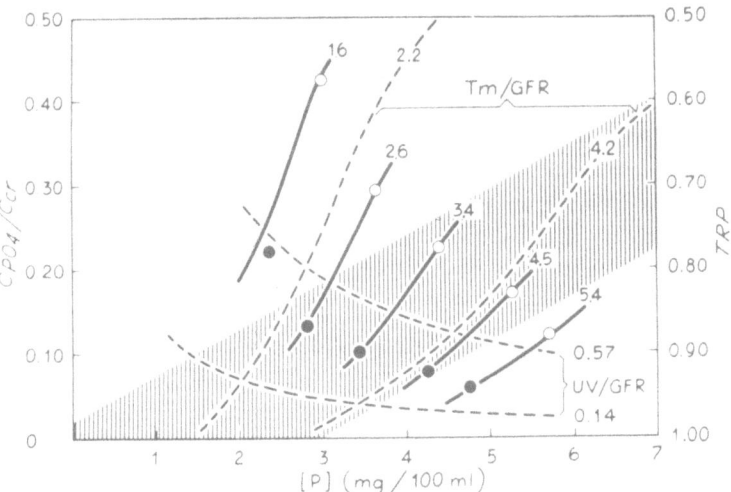

Fig. 11. The relationship between C_{PO_4}/C_{cr} (= UV/L) and plasma phosphate ([P]; mg/100 ml) in 100 persons grouped according to Tm/GFR, calculated from the relationship between UV/L and (Tm/GFR)/[P] shown in Fig. 9. The closed circles are the average values for the groups from Fig. 5 during fasting and the open circles, when UV was 1 mg/min. The dashed lines show the 95% range of values in healthy persons of Tm/GFR (2.2–4.2 mg/100 ml) and UV/GFR (0.14–0.57/100 ml). The shaded area indicates the normal range of the phosphate excretion index (PEI) as given by Nordin and Fraser (1960). (From Bijvoet et al., 1969.)

Crawford and co-workers (1950) reconsidered the suggestion by Smith *et al.* (1943) that there was a constant fractional reabsorption of phosphate and reasoned that animals would react to phosphate administration with a parathyroid-mediated decrease of reabsorption and that parathyroidectomy would fix the parameter on which parathyroid hormone acts. Indeed, they found that in parathyroidectomized rats, C_{PO_4}/C_{cr} is very low and hardly rises with phosphate infusion, but recalculation of their data shows, indeed, an excellent conformity with the Tm_{PO_4}/GFR model. When the phosphate threshold concentration (Tm_{PO_4}/GFR) is low (hyperparathyroidism), the slope of C_{PO_4}/C_{cr} against plasma PO_4 is steep (Fig. 11), and C_{PO_4}/C_{cr} changes more rapidly during dietary manipulations than in normal controls. In contrast, when the phosphate threshold concentration is high (hypoparathyroidism), the slope of C_{PO_4}/C_{cr} against plasma PO_4 is shallow, and there are only small changes of C_{PO_4}/C_{cr} in the face of big changes of phosphate load (Chambers *et al.*, 1956) (Table 2). The sensitivity to phosphate load makes the clearance ratio unattractive as index of renal phosphate handling. In those cases in which Tm_{PO_4}/GFR cannot be derived because splay has not been quantitated, effects on phosphate handling can be better discerned by charting the relation between $U_{PO_4}V/GFR$ and plasma PO_4 at various values of the latter in any of the conditions to be tested. A shift in the relationship is then attributable to altered renal phosphate handling. Relating $U_{PO_4}V/GFR$ to plasma PO_4 has an advantage over relating C_{PO_4}/C_{cr} to plasma PO_4 in that the latter term contains plasma PO_4 and, therefore, is not an independent variable.

The type of relation between plasma PO_4 and C_{PO_4}/C_{cr} shown in Fig. 11 was already discerned by Pitts (1933). This prompted Milne *et al.* (1952) to define the normal relation between C_{PO_4}/C_{cr} and plasma PO_4. They based their chart on data of Lambert *et al.* (1947) with erroneously low

Table 2. Effect of Phosphate Depletion on Plasma PO_4, TRP, and Renal Phosphate Threshold Concentration (Tm_{PO_4}/GFR)[a]

	n	Days	Plasma PO_4 (mg/100 ml)	TRP	Tm_{PO_4}/GFR (mg/100 ml)
Healthy adults	5	0	3.8	0.85	3.3
		3	3.3	0.92	3.4
		6	3.3	0.90	3.3
Hyperparathyroidism	6	0	2.7	0.63	1.7
		3	2.5	0.76	1.9
		6	2.3	0.82	1.9

[a] After Chambers *et al.* (1956).

values for C_{PO_4}/C_{cr} at high values of plasma PO_4 (Bijvoet et al., 1969). McGeown (1961), too, defined the normal relationship and noted that her values were higher than those of Milne et al. Actually, her normal data do perfectly coincide with the normal range for Tm_{PO_4}/GFR given in Fig. 11 and support the concept of the primacy of threshold concentration (Tm_{PO_4}/GFR) as the fundamental parameter describing tubular reabsorption activity.

In addition to changes in phosphate intake, C_{PO_4}/C_{cr} and TRP are also sensitive to changes in GFR (Fig. 11), because a change in GFR without a proportional change in $U_{PO_4}V$ will change UV/GFR. Any increase of $U_{PO_4}V$ will have the same effect as a proportional decrease of GFR. Variations of both $U_{PO_4}V$ and GFR will, therefore, obscure differences between normal and hypo- or hyperparathyroid persons with respect to differences of tubular phosphate reabsorption activity (Tm_{PO_4}/GFR). Kleeman and Cooke (1951) found, as can be expected, that parathyroid hormone administration decreases TRP in healthy persons, and Sirota (1953) found low values in hyperparathyroid patients. Schaaf and Kyle (1954) and Talpers and Stein (1959) established a normal range for TRP of 0.73–0.97. They found lower values in hyperparathyroidism, but Reynolds et al. (1960) then found that TRP alone insufficiently distinguishes hyperparathyroid patients from normals. For that reason, Chambers et al. (1956) used the effect of phosphate deprivation on TRP as the basis for a phosphate deprivation test (Table 2). Table 2, however, shows that Tm_{PO_4}/GFR (normal range 2.5–4.2 mg/100 ml) and plasma PO_4 discern the patients equally well. Reiss and Alexander (1956) and Goldman and Bassett (1958) pointed out that the data of Chambers et al. (1956) were perfectly compatible with the Tm_{PO_4}/GFR model. The sensitivity of TRP to changes in dietary phosphate induced Bernstein et al. (1956) to measure TRP during a standard 600 mg phosphate diet, but direct measurement of Tm_{PO_4}/GFR makes this measure superfluous.

The shaded area in Fig. 11 represents the phosphate excretion index (PEI), which is a regression line through normal data from patients infused with phosphate (Nordin and Fraser, 1960). Deviations from the regression line are expressed in units of C_{PO_4}/C_{cr} exceeding ± 0.09 above or below the mean value for a given plasma PO_4. The discrepancy from the normal range, as defined by the normal range for Tm_{PO_4}/GFR, is caused by the clearance data being based on midpoint plasma PO_4 determinations during an exponential decrease of the latter. This causes overestimation of high plasma PO_4 values and underestimation of high C_{PO_4}/C_{cr} values (Bijvoet et al., 1969). PEI (Nordin and Fraser, 1956, 1960), like another index, "EPI," which is a regression line through the normal relation between $U_{PO_4}V/GFR$ and plasma PO_4 (Nordin and Bulusu, 1968), is a linear approximation of splay and should be replaced by the more direct measurement in terms of Tm_{PO_4}/GFR based on measurement of splay.

4.4. The Excretion Rate of Phosphate

At the turn of the century, after Moleschott (1863) had coined the slogan "without phosphate no thought," experiments were devised to discern the effect of thinking and sleep on phosphate excretion. This was the setting in which a circadian variation in phosphate excretion was observed (Kleitman, 1925; Wesson, 1964). Excretion is lowest in the morning, with a minimum at about 11 hr, and thereafter increases, becoming maximal between 18 and 24 hr. Early authors assumed that the rhythm was not due to feeding habits, but Albright and Reifenstein (1948) pointed out that phosphate feeding is always followed by an increase in excretion rate. Dossetor et al. (1963) showed that the rhythm could be reversed by feeding at night. However, this rhythm is not abolished completely when phosphate intake is distributed equally throughout the day, although its timing may change (Birkenhäger et al., 1957). Therefore, other factors, such as muscular activity, may be influential. Because of this discontinuous nature of phosphate excretion, sequential studies need control measurements over comparable periods.

The daily phosphate excretion is closely correlated with the diet (Robertson, 1976). There is a wide variation in excretion rate within and between populations, which is due mainly to the marked influence of the dietary intake. The excretion rate ranges between 12 and 400 mg/24 hr. The daily phosphate excretion increases with age until the second or third decade and thereafter falls progressively; again, much of this pattern is attributable to variation of dietary intake, but reduced absorption makes some contribution in elderly subjects.

Phosphate deprivation (Chambers et al., 1956) or binding of dietary phosphate with aluminum hydroxide gel (Fauley et al., 1941) considerably reduces phosphate excretion, and a combination of both may virtually abolish it (Lotz et al., 1968). Administration of extra phosphate has the opposite effect.

The equality of phosphate input and renal output is a prerequisite for a steady state of whatever extracellular phosphate concentration—low, normal, or high. In hyperparathyroidism, the low renal phosphate threshold concentration lowers the prevailing plasma PO_4, yet even hyperparathyroid patients excrete phosphate at the same rate as healthy persons when they eat the same diet and show similar changes of phosphate output when the dietary intake is varied. The terms "hyperphosphaturia" and/or "hypophosphaturia" in relation to the parathyroid state refer to the transient increase or decrease occurring after a sudden increase or decrease of the parathyroid hormone level in the blood (Albright and Reifenstein, 1948). These transient changes persist until a new level of plasma PO_4 has been obtained at which excretion again equals input. The widespread use in experimental medicine of TRP as an index of exquisite sensitivity to changes in phosphate input into the extracellular fluid and in GFR has led to misconceptions concerning the role of parathyroid hormone in the adaptation to phosphate intake or to altered GFR.

This point has been discussed by Goldman and Bassett (1958) (Table 3). The excreted fraction of the phosphate load immediately increases with phosphate feeding and continues to increase when this new situation persists. On the basis of these data, Crawford et al. (1950) concluded that this is an exquisitely sensitive phenomenon and represents an immediate response in renal phosphate handling, probably mediated through the parathyroid glands. Goldman and Bassett, however, recognized that the phenomenon is a purely passive and automatic sequel to altered filtered load, without any change in Tm_{PO_4}/GFR; only later will a decrease in the phosphate threshold concentration ensue that may be dependent on the parathyroid glands, but it may also occur independent of any change in the secretion of parathyroid hormone (Parfitt and Frame, 1976).

4.5. The Plasma Phosphate Concentration

The plasma PO_4 concentration is influenced by three distinct factors: (1) the renal phosphate threshold concentration (Tm_{PO_4}/GFR), (2) the net input of phosphate into the extracellular fluid from the gut, cells, and bone, and (3) the efficiency of the kidney in modulating plasma PO_4, determined by the fraction of extracellular fluid processed per unit time, which is proportional to GFR. Of these three factors, the renal threshold concentration is the most important. When GFR is in the normal range

Table 3. Effect of Phosphate Intake on Renal Excretion of Phosphorus[a]

PO_4 intake (24 hr)	Day of study	Plasma PO_4	$U_{PO_4}V$	C_{cr}	C_{PO_4}/C_{cr}	Tm_{PO_4}/GFR
400 mg—10th day	10	3.74	0.46	148	0.083	3.9
1900 mg—1st day	11	4.52	1.63	165	0.218	3.6
1900 mg—10th day	20	4.16	1.80	122	0.354	2.7
400 mg—1st day	21	3.52	0.82	129	0.180	2.9
400 mg—10th day	30	3.52	0.35	152	0.065	3.9
3400 mg—1st day	31	4.67	1.84	160	0.248	3.4
3400 mg—10th day	40	4.62	3.02	167	0.392	2.8
400 mg—1st day	41	3.29	1.09	157	0.212	2.6

[a] After Goldman and Bassett (1958).

and dietary conditions are normal, a measurement of the fasting plasma phosphate concentration is generally sufficient to obtain a good impression of renal phosphate reabsorption. Measurements of Tm_{PO_4}/GFR are generally useful when a more precise assessment is needed in sequential studies or when groups of patients are compared.

4.5.1. The Role of the Threshold Concentration in the Setting of the Plasma Phosphate Concentration

The influence of the threshold concentration for phosphate (Tm_{PO_4}/GFR) on the setting of the plasma PO_4 is illustrated in Fig. 12. The figure compares the fasting plasma PO_4 with Tm_{PO_4}/GFR, measured during phosphate infusion in 100 persons with widely different threshold values (Bijvoet, 1969). There is a close correlation between both values. The variance of plasma PO_4 was reduced by 70% when Tm_{PO_4}/GFR was taken into account. Figure 12 illustrates to what degree a simple measurement of plasma PO_4 reflects the renal reabsorptive activity. In fact, Harrison and Harrison had already suggested in 1941 that the threshold was the main determinant of the plasma PO_4 concentration. Most factors that influence the plasma PO_4 do this through an effect on Tm_{PO_4}/GFR. There is a considerable age-related variation in Tm_{PO_4}/GFR. It increases in children and adolescents (Corvilain, 1972; Stalder et al., 1957; Thalassinos et al., 1970). In adults, it varies between 2.5 and 4.2 mg/100 ml (Bijvoet, 1977). It is higher in women after the menopause and then correlates with growth hormone concentration (Aitken et al., 1973). Many other hormones influence Tm_{PO_4}/GFR, one of the best known of which is parathy-

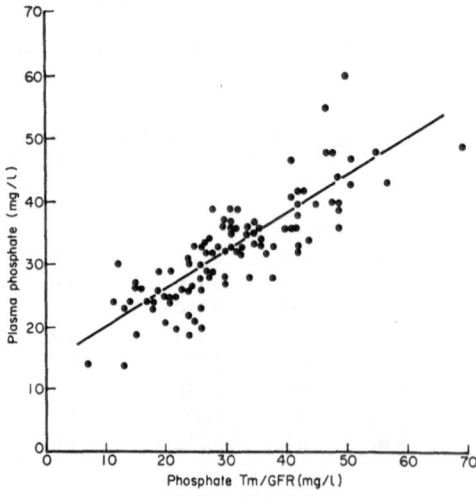

Fig. 12. The relationship between fasting plasma phosphate concentration and maximum tubular reabsorption per 100 ml of glomerular filtrate (Tm/GFR) in 100 experiments. The equation of the regression line is $y = 0.60x + 14$; $r = 0.84$. (From Bijvoet, 1969.)

roid hormone (Bijvoet, 1977). Phosphate reabsorption is decreased in primary and secondary hyperparathyroidism and increased in hypoparathyroidism (Fig. 4), and this fact has formed the basis for many clinical tests for the diagnosis of parathyroid disorders (Bijvoet *et al.*, 1969). Drezner *et al.* (1973) have demonstrated that a very useful refinement of the Ellsworth–Howard test (Ellsworth and Howard, 1934) for hypoparathyroidism is obtained by using Tm_{PO_4}/GFR rather than phosphate excretion as a parameter of the effect of parathyroid hormone on renal function. The inhibitory effect of parathyroid hormone on the renal tubular reabsorption of phosphate was the first action of the hormone to be well documented (Albright *et al.*, 1929; Greenwald, 1911; Greenwald and Gross, 1925; Pullman *et al.*, 1960; Vereecke, 1898) and was once considered to be its most immediate physiological effect. However, an increase in cyclic ÁMP (cAMP) excretion (Aurbach and Chase, 1970; Chase and Aurbach, 1967; Kaminsky *et al.*, 1970; Nelson *et al.*, 1970) precedes the phosphaturia, and it has, therefore, been assumed that the parathyroid-hormone-induced inhibition of tubular phosphate reabsorption is due to adenyl cyclase activation (Aurbach and Chase, 1970). This hypothesis is supported by the rise in phosphate excretion observed in thyroparathyroidectomized rats after infusion of dibutyryl cAMP (Agus *et al.*, 1971). Walker and co-workers (1977) have shown that there is a maximum parathyroid infusion rate above which no additional effect on Tm_{PO_4}/GFR can be seen. There is also a lower rate that still does influence Tm_{PO_4}/GFR but does not produce detectable changes in plasma or urinary cAMP.

4.5.2. The Effects of Phosphate Intake and of Glomerular Filtration Rate on the Plasma Phosphate Concentration

The setting of phosphate reabsorption is not the only factor that influences the plasma PO_4. Additional factors are the net influx of phosphate into the extracellular fluid and the integrity of renal function. Figure 13 illustrates the effects of altered input (equal to $U_{PO_4}V$ in the steady state) and/or GFR on the plasma PO_4 when Tm_{PO_4}/GFR is constant. A change in GFR at a set value of Tm_{PO_4}/GFR will reduce the slope of the line relating excretion to the plasma PO_4. The dashed lines indicate the normal limits of $U_{PO_4}V$. At a GFR of 100 ml/min, a $U_{PO_4}V$ of 0.25 mg/min, and an average normal Tm_{PO_4}/GFR of 3.2 mg/100 ml, the plasma PO_4 will be maintained at about 3.0 mg/100 ml. A 50% reduction of GFR will result in a rise in plasma PO_4 to about 3.6 mg/100 ml. A doubling of intake and, hence, a doubling of steady-state $U_{PO_4}V$ will have the same effect. Proportional, but inverse, changes of $U_{PO_4}V$ and of GFR will, therefore, have identical effects on the plasma PO_4.

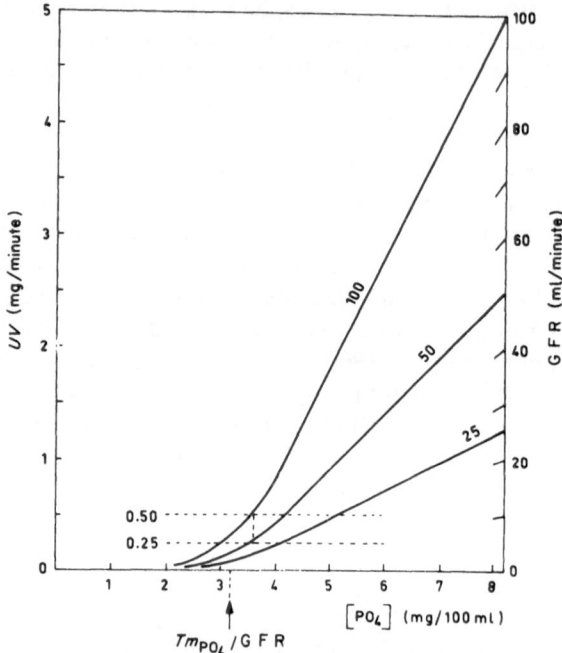

Fig. 13. The relationship between urinary excretion rate of phosphate ($U_{PO_4}V$; mg/min) and plasma phosphate concentration ($[PO_4]$; mg/100 ml) with respect to glomerula filtration rate (GFR; ml/min). In a steady state, UV equals the phosphate absorbed from the diet. Note that a proportional reduction of GFR and of phosphate absorbed from the diet will leave $[PO_4]$ unaffected and that the increase in $[PO_4]$ due to a given increase in phosphate intake (UV) is inversely proportional to GFR even at very low values of GFR (Arner, 1964); splay was calculated according to Bijvoet (1969). (From Bijvoet, 1976.)

The joint influences of Tm_{PO_4}/GFR, $U_{PO_4}V$, and GFR on the plasma PO_4 has been studied by multiple regression analysis of the variance in the fasting plasma PO_4 concentrations in 100 persons (Bijvoet, 1969) (Table 4). It must be emphasized that these persons were fasting and that the GFR in all persons was more than 40 ml/min. The table conclusively shows that nearly 70% of the variance in the plasma PO_4 concentration in a fasting person is determined by the activity of renal phosphate reabsorption, measured as Tm_{PO_4}/GFR. Figure 12 illustrates this relation. It also shows that the average concentration around which the concentration of phosphate varies depends on Tm_{PO_4}/GFR. Thus, at GFR values above 40 ml/min, and in the fasting state, Tm_{PO_4}/GFR is the main determinant of the plasma PO_4 concentration. At these values of GFR, the contribution of glomerular filtration to the setting of serum phosphate is small but significant.

Table 4. Multiple Regression Analysis of Variance in Fasting Plasma PO_4 Concentrations[a,b]

Regression equation[c]	Residual variance
$[PO_4] = 3.3$	0.708
$[PO_4] = 1.4 + 0.60 \ (Tm_{PO_4}/GFR)$	0.215
$[PO_4] = 1.7 + 0.62 \ (Tm_{PO_4}/GFR) - 0.0064 \ (GFR)$	0.201
$[PO_4] = 1.1 + 0.69 \ (Tm_{PO_4}/GFR)** - 0.0062 \ (GFR)* + 1.5 \ (U_{PO_4}V)**$	0.142

[a] From Bijvoet (1969).
[b] Dependent variable: fasting plasma phosphate concentration ($[PO_4]$; mg/100 ml); independent variables: tubular phosphate reabsorption (Tm_{PO_4}/GFR; mg/100 ml), glomerular filtration rate (GFR; ml/min), and extrarenal load ($= U_{PO_4}V$; mg/min).
[c] p values: *0.005–0.001; **0.001.

The consideration of the effect of GFR is interesting in relation to Section 2.2 of this chapter. The lower vertebrates probably have a mechanism for tubular secretion of phosphate that serves to maintain a normal phosphate concentration, despite a relative excess of dietary phosphate. Humans may not possess this mechanism, and even if they do, it is not sufficient to counterbalance an effect of reduced glomerular filtrate. Loss of renal function has three interesting sequelae that serve to highlight what the kidney normally achieves: (1) The fasting serum phosphate concentration rises as first described by Goldman *et al.* (1954) and illustrated in Fig. 14; (2) when GFR falls below 25 ml/min, the plasma PO_4 becomes abnormally sensitive to variations in phosphate intake (Friis *et al.*, 1968) and (3) parathyroid hormone, by its action on bone, which is now unopposed by that on the kidney, may actually raise the serum PO_4 instead of decreasing it (Stanbury *et al.*, 1960). The effect of renal failure on the renal handling of phosphate is discussed in detail in Chapter 12.

4.6. The Choice between Indices

This chapter has given an overview of the various known indices for the measurement of the renal handling of phosphate. These indices are listed in Table 5 with their respective normal ranges. The choice of index does depend on the situation and the sort of question asked. Section 2 made it clear that simple comparison of excretion rate with filtered load gives information about the possibility of net secretion or reabsorption as the operative mechanism in maintaining homeostasis. At a set phosphate level, transient changes of $U_{PO_4}V$ will indicate opposite changes of reabsorption. For sequential studies in adult humans, Tm_{PO_4}/GFR can be

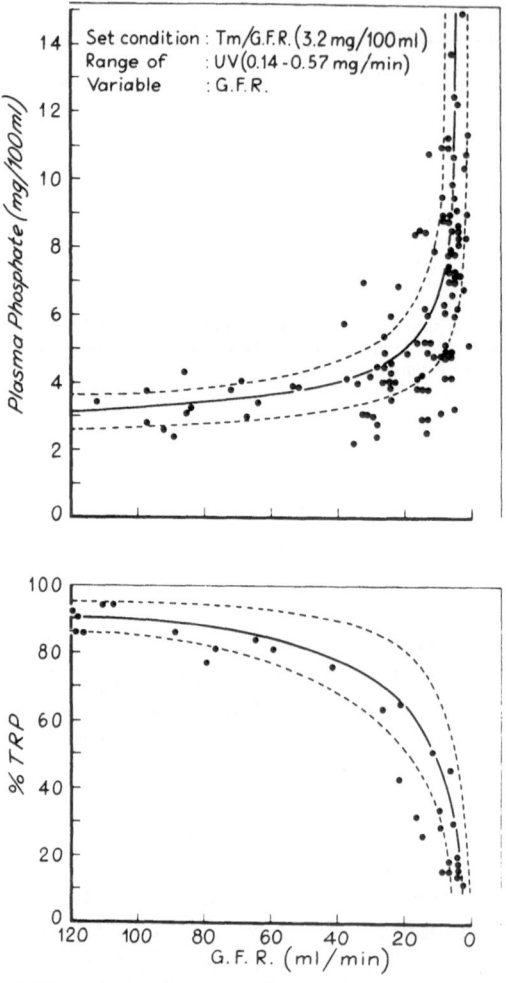

Fig. 14. Upper half: The relation between plasma phosphate and GFR in healthy individuals and in patients with chronic renal disease. The dots represent actual observations. The continuous line is the predicted relation when Tm/GFR remains constant. The dashed lines show the predicted range of plasma phosphate at a given value of GFR due to normal variations in phosphate load (= UV). Lower half: The relation between percent TRP and GFR under the same conditions. Note that TRP may decrease despite constant Tm/GRF. (From Bijvoet and Morgan, 1971.)

used with advantage; the use of Tm_{PO_4}/GFR also gives quantitative information about normality or abnormality of phosphate transport. When splay is not known, for instance, in infants or in animal experiments, Tm_{PO_4}/GFR cannot be sequentially assessed. Use of TRP or C_{PO_4}/C_{cr} is then not advisable, because they contain a term for plasma PO_4 and cannot

Table 5. Variables Which Influence the Tubular Reabsorption of Phosphate[a]

Variable	Symbol	Calculation	Dimensions	Average	Range
Plasma phosphate	PO_4		mass/vol; mg/100 ml	3.2	2.3–4.4
Glomerular filtration rate	GFR		vol/time; ml/min	100	80–120
Filtered load	L_{PO_4}	$[PO_4] \times GFR$	mass/time; mg/min	3.2	
Urinary excretion rate	$U_{PO_4}V$		mass/time; mg/min	0.36	0.14–0.57
Tubular reabsorption rate	T_{PO_4}	$L_{PO_4} - U_{PO_4}V$	mass/time; mg/min	2.84	
Maximum tubular reabsorption rate	Tm	See Fig. 1	mass/time; mg/min	3.2	
Limit or threshold phosphate concentration	Tm_{PO_4}/GFR	See Figs. 1, 2, and 10	mass/vol; mg/100 ml	3.2	2.5–4.2
Phosphate clearance	C_{PO_4}	$U_{PO_4}V/[PO_4]$	vol/time; ml/min	12	
Phosphate/creatinine clearance	C_{PO_4}/C_{Cr}	$U_{PO_4}V/L_{PO_4}$	No dimension	0.12	
Fractional reabsorption of filtered load	TRP	$T_{PO_4}/L_{PO_4} = 1 - U_{PO_4}V/L_{PO_4}$	No dimension	0.88	
Phosphate excretion index	PEI	[b]	Dimension?		±0.09
Index of phosphate excretion	IPE	[c]	mass/vol; mg/100 ml		±0.50

[a] From Bijvoet and Morgan (1971).
[b] $PEI = C_{PO_4}/C_{Cr} - 0.055\,[PO_4] + 0.07$; $[PO_4]$ is expressed in mg/100 ml.
[c] $IPE = U_{PO_4}V/GFR - ([PO_4] - 2.5)/2$; $[PO_4]$ is expressed in mg/100 ml.

then be compared with the plasma PO_4. In these cases, $U_{PO_4}V/GFR$ compared with the plasma PO_4 will allow independent comparison of terms of similar dimension, relatively independently of GFR.

Measurement of phosphate handling in renal failure poses problems of its own, but then the efficiency of the kidney in setting the plasma PO_4 becomes a minor factor, and management of phosphate intake and bone turnover are the major factors that deserve consideration.

It should not be forgotten that a simple series of measurements of the fasting plasma PO_4 can indicate whether renal handling is abnormal or not, provided GFR and phosphate intake are normal. However, the best differentiation between the various causes of abnormal plasma PO_4 concentration is given by a simple estimate of Tm_{PO_4}/GFR, the renal threshold concentration for phosphate.

5. REFERENCES

Adolph, E. F., 1925, The chemical sensitiveness of the kidneys, Am. J. Physiol. 74:93.

Agus, Z. S., Puschett, J. B., Senesky, D., and Goldberg, M., 1971, Mode of action of parathyroid hormone and cyclic adenosine 3',5'-monophosphate on renal tubular phosphate reabsorption in the dog, J. Clin. Invest. 50:617.

Aitken, J. M., Hart, D. M., Anderson, J. B. J., Lindsay, R., Smith, D. A., and Speirs, C. F., 1973, Osteoporosis after oophorectomy for nonmalignant disease in premenopausal women, Br. Med. J. 2:325.

Albright, F., and Reifenstein, E. C., 1948, The Parathyroid Glands and Metabolic Bone Disease, Williams and Wilkins, Baltimore.

Albright, F., Bauer, W., Ropes, M., and Aub, J. C., 1929, Studies of calcium and phosphorus metabolism. VI. The effect of parathyroid hormone, J. Clin. Invest. 7:139.

Ambard, L., and Weil, A., 1912, Les lois numériques de la sécrétion rénale de l'urée et du chlorure du sodium, J. Physiol. Pathol. 14:753.

Anderson, J., and Parsons, V., 1963, The tubular maximal resorptive rate for inorganic phosphate in normal subjects, Clin. Sci. 25:431.

Arner, B., 1964, Phosphate disappearance from plasma and the renal handling of phosphate after intravenous loading in man, Acta Med. Scand. Suppl. 176:415.

Aurbach, G. D., and Chase, L. R., 1970, Cyclic 3',5'-adenylic acid in bone and the mechanism of action of parathyroid hormone, Fed. Proc. Fed. Am. Soc. Exp. Biol. 29:1179.

Bernstein, M., Yamahiro, H. S., and Reynolds, T. B., 1965, Phosphorus excretion tests in hyperparathyroidism with controlled phosphorus intake, J. Clin. Endocrinol. 25:895.

Bijvoet, O. L. M., 1969, Relation of plasma phosphate concentration to renal tubular reabsorption of phosphate, Clin. Sci. 37:23.

Bijvoet, O. L. M., 1976, The importance of the kidneys in phosphate homeostasis, in: Phosphate Metabolism, Kidney and Bone (L. Avioli, P. Bordier, H. Fleisch, S. Massry, and E. Slatopolsky, eds.), pp. 421–474, Nouvelle Imprimerie Fournié, Toulouse.

Bijvoet, O. L. M., 1977, Kidney function in calcium and phosphate metabolism, in: Metabolic Bone Disease, Vol. 1 (L V. Avioli and S. Krane, eds.), pp. 49–140, Academic Press, New York.

Bijvoet, O. L. M., and Morgan, D. B., 1971, The tubular reabsorption of phosphate in man, in: Phosphate et Métabolisme Phosphocalcique (D. J. Hioco, ed.), pp. 153–180, L'Expansion Scientifique Française, Paris.

Bijvoet, O. L. M., and Reitsma, P. H., 1977, Phylogeny of renal phosphate transport in the vertebrates, in: *Phosphate Metabolism* (S. G. Massry and E. Ritz, eds.), pp. 41–53, Plenum Press, New York.

Bijvoet, O. L. M., Morgan, D. B., and Fourman, P., 1969, The assessment of phosphate reabsorption, *Clin. Chim. Acta* **26**:15.

Birkenhäger, W. H., Hellendoorn, H. B. A., and Gerbrandy, J., 1957, Enkele aspecten van de calcium- en fosfaatstofwisseling, in het bijzonder na intraveneuze injektie van calcium-levulinaat, *Ned. Tijdschr. Geneeskd.* **101**:1294.

Brain, R. T., Kay, H. D., and Marshall, P. G., 1928, Observations on phosphates in blood and on the urinary excretion of phosphates, *Biochem. J.* **22**:628.

Brenner, B. M, Troy, J. L., Daugharty, T. M., Deen, W. M., and Robertson, C. R., 1972, Dynamics of glomerular ultrafiltration in the rat. II. Plasma-flow dependence of GFR, *Am. J. Physiol.* **223**:1184.

Burgen, A. S. V., 1956, A theoretical treatment of glucose reabsorption in the kidney, *Can. J. Biochem.* **34**:466.

Chambers, E. L., Gordan, G. S., Goldman, L., and Reifenstein, E. C., 1956, Tests for hyperparathyroidism: Tubular reabsorption of phosphate, phosphate deprivation, and calcium infusion, *J. Clin. Endocrinol.* **16**:1507.

Chase, L. R., and Aurbach, G. D., 1967, Parathyroid function and the renal excretion of 3′,5′-adenylic acid, *Proc. Natl. Acad. Sci. U.S.A.* **58**:518.

Corvilain, J., 1972, Growth and renal control of plasma phosphate, *J. Clin. Endocrinol. Metab.* **34**:452.

Crawford, J. D., Osborne, M. M., Talbot, N. B., Terry, M. L., and Morrill, M. F., 1950, The parathyroid glands and phosphorus homeostasis, *J. Clin. Invest.* **29**:1448.

Cushny, A. R., 1917, *The Secretion of the Urine*, Longmans and Green, London.

Dean, R. F. A., and McCance, R. A., 1948, Phosphate clearances in infants and adults, *J. Physiol. (London)* **107**:182.

Dossetor, J. B., Gorman, H. M., and Beck, J. C., 1963, The diurnal rhythm of urinary electrolyte excretion. I. Observations in normal subjects, *Metabolism* **12**:1083.

Drezner, M., Neelon, F. A., and Lebovitz, H. E., 1973, Pseudohypoparathyroidism type II: A possible defect in the reception of the cyclic AMP signal, *N. Engl. J. Med.* **289**:1056.

Ellsworth, R., and Howard, J. E., 1934, Studies on the physiology of the parathyroid gland. VII. Some responses of the normal human kidney and blood to intravenous parathyroid extract, *Bull. Johns Hopkins Hosp.* **55**:296.

Fauley, G. B., Freeman, S., Ivy, A. C., Atkinson, A. J., and Wigodsky, H. S., 1941, Aluminium phosphate in therapy of peptic ulcer. Effect of aluminium hydroxyde on phosphate absorption, *Arch. Intern. Med.* **67**:563.

Friis, T., Hahnemann, S., and Weeke, E., 1968, Serum calcium and serum phosphorus in uremia during administration of sodium phytate and aluminium hydroxyde, *Acta Med. Scand.* **183**:497.

Fuchs, A. R., and Fuchs, F., 1954a, Investigations on the plasma phosphate, *Acta Physiol. Scand.* **30**:191.

Fuchs, A. R., and Fuchs, F., 1954b, Investigations on the plasma phosphate. II. Diffusibility of the inorganic phosphate of guinea pig serum, *Acta Physiol. Scand.* **32**:363.

Goldman, R., and Bassett, S. H., 1958, Renal regulation of phosphorus excretion, *J. Clin. Endocrinol.* **18**:981.

Goldman, R., Bassett, S. H., and Duncan, G. B., 1954, Phosphorus excretion in renal failure, *J. Clin. Invest.* **33**:1623.

Govaerts, J., 1947, Etude de l'état physico-chimique de l'ion phosphorique dans le plasma à l'aide du radiophosphore 32/15 P en rapport avec le seuil de l'élimination urinaire de l'ion phosphorique, *Arch. Int. Pharmacodyn. Thér.* **75**:261.

Govaerts, P., 1950, Interprétation des relations mathématiques entre le taux du glucose sanguin et le débit urinaire de cette substance, *Acta Clin. Belg.* **5**:1.

Greenwald, I., 1911, Effect of parathyroidectomy on metabolism, *Am. J. Physiol.* **28**:103.

Greenwald, I., and Gross, J., 1925, The effect of the administration of a potent parathyroid extract upon the excretion of nitrogen, phosphorus, calcium and magnesium, with some remarks on the solubility of calcium phosphate in serum and on the pathogenesis of tetany, *J. Biol. Chem.* **66**:217.

Handley, C. A., and Moyer, J. H., 1955, Significance of the GFR/Tm ratio, *Am. J. Physiol.* **180**:151.

Harris, C. A., Balr, P. G., Chirito, E., and Dirks, A. J. H., 1974, Composition of mammalian glomerular filtrate, *Am. J. Physiol.* **227**:972.

Harrison, H. E., and Harrison, H. C., 1941, The renal excretion of inorganic phosphate in relation to the action of vitamin D and parathyroid hormone, *J. Clin. Invest.* **20**:47.

Hellman, D., Baird, H. P., and Bartter, F. C., 1964, Relationship of maximal tubular phosphate resorption to filtration rate in the dog, *Am. J. Physiol.* **207**:89.

Henry, J. A., Jacobs, E., and Verbanck, M., 1953, Study of renal permeability to plasma inorganic phosphorus by means of P 32, *Arch. Int. Pharmacodyn. Thér.* **94**:235.

Hodgkinson, A., 1961, Renal phosphate excretion indices in the diagnosis of hyperparathyroidism, *Clin. Sci.* **21**:125.

Hyde, R. D., Vaughan Jones, R., McSwiney, R. R., and Prunty, F. T. G., 1960, Investigation of hyperparathyroidism in the absence of bone disease, *Lancet* **1**:250.

Kaminski, N. I., Broadus, A. E., Hardman, J. G., Jones, D. J., Jr., Ball, J. H., Sutherland, E. W., and Liddle, G. W., 1970, Effects of parathyroid hormone on plasma and urinary adenosine 3′,5′-monophosphate in man, *J. Clin. Invest.* **49**:2387.

Kleeman, C. R., and Cooke, R. E., 1951, The acute effects of parathyroid hormone on the metabolism of endogenous phosphate, *J. Lab. Clin. Med.* **38**:112.

Kleitman, N., 1925, Studies on the physiology of sleep. III. The effect of muscular activity, rest and sleep on the urinary excretion of phosphorus, *Am. J. Physiol.* **74**:225.

Kyle, L. H., Schaaf, M., and Canary, J. J., 1958, Phosphate clearance in the diagnosis of parathyroid dysfunction, *Am. J. Med.* **24**:240.

Lambert, P. P., Van Kessel, E., and LePlat, C., 1947, Etude sur l'élimination des phosphates inorganiques chez l'homme, *Acta Med. Scand.* **128**:386.

Lewis, J., and Ford, R. V., 1961, Correlation of glomerular filtration rate and tubular reabsorption of phosphate and the interrelationships of phosphate and para-aminohippurate clearance in man, *J. Lab. Clin. Med.* **57**:546.

Liljestrand, A., and Swedin, B., 1952, The urinary excretion of phosphate in the dog, *Acta Physiol. Scand.* **25**:168.

Lotz, M., Zisman, E., and Bartter, F. C., 1968, Evidence for a phosphorus-depletion syndrome in man, *N. Engl. J. Med.* **278**:409.

Ludwig, C., 1844, Nieren und Harnbereitung, in: *Handwörterbuch der Physiologie mit Rücksicht auf physiologische Pathologie*, Vol. 2 (R. Wagner, ed.), p. 629, Bieweg und Sohn, Braunschweig.

Marshall, D. H., 1976, Calcium and phosphate kinetics, in: *Calcium, Phosphate and Magnesium Metabolism* (B. E. C. Nordin, ed.), pp. 257–297, Churchill Livingstone, Edinburgh.

Marshall, E. K., and Smith, H. W., 1930, The glomerular development of the vertebrate kidney in relation to habitat, *Biol. Bull.* **59**:135.

McGeown, M. G., 1961, The values of the calcium infusion test, tests of renal tubular function and changes in the serum proteins in the diagnosis of hyperparathyroidism, *Proc. R. Soc. Med.* **54**:642.

Milne, M. D., 1951, Observations on the action of parathyroid hormone, *Clin. Sci.* **10**:471.

Milne, M. D., Stanbury, S. W., and Thomson, A. E., 1952, Observations on the Fanconi syndrome and renal hyperchloremic acidosis in the adult, *Q. J. Med.* **21**:61.

Moleschott, J., 1863, *Der Kreislauf des Lebens*, V. Zabern, Mainz.

Needham, A. E., 1965, *The Uniqueness of Biological Materials*, pp. 401–415, Pergamon Press, Oxford.

Nelson, G. L., Chase, L. R., and Aurbach, G. D., 1970, Parathyroid hormone sensitive adenyl cyclase in isolated renal tubules, *Endocrinology* **86**:511.

Nordin, B. E. C., and Bulusu, L., 1968, A modified index of phosphate excretion, *Postgrad. Med. J.* **44**:93.

Nordin, B. E. C., and Fraser, R., 1956, The indirect assessment of parathyroid function, in: *Ciba Foundation Symposium on Bone Structure and Metabolism*, pp. 222–232, Churchill, London.

Nordin, B. E. C., and Fraser, R., 1960, Assessment of urinary phosphate excretion, *Lancet* **1**:947.

Nordin, B. E. C., and Smith, D. A., 1965, *Diagnostic Procedures in Disorders of Calcium Metabolism*, Churchill, London.

Oliver, J., and McDowell, M., 1961, The structural and functional aspects of the handling of glucose by the nephrons and the kidney and their correlation by means of structural–functional equivalents, *J. Clin. Invest.* **40**:1093.

Parfitt, A. M., and Frame, B., 1976, Phosphate loading and depletion in vitamin D treated hypoparathyroidism, in: *Phosphate Metabolism, Kidney and Bone* (L. Avioli, P. Bordier, H. Fleisch, S. Massry, and E. Slatopolsky, eds.), pp. 179–196, Nouvell Imprimerie Fournié, Toulouse.

Partington, J. R., 1961–1962, *A History of Chemistry*, Vols. II and III, Macmillan, New York.

Pitts, R. F., 1933, The excretion of urine in the dog. VII. Inorganic phosphate in relation to plasma phosphate level, *Am. J. Physiol.* **106**:1.

Pitts, R. F., and Alexander, R. S., 1944, The renal reabsorption mechanism for inorganic phosphate in normal and acidotic dogs, *Am. J. Physiol.* **142**:648.

Pronovo, P., and Bartter, F. C., 1961, Diagnosis of hyperparathyroidism, *Metabolism* **10**:349.

Pullman, T. N., Lavender, A. R., Aho, I., and Rasmussen, H., 1960, Direct renal action of a purified parathyroid extract, *Endocrinology* **67**:570.

Pyrah, L. N., Hodgkinson, A., and Anderson, C. K., 1966, Primary hyperparathyroidism, a critical review, *Br. J. Surg.* **53**:245.

Reiss, E., and Alexander, F., 1959, The tubular reabsorption of phosphate in the differential diagnosis of metabolic bone disease, *J. Clin. Endocrinol.* **19**:1212.

Reubi, F. C., 1954, Glucose titration in renal glucosuria, in: *Ciba Foundation Symposium on the Kidney* (G. E. W. Wolstenholme and M. O'Connor, eds.), pp. 96–106, Churchill, London.

Reynolds, T. B., Lanman, H., and Tupikova, N., 1960, Reevaluation of phosphate excretion tests in the diagnosis of hyperparathyroidism, *Arch. Intern. Med.* **106**:48.

Robertson, W. G., 1976, Urinary excretion, in: *Calcium, Phosphate and Magnesium Metabolism* (B. E. C. Nordin, ed.), pp. 113–161, Churchill Livingstone, London.

Schaaf, M., and Kyle, L. H., 1954, Measurement of per cent renal phosphorus reabsorption in the diagnosis of hyperparathyroidism, *Am. J. Med. Sci.* **228**:262.

Schiess, W. A., Ayer, J. L., Lotspeich, W. D., and Pitts, R. F., 1948, The renal regulation of acid–base balance in man. II. Factors affecting the excretion of titratable acid by the normal human subject, *J. Clin. Invest.* **27**:57.

Schmitt, F. O., and White, H. L., 1928, Th phosphate content of renal capsular fluid in *Necturus*, *Am. J. Physiol.* **84**:401.

Shannon, J. A., and Fisher, S., 1938, The renal tubular reabsorption of glucose in the normal dog, *Am. J. Physiol.* **122**:765.

Sirota, J. H., 1953, Renal tubule reabsorption of phosphate in hyperparathyroidism before and after removal of parathyroid adenoma, *Fed. Proc. Fed. Am. Soc. Exp. Biol.* **12**:133.

Smith, H., 1961, *From Fish to Philosopher,* Anchor Books, Garden City, New York.

Smith, H. W., 1930, The absorption and excretion of water and salts by marine teleosts, *Am. J. Physiol.* **93**:480.

Smith, H. W., Goldring, W., Chasis, H., Ranges, H. A., and Bradley, S. E., 1943, The application of saturation methods to the study of glomerular and tubular function in the human kidney, *J. Mt. Sinai Hosp. N.Y.* **10**:59.

Smith, P. K., Ollayos, R. W., and Winkler, A. W., 1943, Tubular reabsorption of phosphate in the dog, *J. Clin. Invest.* **22**:143.

Stalder, G., Schmidt, R., and Gerstner, I., 1957, Die maximale tubuläre Phosphat Rückresorption (TmP) in den Nieren des gesunden Kindes, *Ann. Paediatr. (Basel)* **189**:293.

Stamp, T. C., and Stacey, T. E., 1970, Evaluation of theoretical renal phosphorus threshold as an index of renal phosphorus handling, *Clin. Sci.* **39**:506.

Stanbury, S. W., Lumb, G. A., and Nicholson, W. F., 1960, Elective subtotal parathyroidectomy for renal hyperparathyroidism, *Lancet* **1**:793.

Strickler, J. C., Thompson, D. D., Klose, R., and Giebisch, G., 1964, Micropuncture study of inorganic phosphate excretion in the rat, *J. Clin. Invest.* **43**:1956.

Talpers, S. J., and Stein, J. D., Jr., 1959, Tubular reabsorption of phosphorus as a measure of parathyroid activity, *Metabolism* **8**:170.

Thalassinos, N. C., Leese, B., Latham, S. C., and Joplin, G. F., 1970, Urinary excretion of phosphate in normal children, *Arch. Dis. Child.* **45**:269.

Thomas, W. F., Connor, T. B., and Morgan, H. G., 1958, Some observations on patients with hypercalcemia exemplifying problems in differential diagnosis especially in hyperparathyroidism, *J. Lab. Clin. Med.* **52**:11.

Thompson, D. D., and Hiatt, H. H., 1957, Renal reabsorption of phosphate in normal human subjects and in patients with parathyroid disease, *J. Clin. Invest.* **36**:550.

Van Slyke, D. D., Wu, H., and McLean, F. C., 1923, Studies of gas and electrolyte equilibria in the blood. V. Factors controlling the electrolyte and water distribution in the blood, *J. Biol. Chem.* **56**:765.

Vereecke, A., 1898, Etude de l'influence de la sécrétion interne du corps thyroïde sur les échanges organiques, *Arch. Int. Pharmacodyn. Thér.* **4**:81.

Walker, A. M., 1933, Quantitative studies on the composition of glomerular urine. X. The concentration of inorganic phosphate in glomerular urine from frogs and necturi determined by an ultramodification of the Bell–Doisy method, *J. Biol. Chem.* **101**:239.

Walker, D. A., Davies, S. J., Siddle, K., and Woodhead, J. S., 1977, Control of renal tubular phosphate reabsorption by parathyroid hormone in man, *Clin. Sci. Mol. Med.* **53**:431.

Walser, M., 1961, Ion association. VI. Associations between calcium, magnesium, inorganic phosphate, citrate and protein in normal human plasma, *J. Clin. Invest.* **40**:723.

Walser, M., Ford, M. J., and Butler, S., 1960, Protein-binding of inorganic phosphate in plasma of normal subjects and patients with renal disease, *J. Clin. Invest.* **39**:501.

Walton, R. J., and Bijvoet, O. L. M., 1975, Nomogram for the derivation of renal threshold phosphate concentration, *Lancet* **2**:309.

Wearn, J. T., and Richards, A. N., 1924, Observations on the composition of glomerular urine, with particular reference to the problem of reabsorption in the renal tubules, *Am. J. Physiol.* **71**:209.

Wesson, L. G., 1964, Electrolyte excretion in relation to diurnal cycles of renal function, *Medicine* **43:**547.
White, H. L., 1932, Further observations on glomerular function, *Am. J. Physiol.* **102:**222.
Wigglesworth, V. B., and Woodrow, C. E., 1924, The relation between phosphate in blood and urine, *Proc. R. Soc. London Ser. B* **95:**558.

2

Sites of Renal Tubular
Reabsorption of Phosphate

CLAUDE AMIEL

1. INTRODUCTION

When tubular phosphate reabsorption was first studied with micropuncture techniques by Strickler *et al.* (1964), one would have expected the question "Where is phosphate reabsorbed in the nephron?" to be answered quickly, easily, and definitively. Sixteen years later, and despite a considerable number of publications on the subject, it still appeared timely to the editors of this volume to ask for a discussion of site(s) of phosphate reabsorption along the nephron. Is this the consequence of a failure of the micropuncture technique, of inadequate protocol design, or of insufficient interpretation of the data? A critical evaluation of the available data on the sites of phosphate reabsorption along the nephron is presented in this chapter.

2. PHOSPHATE TRANSPORT BETWEEN THE GLOMERULUS AND THE LATE ACCESSIBLE PROXIMAL CONVOLUTION OF THE SUPERFICIAL NEPHRON

2.1. Phosphate Reabsorption in the Intact Animal

The bulk of phosphate reabsorption in the superficial nephron occurs between the glomerulus and the late proximal tubule accessible to micropuncture. Indeed, 60–70% of the filtered phosphate is already reabsorbed when the filtrate reaches this site (Tables 1 and 2). Phosphate reabsorption in the accessible segment, however, is not homogeneous.

39

Table 1. Phosphate Delivery (Percentage of Filtered Load) in Late Accessible Proximal Tubule and Early Accessible Distal Tubule Sampled at Random[a]

Reference	Experimental condition	Proximal	Distal	Loop[c]
Strickler et al.	Intact	25	25	NS
(1964)	Pi load	79	71	NS
Amiel et al.	Intact	34	41	NS
(1970)	Chronic PTX	40	36	NS
	Acute TPTX	34	10	24
Le Grimellec et al.	Intact	34	35	NS
(1973a)	Intact	44	48	NS
Le Grimellec et al.	Control	32	33	NS
(1973b)	Mg load	35	34	NS
	Post Mg load	35	41	NS
Le Grimellec et al.	Control	35	36	NS
(1974a)	Ca load	32	37	NS
	Post Ca load	29	40	−11
Le Grimellec et al.	Control	37	36	NS
(1974b)	Pi load	77	70	NS
	Post Pi load	52	54	NS
de Rouffignac et al.	Psammomys	39	25	14
(1973)				
Boudry et al.	Control	30	31	NS
(1975)	Pi load	50	48	NS
Poujeol et al.	Nondiuretic	34	34	NS
(1976)	Saline diuresis	49	46	NS
Greger et al.	Intact	38	37	NS
(1977a)	Acute TPTX	14	4	10

[a] Not from the same nephron.
[b] Unless otherwise indicated.
[c] NS, not significant

It has been shown that the intratubular phosphate concentration at a point where no more than 14% of the glomerular filtrate is reabsorbed is already the same as the concentration measureable along the whole accessible proximal tubule (Amiel et al., 1970). This observation confirmed earlier reports of phosphate concentrations that were within 1 SD of the mean for the whole accessible proximal tubule at sites where no more than 20% of glomerular filtrate was reabsorbed (Morel et al., 1969; Strickler et al., 1964). The implication of these observations is that in the early part of the proximal tubule, where up to 15–20% of glomerular filtrate is reabsorbed, absolute phosphate reabsorption is more than twice that in all the remaining parts of the accessible proximal tubule (Amiel et al., 1970). Similar information was obtained from studies of the accessible proximal tubule of the dog (Agus et al., 1971). The more avid phosphate reabsorption in the very early superficial proximal tubule, which usually is not accessible to micropuncture, was studied in the Munich–Wistar strain of rats; a linear decrease of intratubular phosphate concentration, expressed as a function of tubular fluid/glomerular filtrate inulin ratio, was demonstrated from the glomerulus to a point where the inulin ratio equals 1.15 (Le Grimellec, 1975). It can be concluded, therefore, that whatever the cellular mechanisms by which such a difference is achieved, the con-

Table 2. Phosphate Delivery in Late Accessible Proximal Tubule and in Urine in Studies in Which Distal Tubule Micropuncture Was Not Performed

Reference	Experimental animal	Experimental condition[a]		Phosphate delivery (% of filtered load)		
				Late proximal	Urine	Difference
Agus et al. (1971)	Dog	PTH	C	60	4	56
			R	59	8.5	50.5
			C	42	3.9	38.1
			R	54	2.4	51.6
		BT$_2$ cAMP (systemic)	C	58	7	51
			R	74	34	40
		Bt$_2$ cAMP (renal artery)	C	31	5	26
			R	59	24	35
		Expansion	C	53	8.2	44.8
			R	68	17	51
Frick (1972)	Rat	Intact		60.8	36.5	24.3
		Acute PTX		38.1	4.8	33.3
		Acute PTX + PTH		69.8	37.9	31.9
Puschett et al. (1972)	Dog	Intact		47	9.6	37.4
		Expansion		62	18.6	43.4
Maesaka et al. (1973)	Rat	Intact (control)		10.8	0.7	10.1
		Expansion		38	7.1	30.9
		Acute TPTX				
		Control		1.8	0.1	1.7
		Expansion		9.6		9.5
					0.1	
Agus et al. (1973)	Dog	PTH	C	49	8.4	40.6
			R	69	29.2	39.8
		Bt$_2$ cAMP	C	44	2.4	41.6
			R	75	30.4	44.6
Beck and Goldberg (1973)	Dog	Intact		36.4	1.3	35.1
		Idem + acetazolamide		54.7	11	43.7
		24–72 hr TPTX		17.5	0.8	16.7
		Idem + acetazolamide		38.5	3.4	35.1

(continued)

Table 2. (*Continued*)

Reference	Experimental animal	Experimental condition[a]		Phosphate delivery (% of filtered load)		
				Late proximal	Urine	Difference
Wen	Dog, 24–72 hr	Control		41	2.9	38.1
(1974)	TPTX	PTH		62	26.4	35.6
		Control		45	4.5	40.5
		Expansion		67	18.2	48.8
		Control		46	5.5	40.5
		Acetazolamide		68	31.2	36.8
Beck and	Dog	Intact	C	34	4.63	29.37
Gold-			R	37	6.91	30.09
berg						
(1974)						
		Acute TPTX	C	23	0.37	22.63
			R	28	0.24	27.76
		Intact + saline	C	36	2.41	33.59
			R	65	25.51	39.49
		Acute TPTX +	C	22	0.26	21.74
		saline	R	56	3.06	52.94
		24 hr TPTX + saline	C	24	1.63	22.37
			R	58	3.93	54.07
Knox and	Dog, acute	Control		26	2.3	23.7
Lechêne	TPTX	PTH		37	21.4	15.6
(1975)		Control		27	5.1	21.9
		Expansion		36	9.8	26.2
Knox *et*	Dog, acute	Control		28	3.8	24.2
al.	TPTX	PTH		38	19.9	18.1
(1976)		Acetazolamide		50	8.7	41.3
		Acetazolamide + PTH		58	31	27

[a] Abbreviations: C, collection; R, recollection; Bt$_2$ cAMP, dibutyryl cyclic AMP.

voluted proximal tubule includes at least two portions with distinctly different reabsorptive characteristics for phosphate.

2.2. Phosphate Reabsorption in the Absence of Parathyroid Hormone

In contrast to that in normal animals, phosphate reabsorption is evenly distributed along the whole accessible proximal tubule in rats deprived of parathyroid glands either at the beginning of the experiment (acute PTX) or several days before it (chronic PTX). Amiel *et al.* (1970) have shown that in those two situations the intratubular phosphate concentration declined linearly when plotted as a function of water reabsorption along the proximal tubule (Fig. 1). This was confirmed by others in the rat (Gekle *et al.*. 1971) and in the dog (Beck and Goldberg, 1974). In the absence of parathyroid hormone (PTH), therefore, it appears that the absolute phosphate reabsorption is constant, whatever the location in the proximal convoluted tubule. At variance with these data are results obtained with the use of capillary microperfusion and stationary droplet techniques in rats 48–72 hr after PTX. These studies disclosed faster phosphate transport rates in the early than in the late convolutions (Baumann *et al.*, 1975).

2.3. Phosphate Secretion in the Proximal Tubule

Three studies have reported mean fractional phosphate deliveries slightly higher than 100% in the early convoluted proximal tubule either at high-phosphate filtered load (Boudry *et al.*, 1975; Mühlbauer *et al.*, 1977) or at normal filtered load (Le Grimellec, 1975).

The possibility of phosphate entry into the proximal tubular lumen has been evaluated by widely different experimental protocols. Murayama *et al.* (1972) concluded from microperfusions in intact rats that no phos-

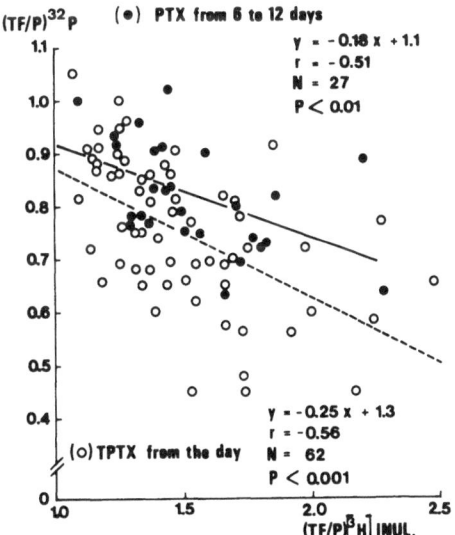

Fig. 1. Evolution of phosphate concentration along the proximal tubule as a function of water reabsorption in acute TPTX (○) and chronic PTX (●) rats. Ordinate: ratio of tubular fluid to plasma ^{32}P. Abscissa: ratio of tubular fluid to plasma [^3H]inulin. (Adapted from Amiel *et al.*, 1970.)

phate addition occurred when intratubular concentration was normal but that some phosphate backflux took place when the phosphate concentration was low in the perfusate. Boudry *et al.* (1975) demonstrated net entry of phosphate into the proximal tubule during microperfusion studies in rats with and without phosphate load. A similar result was reported by Shirley *et al.* (1976) with the use of a modified split-drop technique, and the authors suggested that the phosphate which entered the lumen had diffused from the tubular cells. Greger *et al.* (1977b), however, did not observe any net phosphate secretion in the proximal microperfused tubule of the intact dog, intact rat, and acute thyroparathyroidectomized (TPTX) rat. It should be noted that these studies were not performed with plasma ultrafiltrate but rather with artificial solutions of quite different composition and that the earliest part of the proximal tubule, which could be the site of phosphate secretion according to the micropuncture experiments mentioned above, was not explored. During *in vitro* micro-

Table 3. Phosphate Reabsorption by the Loop: Information Obtained from Microperfusions

1. Microperfusion of Late Proximal Tubule and Collection in Early Distal Tubule of the Same Nephron in the Rat (Murayama *et al.*, 1972)

Pi in perfusate (mM)	Loop reabsorption (pmol·min^{-1})
2.05	5
0.56	0

2. Comparison of Radioactive Phosphate Recoveries (Percentage of Injected Radioactivity) after Microperfusion in Late Proximal or Early Distal Tubule of the Rat (Greger *et al.*, 1977a)

Experimental condition	Late proximal	Early distal	Loop
Intact	58.7	101	42.3[a]
Acute TPTX	4.8	94.6	89.8[b]

3. Phosphate Fluxes in *in Vitro* Microperfusion of Rabbit Kidney Pars Recta

	Flux (pmol·mm^{-1}·min^{-1})	Pars recta		Convoluted segment	
Dennis *et al.* (1976)	Lumen to bath	2.22 ± 0.48		6.60 ± 1.41	
	Bath to lumen	0.31 ± 0.05		0.45 ± 0.08	
		Control	PTH	Control	PTH
Dennis *et al.* (1977)	Lumen to bath	2.64 ± 0.41	1.90 ± 0.34	5.45 ± 0.97	5.79 ± 1.10
	Bath to lumen	0.74 ± 0.14	0.33 ± 0.17	0.50 ± 0.08	0.46 ± 0.08

[a] To be compared with 1% obtained in the same animals by micropuncture at both sites (see Table 1)
[b] To be compared with 10% obtained in the same animals by micropuncture at both sites (see Table 1).

perfusion of proximal convoluted tubules with plasma ultrafiltrate, Dennis *et al.* (1976, 1977) noted that bath-to-lumen fluxes were about one-tenth those from lumen to bath (Table 3) The issue of phosphate secretion by the nephron is discussed in detail in Chapter 3.

3. PHOSPHATE TRANSPORT IN THE LOOP*

3.1. Evaluation by Micropuncture of the Late Accessible Proximal and Early Accessible Distal Convolutions Sampled at Random†

Comparison of phosphate deliveries to late proximal and to early distal tubules sampled at random fails to disclose any significant loop reabsorption in the intact rat (Table 1). Reabsorption is detectable only in acute PTX or TPTX animals or in the intact psammomys (Table 1). For this reason, loop reabsorption has received little credit.

3.2. Evaluation by Micropuncture of the Late Accessible Proximal and Early Accessible Distal Convolutions of the Same Nephron

Sampling of late proximal and early distal sites of the same nephron allowed us the calculation of a significant reabsorption in the loop in all the experimental conditions tested, including the normal rat (Table 4). The loop fractional phosphate reabsorption was highest in acute PTX rats, intermediate in chronic PTX rats, and lowest, although significant, in intact rats.

---

* Loop is defined as the segments of the nephron between the late accessible proximal and early accessible distal convolutions of superficial nephrons.

† Numerous works in which only late proximal but not distal phosphate delivery in superficial nephrons was evaluated have not been considered in detail in this chapter (Table 2). Indeed, late proximal delivery compared to fractional urinary excretion does not allow conclusions on sites of reabsorption beyond the accessible proximal tubule, as the respective contributions of the loop and of terminal segments cannot be evaluated. Some of the workers in this field have concluded that the difference between late proximal and urine phosphate delivery is likely to be accounted for by reabsorption in the pars recta (Agus *et al.*, 1971; Beck and Goldberg, 1973; Puschett *et al.*, 1972), while others have proposed that reabsorption beyond the distal tubule was likely in normal and/or in PTX animals (Beck and Goldberg, 1974; Frick, 1972; Maesaka *et al.*, 1973; Wen, 1974). In one study (Knox *et al.*, 1976), it was concluded that PTH inhibited phosphate reabsorption beyond the point of micropuncture in the late proximal tubule. Results of stop-flow experiments indicated that PTH decreased phosphate reabsorption in the distal nephron (Knox and Lechêne, 1975).

Table 4. Phosphate Reabsorption by the Loop of Superficial Nephrons: Information Obtained from Micropuncture of Late Accessible Proximal and Early Accessible Distal Convolutions of the Same Nephron in the Rat (Mean ± SEM)

Reference	Experimental condition	Individual loop reabsorption	p	Fractional delivery (% of filtered load)		
				Late proximal	Early distal	p
Küntziger et al. (1974)	Nondiuretic	7.54 ± 1.65	<0.001	39.11 ± 2.00	31.57 ± 1.62	<0.01
	Saline diuresis	18.66 ± 2.01	<0.001	43.24 ± 2.19	24.58 ± 1.65	<0.001
Küntziger et al. (1974)	Acute PTX	22.73 ± 2.96	<0.01	24.94 ± 2.84	1.21 ± 0.17	<0.001
	Acute PTX + cAMP	13.12 ± 0.76	<0.001	43.32 ± 1.39	30.13 ± 1.65	<0.001
Amiel et al. (1976)	Chronic PTX	16.77 ± 2.15	<0.001	42.52 ± 3.79	25.60 ± 3.58	<0.01
	Chronic PTX + Ca	20.08 ± 1.27	<0.001	28.90 ± 1.91	8.82 ± 2.07	<0.001
	Chronic PTX + cAMP	11.40 ± 2.93	<0.02	44.02 ± 2.22	32.62 ± 3.09	<0.02
	Chronic PTX + Ca + cAMP	13.54 ± 1.24	<0.001	33.58 ± 2.78	20.27 ± 3.52	<0.02

3.3. Evaluation by Microinjections into the Late Accessible Proximal and Early Accessible Distal Convolutions

Loop phosphate reabsorption has also been evaluated from the recovery of radioactive phosphate microinjected into either the late proximal or the early distal tubule (Table 5). The microinjections were not performed at both sites of the same nephron. Results are summarized in Table 5. In two of the three reports (Poujeol and de Rouffignac, 1976; Staum et al., 1972), no significant reabsorption was detected in the intact animal. The two works using acute TPTX rats (Brunette et al., 1973; Poujeol and de Rouffignac, 1976) revealed a reabsorption in this experimental condition.

3.4. Evaluation by in Vivo Microperfusion

Loop reabsorption has also been studied by in vivo microperfusion (Table 3). The first study showed a significant reabsorption when the perfusate was 2.05 mM phosphate but no reabsorption when it was 0.56 mM phosphate (Murayama et al., 1972). It must be pointed out that the intratubular phosphate concentration in the late proximal tubule is about 1.4 mM, a value intermediate between those used. In a subsequent study by microperfusion (Greger et al., 1977a), the fractional reabsorption of the radioactive tracer was far above the fractional phosphate reabsorption observed in the same work by micropuncture at random of late proximal and early distal accessible sites. This observation was attributed by the authors to the artificial composition of the microinfused fluid, to the possibility that a unidirectional flux and not a net flux was measured, and to the proximal oil blockade of the tubule.

Table 5. Phosphate Reabsorption by the Loop: Mean Fractional Recovery (Percentage of Injected Radioactive Phosphate) after Microinjections into Late Accessible Proximal and Early Accessible Distal Tubules in the Rat

Reference	Experimental condition	Proximal	Distal	"Loop"
Staum et al. (1972)	Intact	>95	100	
Brunette et al. (1973)	Saline diuresis	77.9	95.1	17.2
	PTH	85.6	103.3	17.7
	Acute TPTX	49.5	98.9	49.4
Poujeol and de Rouffignac (1976)	Intact	77	82.6	NS[a]
	Acute TPTX	65.8	92	26.2
	TPTX + PTH	73.3	85.4	12.1

[a] NS, not significant.

3.5. Evaluation by *in Vitro* Microperfusion

Undoubtedly, the most elegant and informative studies on phosphate reabsorption in one segment of the loop were performed by *in vitro* microperfusion of rabbit kidney pars recta (Table 3). An absolute phosphate reabsorption was observed in the straight portion (Dennis *et al.*, 1976). It was about one-third that in the convoluted segment per unit of length. It was also pointed out that when PTH is added, phosphate reabsorption is significantly decreased only in the pars recta and not in the convoluted segment, despite the fact that in the latter, the inhibition of fluid reabsorption was significant (Dennis *et al.*, 1977). These observations, although made in a species which has not been extensively studied by micropuncture techniques, point to the straight portion as a major site of PTH action on phosphate reabsorption.

As far as other segments of the loop are concerned, the *in vitro* microperfusion of thin descending limbs, thin ascending limbs, and thick ascending limbs of the rabbit kidney did not show any significant phosphate reabsorption (Rocha *et al.*, 1977).

3.6. Characteristics of Loop Phosphate Reabsorption

Additional information on loop reabsorption was provided by our studies in which the same superficial nephron was sampled at both late proximal and early distal accessible sites. In all of these experiments, phosphate reabsorption was significantly correlated to water reabsorption (Table 6). Such a correlation may indicate that phosphate reabsorption is likely to take place at a site where water subtraction occurs as well, which points to the pars recta. The ordinate intercepts of regression lines listed in Table 6 could represent the behavior of segments where little or no water reabsorption takes place. Positive values would correspond to phosphate reabsorption, and negative ones would suggest phosphate addition. However, the latter possibility is not supported by either microperfusion experiments (Murayama *et al.*, 1972) or loop micropunctures (de Rouffignac *et al.*, 1973), although phosphate secretion might occur after a calcium load (Le Grimellec *et al.*, 1973a) (Table 1).

Analysis of the relationship between the phosphate load entering the loop (delivery to the late proximal tubule) and the phosphate load escaping from it (delivery to the early distal tubule) showed that there was a significant linear correlation between them in all of the experimental circumstances studied, with the exception of the acute PTX rat (Table 6). This suggests that phosphate reabsorption in the loop was limited by a gradient in the acute PTX animal, while in the other situations it was in proportion to the load.

Table 6. Phosphate Reabsorption by the Loop: Correlation between Phosphate and Water Reabsorption in the Loop and between Phosphate Escaping the Loop and Phosphate Delivered to the Loop

Reference	Experimental condition	Pi reabsorption vs. water reabsorption (% of filtered load)			Pi escaping the loop vs. Pi delivered to the loop (% of filtered load)		
		Slope	Ordinate	p	Slope	Ordinate	p
Küntziger et al. (1972)	Nondiuretic	0.57	− 8.5	<0.01	0.46	+13.7	<0.01
	Saline diuresis	0.95	− 10.2	<0.001	0.65	− 3.2	<0.001
Küntziger et al. (1974)	Acute PTX	0.54	+10	<0.05	NS[a]	NS[a]	NS[a]
	Acute PTX + cAMP	0.72	+ 6.2	<0.001	0.55	+ 6.3	<0.001
Amiel et al. (1976)	Chronic PTX	0.46	+ 6.1	<0.01	0.46	+ 6.2	<0.05
	Chronic PTX + Ca	0.45	− 3.8	<0.001	0.45	− 3.8	<0.001
	Chronic PTX + cAMP	0.29	+19.3	<0.05	0.28	+20.1	<0.05
	Chronic PTX + Ca + cAMP	0.76	− 5	<0.001	0.76	− 5.0	<0.001

[a] NS, not significant.

4. PHOSPHATE TRANSPORT IN THE TERMINAL NEPHRON*

4.1. Evaluation by Micropuncture

We have shown that fractional phosphate delivery to the distal tubule is higher than in ureteral urine in intact, chronic PTX, and acute PTX rats (Amiel *et al.*, 1970). This fact has been confirmed by all of the subsequent micropuncture studies which included distal tubular sampling, with the exception of two out of the three in which phosphate-loaded rats were studied (Table 7).

The heterogeneity of the nephron population was a possible explanation for the discrepancy between phosphate delivery in the distal tubule and in urine. We have examined that hypothesis, namely that deep nephrons may reabsorb all the filtered phosphate in their proximal tubules and, therefore, account for a urine mixture of high-phosphate fluid delivered by superficial nephrons and of phosphate-free fluid delivered by deep nephrons. It was calculated that deep nephrons should account for 36, 68, and 83%, respectively, of the entire glomerular filtration in intact, chronic PTX, and acute PTX rats. Therefore, we concluded that in intact rats, there was a theoretical possibility of spurious reabsorption accounted for by the heterogeneity of the nephron population but that in chronic and acute PTX rats, the high figures (68% and 83%) were incompatible with such a postulate (Amiel *et al.*, 1970). This kind of hypothesis, moreover, would implicate a different heterogeneity in normal, chronic PTX, and acute PTX rats. Therefore, it appears from a critical study of superficial distal tubule micropuncture data that terminal reabsorption must exist, although it may be less important than suggested by the calculation of the difference between phosphate delivery in the distal superficial tubule and in urine if deep nephrons reabsorb proportionally more phosphate than superficial ones.

A recent study attempted to evaluate directly the behavior of deep nephrons by sampling the ascending limbs of Henle's loop at the papilla in either acute or chronic PTX Munich–Wistar rats (Haas *et al.*, 1978). Superficial distal tubules were punctured in the same animals. In chronic PTX animals, it was found that phosphate delivery not only to the superficial distal tubule but also to the ascending limb of deep nephrons was higher than in urine. These results confirm, in the chronic PTX model, terminal phosphate reabsorption in superficial nephrons and also indicate a reabsorption beyond the ascending limb in deep nephrons. As far as the acute PTX model is concerned, the results indicated that phosphate delivery to superficial distal tubules was significantly higher than in urine,

---

* Terminal nephron is defined as the segments of nephron between the early accessible distal tubule and the end of the collecting duct.

Table 7. Phosphate Delivery (Percentage of Filtered Load) in Distal Tubules of Superficial Nephrons and in Urine of the Rat[a]

Reference	Experimental condition	Distal	Urine	Difference
Amiel et al.	Intact	35[b]	21	14
(1970)	Chronic PTX	33[b]	11	22
	Acute TPTX	9[b]	2.5	6.5
Küntziger et al.	Nondiuretic	32	22	10
(1972)	Saline diuresis	25	16	8
Le Grimellec et al.	Intact	35	23	12
(1973a)	Intact	48	28	20
Le Grimellec et al.	Control	33	23	10
(1973b)	Mg load	34	17	17
	Post Mg load	41	10	31
Le Grimellec et al.	Control	37	22	15
(1974a)	Ca load	55	23	32
	Post Ca load	46	5	41
Le Grimellec et al.	Control	36	24	12
(1974b)	Pi load	70	57	13
	Post Pi load	54	37	17
de Rouffignac et al.	Psammomys	25	7	18
(1973)				
Küntziger et al.	Acute PTX	1.21	0.23	0.98
(1974)	Acute PTX + cAMP	30	20	10
Boudry et al.	Intact	31	17	14
(1975)	Pi load	48	66	−18
	Pi load + PTH	43	70	−27
Poujeol et al.	Nondiuretic	34	18	16
(1976)	Saline diuresis	46	25	21
Amiel et al.	Chronic PTX	26	8	17
(1976)	Chronic PTX + Ca	9	3	6
	Chronic PTX + cAMP	33	19	13
	Chronic PTX + Ca + cAMP	20	15	5
Greger et al.	Intact	37	24	13
(1977a)	Acute PTX	4	1.7	2.3
Knox et al.	Pi load + PTH	56	67	11
(1977a)	Pi load + PTH	51	72	21
Mülhbauer et al.	Low-Pi diet + Pi load	21	21	0
(1977)	High-Pi diet + Pi load	64	39	25
Haas et al.	Acute PTX	8.6	0.6	8
(1978)	Chronic TPTX	19.3	3.6	15.7

[a] Unless otherwise indicated.
[b] All distal tubule values.

while the difference between delivery to deep-nephron ascending limbs (3.6 ± 1.6 SEM, percentage of filtered load) and urine (0.6 ± 0.3 SEM) did not achieve significance. Even if one assumes that delivery to ascending limbs in acute PTX animals was equal to that in urine, one cannot see how deep nephrons could explain the observed difference between the superficial distal tubule and urine. Obviously, to account for such a difference, deep nephrons should deliver less phosphate than that in urine. This work, therefore, confirms a terminal reabsorption of phosphate in superficial nephrons of both chronic and acute PTX rats and a phosphate reabsorption beyond the ascending limb in chronic if not in acute PTX animals.

4.2. Evaluation by Distal Tubular Microperfusion and Microinjection

In order to avoid the inherent difficulties in interpretation due to the heterogeneity of the nephron population, several studies were performed with distal tubular microinjections or microperfusions. Results of these are listed in Table 8. It can be seen that the results are discrepant. Three groups did not observe any significant phosphate reabsorption beyond the distal tubule.

One of these three works comes from the same laboratory in which the aforementioned ascending-limb micropunctures were performed. Thus, with the same Munich–Wistar rat strain, in the same acute PTX condition, one work concludes that "phosphate reabsorption is confined in the proximal tubule and the loop of Henle" (Greger et al., 1977a), while the other (Haas et al., 1978), as discussed above, brings clear evidence that the differences in phosphate deliveries in superficial distal tubules and urine cannot be accounted for by deep-nephron function. This apparent contradiction highlights the difficulties inherent in this field.

Table 8. Phosphate Reabsorption by the Terminal Nephron: Fractional Recovery (Percentage of Injected Radioactive Phosphate) after Distal Tubular Microinjections or Microperfusions in the Rat

Reference	Experimental condition	Recovery
Staum et al. (1972)	Intact	100
Brunette et al. (1973)	Control	99
	PTH	99
	Acute PTX	100
Poujeol and de Rouffignac (1976)	Control	82.6
	Acute TPTX	92
	Acute TPTX + PTH	85.4
Poujeol et al. (1977)	Saclay–Wistar strain	82.6
	Bordeaux–Wistar strain	88.2
	Munich–Wistar strain	99
Greger et al. (1977a)	Control	101
	Acute TPTX	94.6

Another group (Poujeol *et al.*, 1977) cast some light on the complexity of interpreting results of microinjection or microperfusion studies when they demonstrated that there was no reabsorption of the radioactive tracer beyond the distal tubule in the intact Munich–Wistar rat—an observation which is in agreement with the absence of phosphate reabsorption in the same strain during either stationary microperfusion of the distal tubule (performed by Lang *et al.*, 1977) or free-flow microperfusion (performed by Greger *et al.*, 1977a)—but a significant reabsorption in two other Wistar strains (Bordeaux and Saclay). In the same work, direct evidence of heterogeneity of the nephron population was provided. In Munich–Wistar rats, fractional phosphate excretion in urine was 36.4% and fractional phosphate excretion of the radioactive tracer injected into the renal artery was also 36.4%, but fractional excretion of the radioactive tracer injected into surface glomeruli was 55.7%. This clearly shows that deep nephrons must have reabsorbed a greater fraction of filtered phosphate than superficial ones. The same investigators observed that 24% of the radioactive phosphate microinjected into the ascending limb of deep nephrons was reabsorbed downstream in the intact Munich–Wistar rate (P. Poujeol, 1978, personal communication). Thus, the higher reabsorption of deep nephrons may occur, at least in part, in their terminal segments.

It should be noted that neither distal microinjections nor distal microperfusions, in an attempt to detect and evaluate terminal phosphate reabsorption, were performed in what is obviously the best experimental model, that is, the chronic PTX animal. Apparent terminal reabsorption in the chronic PTX animal is about 17–22% of the filtered load, or 62–66% of the load delivered to the distal tubule, and amounts to 25 pmol·min^{-1} (Amiel *et al.*, 1970, 1976).

The results obtained with distal microinjections in the Saclay–Wistar strain (Poujeol and de Rouffignac, 1976; Poujeol *et al.*, 1977) indicate a terminal reabsorption of phosphate of about 17–18% of the load delivered to the distal tubule. The difference between phosphate deliveries in the superficial distal nephron and in urine indicates an apparent reabsorption of 46% of the load in the same strain, studied in the same laboratory (Poujeol *et al.*, 1976). It has been stressed in a recent review (Knox *et al.*, 1977b) that the figures of terminal reabsorption are very low, both in terms of absolute reabsorption (about 1 pmol·min^{-1}) and as a fraction of the filtered load (about 1%). Actually, the figures are nearer 3 pmol·min^{-1} and 6%, and, in terms of tubular homeostatic mechanisms, it is perfectly possible that precise adjustments may be achieved by reabsorption of such small amounts. Analogous to sodium reabsorption, the physiological importance of the distal reabsorptive processes need not be based on their relative magnitude compared to that in the rest of the nephron.

Also quoted against the possibility of terminal reabsorption are observations that no phosphate reabsorption was found in the isolated microperfused rabbit cortical collecting duct (Dennis *et al.*, 1977). However, it has been clearly indicated by the authors that "the cortical collecting segments examined . . .correspond to the light segments designated by Morel *et al.* (1976) . . .who have demonstrated that the light portion of the cortical collecting ducts lacks PTH-sensitive adenylate cyclase activity, an observation consistent with the present absence of PTH-induced changes in fluid or in phosphate absorption in this segment. Although it is not certain that each PTH-sensitive area of the nephron is involved directly in phosphate transport, phosphate absorption may occur in the earlier, so called granular, portion of the cortical collecting duct" (Dennis *et al.*, 1977).

4.3. Possible Sites of Phosphate Reabsorption in the Terminal Nephron

The description of several PTH-sensitive, adenylate-cyclase-containing segments along the nephron (Chabardès *et al.*, 1975; Morel *et al.*, 1976) and their relation to the localization of phosphate reabsorption have been discussed by others (Poujeol *et al.*, 1977), and it was proposed that the arcades connected to distal tubules may well be the main site of terminal phosphate reabsorption.

5. CONCLUSIONS

From the analysis of the preceding data, it appears that the evidence for several sites of phosphate reabsorption along the nephron is quite convincing. These sites include, in the intact rat as well as in acute and chronic PTX animals, (1) the convoluted proximal tubules, (2) the loop, in which the pars recta most certainly plays a dominant role, and (3) the terminal nephron, where the PTH-sensitive, adenylate-cyclase-containing segments may be involved.

The fact that the amounts of phosphate reabsorbed decrease from the beginning to the end of the nephron does not allow one to conclude that the most proximal segments are more important than the terminal ones in terms of homeostatic control of phosphate excretion. It can be suggested, on the contrary, and by analogy with the control of sodium excretion, that the minute, precise adjustments in tubular phosphate handling occur in the terminal segments of the nephron.

Much of the controversy about phosphate reabsorption sites (or about the occurrence and sites of phosphate secretion) is due to the fact that the micropuncture technique has failed to give extensive information on deep-nephron function. As a result, interpretation of the available data from puncture of superficial nephrons often has been burdened by the unlikely behavior sometimes ascribed to deep nephrons. Furthermore, several of the most adequate protocols have not been sufficiently used, the chronic PTX model for the evaluation of terminal reabsorption being an example.

ACKNOWLEDGMENTS. The author is deeply indebted to Adrian I. Katz for his invaluable help in preparation of the manuscript. Much of the author's work cited here was made possible by grants from the Institut National de la Santé et de la Recherche Médicale, the Délégation Générale à la Recherche Scientifique et Technique, and the Unité d'Enseignement et de Recherche Xavier Bichat of the Université Paris 7.

6. REFERENCES

Agus, Z. S., Puschett, J. B., Senesky, D., and Goldberg, M., 1971, Mode of action of parathyroid hormone and cyclic adenosine 3',5'-monophosphate on renal tubular phosphate reabsorption in the dog, J. Clin. Invest. 50:617.

Agus, Z. S., Gardner, L. B., Beck, L. H., and Goldberg, M., 1973, Effects of parathyroid hormone on renal tubular reabsorption of calcium, sodium, and phosphate, Am. J. Physiol. 224:1143.

Amiel, C., Küntziger, H., and Richet, G., 1970, Micropuncture study of handling of phosphate by proximal and distal nephron in normal and parathyroidectomized rat. Evidence for distal reabsorption, Pflügers Arch. 317:93.

Amiel, C., Küntziger, H., Couette, S., Coureau, C., and Bergounioux, N., 1976, Evidence for a parathyroid hormone-independent calcium modulation of phosphate transport along the nephron, J. Clin. Invest. 57:256.

Baumann, K., de Rouffignac, C., Roinel, N., Rumrich, G., and Ullrich, K. J., 1975, Inhomogeneity of local proximal transport rates and sodium dependence, Pflügers Arch. 356:287.

Beck, L. H., and Goldberg, M., 1973, Effects of acetazolamide and parathyroidectomy on renal transport of sodium, calcium, and phosphate, Am. J. Physiol. 224:1136.

Beck, L. H., and Goldberg, M., 1974, Mechanism of the blunted phosphaturia in saline-loaded thyroparathyroidectomized dogs, Kidney Int. 6:18.

Boudry, J.-F., Troehler, V., Touabi, M., Fleisch, H., and Bonjour, J.-P., 1975, Secretion of inorganic phosphate in the rat nephron, Clin. Sci. Mol. Med. 48:475.

Brunette, M. G., Taleb, L., and Carrière, S., 1973, Effect of parathyroid hormone on phosphate reabsorption along the nephron of the rat, Am. J. Physiol. 225:1076.

Chabardès, D., Imbert, M., Clique, A., Montégut, M., and Morel, F., 1975, PTH sensitive adenyl cyclase activity in different segments of the rabbit nephron, Pflügers Arch. 354:229.

Dennis, V. W., Woodhall, P. B., and Robinson, R. R., 1976, Characteristics of phosphate transport in isolated proximal tubule, Am. J. Physiol. 231:979.

Dennis, V. W., Bello-Reuss, E., and Robinson, R. R., 1977, Response of phosphate transport to parathyroid hormone in segments of rabbit nephron, Am. J. Physiol. 233:F29.

de Rouffignac, C., Morel, F., and Roinel, N., 1973, Micropuncture study of water and electrolyte movement along the loop of Henle in Psammomys with special reference to magnesium, calcium and phosphorus, *Pflügers Arch.* **344:**309.

Frick, A., 1972, Proximal tubular reabsorption of inorganic phosphate during saline infusion in the rat, *Am. J. Physiol.* **223:**1034.

Gekle, D., Ströder, J., and Rostock, D., 1971, The effect of vitamin D on renal inorganic phosphate reabsorption of normal rats, parathyroidectomized rats, and rats with rickets, *Pediatr. Res.* **5:**40.

Greger, R., Lang, F., Marchand, G., and Knox, F. G., 1977a, Site of renal phosphate reabsorption, *Pflügers Arch.* **369:**111.

Greger, R. F., Lang, F. C., Knox, F. G., and Lechêne, C. P., 1977b, Absence of significant secretory flux of phosphate in the proximal convoluted tubule, *Am. J. Physiol.* **232:**F235.

Haas, J. A., Berndt, T., and Knox, F. G., 1978, Nephron heterogeneity of phosphate reabsorption, *Am. J. Physiol.* **234:**F287–F290.

Knox, F. G., and Lechêne, C., 1975, Distal site of action of parathyroid hormone on phosphate reabsorption, *Am. J. Physiol.* **229:**1556.

Knox, F. G., Haas, J. A., and Lechêne, C. P., 1976, Effect of parathyroid hormone on phosphate reabsorption in the presence of acetazolamide, *Kidney Int.* **10:**216.

Knox, F. G., Haas, J. A., Berndt, T., Marchand, G. R., and Youngberg, S. P., 1977a, Phosphate transport in superficial and deep nephrons in phosphate-loaded rats, *Am. J. Physiol.* **233:**F150.

Knox, F. G., Osswald, H., Marchand, G. R., Spielman, W. S., Haas, J. A., Berndt, T., and Youngberg, S. P., 1977b, Phosphate transport along the nephron, *Am. J. Physiol.* **233:**F261.

Küntziger, H., Amiel, C., and Gaudebout, C., 1972, Phosphate handling by the rat nephron during saline diuresis, *Kidney Int.* **2:**318.

Küntziger, H., Amiel, C., Roinel, N., and Morel, F., 1974, Effect of parathyroidectomy and cyclic AMP on renal transport of phosphate, calcium, and magnesium, *Am. J. Physiol.* **227:**905.

Lang, F., Greger, R., Marchand, G. R., and Knox, F. G., 1977, Stationary microperfusion study of phosphate reabsorption in proximal and distal nephron segments, *Pflügers Arch.* **368:**45.

Le Grimellec, C., 1975, Micropuncture study along the proximal convoluted tubule. Electrolyte reabsorption in the first convolutions, *Pflügers Arch.* **354:**133.

Le Grimellec, C., Roinel, N., and Morel, F., 1973a, Simultaneous Mg, Ca, P, K, Na and Cl analysis in rat tubular fluid. I. During perfusion of either inulin or ferrocyanide, *Pflügers Arch.* **340:**181.

Le Grimellec, C., Roinel, N., and Morel, F., 1973b, Simultaneous Mg, Ca, P, K, Na and Cl analysis in rat tubular fluid. II. During acute Mg plasma loading, *Pflügers Arch.* **340:**197.

Le Grimellec, C., Roinel, N., and Morel, F., 1974a, Simultaneous Mg, Ca, P, K, Na and Cl analysis in rat tubular fluid. III. During acute Ca plasma loading, *Pflügers Arch.* **346:**171.

Le Grimellec, C., Roinel, N., and Morel, F., 1974b, Simultaneous Mg, Ca, P, K, Na and Cl analysis in rat tubular fluid. III. During acute phosphate plasma loading, *Pflügers Arch.* **346:**189.

Maesaka, J. K., Levitt, M. F. and Abramson, R. G., 1973, Effect of saline infusion on phosphate transport in intact and thyroparathyroidectomized rats, *Am. J. Physiol.* **225:**1421.

Morel, F., Roinel, N., and Le Grimellec, C., 1969, Electron probe analysis of tubular fluid composition, *Nephron* **6:**350.

Morel, F., Chabardès, D., and Imbert, M., 1976, Functional segmentation of the rabbit distal tubule by microdetermination of hormone-dependent adenylate cyclase activity, *Kidney Int.* **9:**264.

Mühlbauer, R. C., Bonjour, J.-P., and Fleisch, H., 1977, Tubular localization of adaptation to dietary phosphate, *Am. J. Physiol.* **233:**F342.

Murayama, Y., Morel, F., and Le Grimellec, C., 1972, Phosphate, calcium and magnesium transfers in proximal tubules and loops of Henle, as measured by single nephron microperfusion experiments in the rat. *Pfluügers Arch.* **333:**1.

Poujeol, P., and de Rouffignac, C., 1976, Microinjection studies of phosphate permeability in rats during mild saline diuresis: Influence of acute thyroparathyroidectomy and parathormore administration, in: *Phosphate Metabolism, Kidney and Bone* (L. Avioli, P. Bordier, H. Fleisch, S. Massry, and E. Slatopolsky, eds.), pp. 111–121, Armour Montagu, Paris.

Poujeol, P., Chabardès, D., Roinel, N., and de Rouffignac, C., 1976, Influence of extracellular fluid volume expansion on magnesium, calcium and phosphate handling along the rat nephron, *Pflügers Arch.* **365:**203.

Poujeol, P., Corman, B., Touvay, C., and de Rouffignac, C., 1977, Phosphate reabsorption in rat nephron terminal segments. Intrarenal heterogeneity and strain differences, *Pflügers Arch.* **371:**39.

Puschett, J. B., Agus, Z. S., Senesky, D., and Goldberg, M., 1972, Effects of saline loading and aortic obstruction on proximal phosphate transport, *Am. J. Physiol.* **223:**851.

Rocha, A. S., Magaldi, J. B. and Kokko, J., 1977, Calcium and phosphate transport in isolated segments of rabbit Henle's loop, *J. Clin. Invest.* **59:**975.

Shirley, D. G., Poujeol, P., and Le Grimellec, C., 1976, Phosphate, calcium, and magnesium fluxes into the lumen of the rat proximal convoluted tubule, *Pflügers Arch.* **362:**247.

Staum, B. B., Hamburger, R. J., and Goldberg, M., 1972, Tracer microinjection study of renal tubular phosphate reabsorption in the rat, *J. Clin. Invest.* **51:**2271.

Strickler, J. C., Thompson, D. D., Klose, E. M., and Giebisch, G., 1964, Micropuncture study of inorganic phosphate excretion in the rat, *J. Clin. Invest.* **43:**1596.

Wen, S. F., 1974, Micropuncture studies of phosphate transport in the proximal tubule of the dog. The relationship to sodium, *J. Clin. Invest.* **53:**143.

3

Is Phosphate Secreted by the Kidney?

EDWARD G. SCHNEIDER, ROBERT C. HANSON,
JENNIFER W. CHILDERS, EDWARD M.
FITZGERALD, and SARAH D. GLEASON

1. INTRODUCTION

The importance of the kidney in the control of phosphate metabolism has long been recognized (Smith, 1932). The kidney is the major excretory organ for phosphate, and, consequently, the removal of excess phosphate from the body is accomplished by the elimination of phosphate via the kidney. The development of various microanalytical techniques capable of measuring phosphate in nanoliter quantities of tubular fluid has increased our understanding of phosphate transport along the mammalian nephron. Despite these technical advances, the question of whether the mammalian kidney can excrete phosphate in excess of the amount of phosphate filtered across the glomerulus (i.e., net phosphate secretion) has not been satisfactorily established.

The ability of an organism to maintain a constant plasma concentration of any substance resides in its ability to adjust the rate of utilization or elimination to the rate of intake or production. Since phosphate is present in the diet in excess of the daily requirements, mechanisms have developed for eliminating this excess from the body. Three models can be used to describe the mechanisms for the elimination of phosphate by vertebrate kidneys. A summary of the three models is shown in Fig. 1.

In model 1, the secretory activity of the tubular cells is the primary determinant of phosphate excretion. The excretion of phosphate into the urine of aglomerular fishes proves the presence of this mechanism in

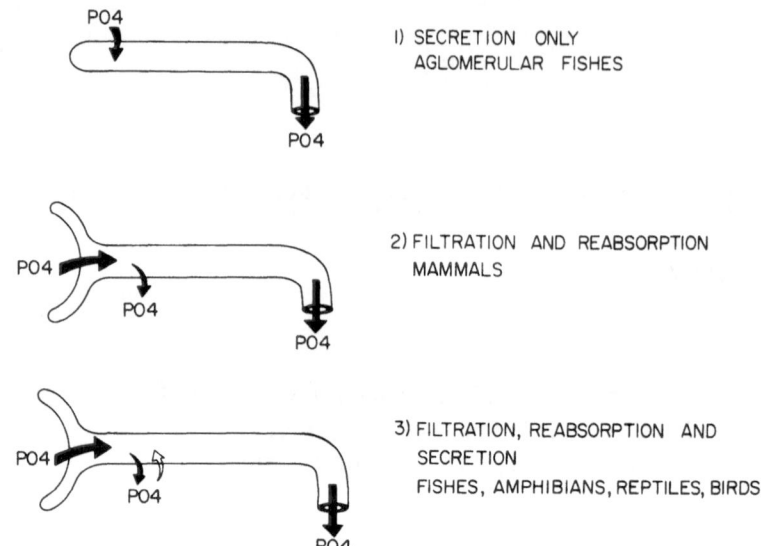

Fig. 1. Renal handling of phosphate: Three models that describe this process in vertebrates.

vertebrates. Two additional models are necessary to describe phosphate excretion in vertebrates that have functional glomeruli.

In model 2, the excretion of phosphate is determined by the amount of phosphate reabsorbed by the tubular cells. In this model, an animal is capable of either excreting no phosphate into the urine (high rate of tubular reabsorption) increasing phosphate excretion until the entire filtered load of phosphate is excreted (inhibition of phosphate reabsorption). This model, filtration and subsequent tubular reabsorption, is considered by many to adequately describe the renal handling of phosphate by humans and other mammals.

Model 3 describes phosphate excretion in the majority of vertebrates. In these vertebrates, the presence of not only filtration at the glomerulus and reabsorption by the tubules, but also secretion of phosphate by the tubules, allows a wide range of phosphate excretions. Thus, when reabsorption is great and secretion is low, little phosphate will be excreted, or, when reabsorption is low and secretion is great, more phosphate can be excreted into the urine than is filtered across the glomerulus. This model describes phosphate handling by the kidneys of fishes, reptiles, birds, and probably amphibians. Clearly, a vast majority of vertebrates on the earth today have developed a system involving a significant phosphate secretory mechanism.

The secretion of phosphate by the kidneys of lower vertebrates is a major factor behind the continued interest in determining whether or not phosphate secretion occurs in the mammalian kidney. Our objective is not to present a comprehensive review of all the work which demonstrates phosphate secretion in lower vertebrates, but to emphasize certain aspects of this secretion which are useful for evaluating the evidence for phosphate secretion and the nephron site at which phosphate secretion may occur in mammals.

2. PHOSPHATE SECRETION BY KIDNEYS OF LOWER VERTEBRATES

2.1. Fishes

Net phosphate secretion by the kidneys of vertebrates was first demonstrated in fish by Clarke and Smith (1932). These authors measured xylose and phosphate excretion in the marine elasmobranch *Squalus acanthias* (spiny dogfish). They found a urine-to-plasma (U/P) ratio for xylose of 3.2 ± 0.5, while the simultaneously measured U/P ratio for phosphate was 42.7 ± 11.5. Thus, 7% of the urinary excreted phosphate could be accounted for by filtration, and 93% of the urinary excreted phosphate was derived from tubular secretion. Although the clearance of xylose may underestimate glomerular filtration rate (GFR), it is unlikely that this error is of sufficient magnitude to alter their conclusion that phosphate was secreted by the renal tubule of the dogfish. Wolbach (1970) reported similar findings in the spiny dogfish when inulin was used to measure GFR.

The hagfish (*Myxine*), the most primitive vertebrate existing today, has also been shown to secrete phosphate (Munz and McFarland, 1964). This species has glomeruli and a mesonephric duct. The cells lining this duct resemble those of the proximal tubular segment I of higher fishes and nonmammalian vertebrates and the proximal convoluted tubule of mammals (Hickman and Trump, 1969). Thus, proximal tubular segment I is thought to secrete phosphate. In addition, proximal tubular segment II is also thought to secrete phosphate. This is based on the observation that the goosefish (*Lophius piscatorius*), a marine fish which lacks both glomeruli and a proximal tubular segment I but has proximal tubular segment II, can secrete phosphate (Marshall and Griffin, 1933).

Further support for the presence of phosphate secretion by both proximal tubular segments I and II has been obtained by Stolte *et al.* (1977). These investigators have measured the tubular fluid to plasma concentration ratio for phosphate [$(TF/P)_{PO_4}$] in the elasmobranch little skate, *Raja erinacea*. The $(TF/P)_{PO_4}$ was 6.7 ± 1.9 in samples obtained from proximal tubular segment I, 24.04 ± 1.4 in samples obtained from proximal tubular segment II, and 56.64 ± 12.07 in samples obtained by microcatheterization of the collecting duct. Since no measurement of water reabsorption was obtained in these experiments, the authors indicated that net phosphate secretion could not be conclusively demonstrated. It is of interest that in clearance studies on the little skate reported by Goldstein and Forster (1971), the U/P inulin ratio averaged 3. If similar values for water reabsorption existed in the micropuncture studies of Stolte et al. (1977), then phosphate would appear to be secreted by at least proximal tubular segments I and II. Since neither late proximal tubular segment II nor early collecting duct samples were obtained, the high $(TF/P)_{PO_4}$ observed at the end of the collecting duct may not indicate secretion of phosphate by this segment. Until simultaneously determined TF/P inulin and phosphate concentration ratios are available, a definite statement about the site of phosphate secretion in fishes cannot be made.

The control of phosphate secretion by the fish kidney has not been extensively studied. Parathyroid hormone (PTH) has not been found in fishes, and administration of mammalian parathyroid gland extract (PTE) is not known to alter phosphate excretion (Hickman and Trump, 1969). Investigators have examined the effects of plasma phosphate concentration on the secretion of phosphate. Marshall and Griffin (1933) reported that infusions of inorganic phosphate into the aglomerular goosefish, L. piscatorius, did not influence phosphate secretion. These authors concluded that secreted phosphate was derived from some unknown organic precursor; however, an already saturated secretory process could also explain these data. Infusion of phosphate into the spiny dogfish increased net phosphate secretion, suggesting that plasma phosphate may determine phosphate secretion in some fishes (Smith, 1939; Wolbach, 1970). In the spiny dogfish, the clearance of phosphate (C_{PO_4}) was ten times the clearance of inulin (C_{in}), but it was always less than the clearance of para-aminohippuric acid (Wolbach, 1970). Thus, inorganic phosphate in the blood perfusing the kidney can account for all of the phosphate excreted, making it unnecessary to hypothesize that secreted phosphate was derived from an organic precursor. At present, it has been shown that the secretion of phosphate occurs in fishes, but the nephron site(s) of this secretion and the control of the secretory process have not been adequately investigated.

2.2. Amphibians

Amphibians, whose kidneys are similar to those of teleosts, are also thought to secrete phosphate; however, we could not find any data which convincingly demonstrate net phosphate secretion. In one of the early micropuncture studies, Walker and Hudson (1937b) measured plasma and tubular fluid phosphate concentrations in the kidneys of frogs and *Necturus*. They concluded (1) that phosphate was freely filtered across the glomerulus and (2) that water reabsorption (measured as the U/P ratio of reducing substances in phlorizin-treated animals) could account for 90% of the increase in phosphate concentration along the nephron. Since the TF/P concentration ratio for reducing substances was known to underestimate the true GFR (Walker and Hudson, 1937a), these results do not demonstrate net phosphate secretion. However, when these authors microperfused proximal tubules with phosphate-free solutions, a $(TF/P)PO_4$ of 0.48 ± 0.10 was obtained in the perfusate (Walker and Hudson, 1937b). Thus, phosphate was shown to enter the proximal tubule down a concentration gradient. Since $(TF/P)PO_4$ was less than 1.0 in the perfusate, passive diffusion of phosphate, rather than active secretion of phosphate, can explain these results.

Trevan (1916) presented evidence for the secretion of phosphate from studies of the perfused frog kidney. When phosphate-free solutions were perfused through both the aortic arch (glomerular perfusion) and the anterior abdominal vein (peritubular perfusion), no acidification of the urine occurred. However, when phosphate was added to either the glomerular perfusion or the peritubular perfusion, acidification of the urine was observed. Trevan interpreted these data to indicate secretion of phosphate by the tubules; however, no measurement of phosphate excretion was reported.

In amphibians, the effect of acute elevations in plasma phosphate concentration on urinary phosphate excretion has not been reported. It is known that PTE and parathyroidectomy (PTX) affect plasma phosphate concentration and urinary phosphate excretion (Cortelyou, 1962; Cortelyou *et al.*, 1967); however, simultaneous measurements of C_{in} and C_{PO_4} have not been reported. Thus, additional studies are needed to determine if the amphibian kidney can excrete phosphate in excess of the amount of phosphate filtered across the glomerulus.

2.3. Reptiles

In one of the few studies of renal phosphate transport in reptiles, Clark and Dantzler (1972) measured C_{PO_4} and C_{in} in catheterized, unanesthetized water snakes of the genus *Natrix*. Several features of these studies are of interest. During control studies in which the animals were given an infusion of a 1.25% mannitol solution, C_{PO_4}/C_{in} was 2.6 ± 0.11, demonstrating net phosphate secretion. When the plasma phosphate concentration was acutely increased, net phosphate secretion increased and appeared to reach a maximum. The maximum rate of phosphate secretion by the reptilian kidney is difficult to evaluate because, at any time, the number of functioning nephrons can vary (Dantzler, 1967). However, this does not negate the conclusion that the kidneys of the snake are capable of secreting phosphate.

In another reptile, the alligator (*Alligator mississippiensis*), the kidneys have also been shown to secrete phosphate. Injections of sodium phosphate into alligators by Hernandez and Coulson (1957) were followed by an increase in the U/P phosphate concentration ratio from 9:1 to approximately 30:1, while the U/P creatinine ratio, a measure of water reabsorption, ranged from 4:1 to 6:1. In alligators cooled to 6°C for six days, the U/P phosphate ratio decreased from 30:1 (28°C) to 5:1 (6°C), while the U/P creatinine ratio remained between 4:1 and 6:1. The U/P phosphate ratio increased to 27:1 after rewarming the alligators to 28°C for 48 hr. These results demonstrate that phosphate secretion by the alligator kidney was reversibly inhibited by cooling, a classical procedure to demonstrate an active process.

The increase in phosphate secretion associated with acute elevations in plasma phosphate concentration may be caused by a direct effect of inorganic phosphate on the tubular cells or by an increase in PTH secretion. Since in both studies the reptiles had intact parathyroid glands, this question cannot be evaluated. Reptiles are the first class of vertebrates in which PTH or PTX has been clearly shown to affect urinary phosphate excretion. In PTX snakes, the C_{PO_4}/C_{in} was 0.32 ± 0.07, compared to a C_{PO_4}/C_{in} of 1.92 ± 0.15 in sham-operated controls. Thus, in the absence of parathyroid glands, the kidneys reabsorbed, rather than secreted, phosphate. The administration of PTE to both PTX and sham-operated snakes resulted in an increase in phosphate excretion. In both cases, a net secretion of phosphate occurred. The injection of saline instead of PTE into either PTX or sham-operated animals did not affect the renal excretion of phosphate. Thus, in the reptile, both net phosphate reabsorption and net phosphate secretion can be demonstrated. PTE has been shown to increase phosphate excretion in both reptiles and mammals; however, in reptiles, PTE has been thought to stimulate phosphate secretion, while in mammals, it inhibits phosphate reabsorption. The secretion of phosphate caused by PTH in reptiles might reflect an inhibition of phosphate reabsorption rather than a stimulation of phosphate secretion. As depicted in Fig. 2, several models can account for the effect of PTH on phosphate excretion by the reptilian kidney.

The first model indicates how PTH could cause net phosphate secretion by stimulating tubular secretion without affecting tubular reabsorption. This model assumes that either the capacity of the tubules to reabsorb phosphate can be exceeded by the secretory process or the site of tubular secretion is distal to the reabsorptive site. The second model

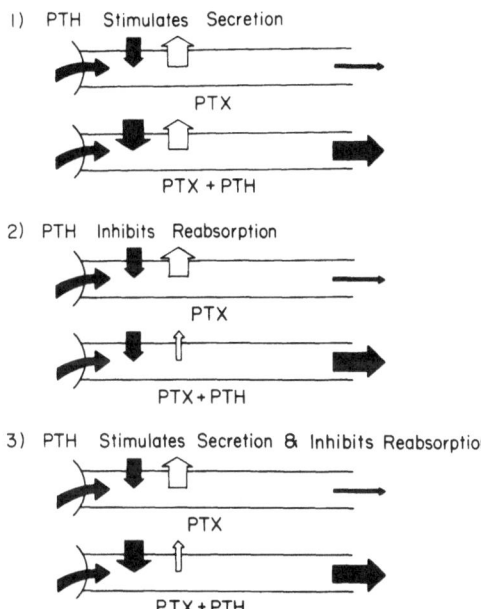

Fig. 2. Parathyroid hormone (PTH) and renal phosphate excretion in reptiles: Three models capable of explaining the phosphaturic effect of parathyroid hormone. PTX, parathyroidectomy.

indicates how PTH could cause net phosphate secretion by inhibiting tubular reabsorption without affecting tubular secretion. This model assumes that the site of secretion is not distal to the site of reabsorption. The third model indicates how PTH could cause net phosphate secretion by inhibiting tubular reabsorption and stimulating tubular secretion. This model makes no assumptions about the sites of secretion and reabsorption. These three models are compatible with the available data and are capable of explaining net reabsorption and secretion of phosphate.

2.4. Birds

The chicken was the first warm-blooded vertebrate shown to secrete phosphate. Levinsky and Davidson (1957) found that net phosphate secretion occurred at both endogenous plasma phosphate concentrations and at elevated plasma phosphate levels. When the peritubular phosphate concentration was selectively increased by infusing phosphate into the renal portal circulation of one kidney, no unilateral increase in phosphate excretion occurred. It could not be determined whether the phosphate secretory mechanism was independent of the peritubular phosphate concentration or was saturated during the control period. However, these investigators reported that following a unilateral infusion of PTE into the renal portal circulation, net phosphate secretion was observed from the perfused kidney, while phosphate excretion by the control kidney was not affected. Since no changes in GFR or plasma phosphate concentration were observed, these data helped demonstrate that the phosphaturia produced by PTE was due to alterations in renal tubular transport rather than to alterations in plasma phosphate or GFR. Martindale (1973) also showed that phosphate infusions into hens that were calcifying eggs caused net phosphate secretion. However, this investigator reported that the infusion of PTE did not cause a net secretion of phosphate. Other investigators have not confirmed these observations; rather, they support the findings of Levinsky and Davidson that PTE causes net phosphate secretion (Clark and Wideman, 1977; Clark *et al.*, 1976; Ferguson and Wolbach, 1967).

The physiological importance of phosphate secretion in birds has been suggested by observations of the phosphate excretion pattern in the laying fowl by Prashad and Edwards (1973). These investigators measured C_{PO_4}/C_{in} before, during, and after active shell calcification. Prior to shell formation, there was net tubular reabsorption of phosphate ($C_{PO_4}/C_{in} = 0.06 \pm 0.03$), while during active calcification, 12–18 hr after the egg reached the isthmouterine junction, net tubular secretion of phosphate ($C_{PO_4}/C_{in} = 2.08 \pm 0.21$) was observed. After oviposition (completion of active calcification), net phosphate reabsorption was again observed. The importance of PTH in causing the net phosphate secretion during shell calcification was suggested by the absence of an increase in C_{PO_4}/C_{in} in hens that received an infusion of calcium levulinate. In these birds, the ultrafilterable calcium concentration was kept above the levels found in non-calcium-infused birds. The calcium infusion also prevented the rise in hydroxyproline excretion, an index of PTH secretion, which was observed to occur during the period of active shell calcification in non-calcium-infused chickens. It appears that calcification of the eggshell (primarily calcium carbonate) is accompanied by a decrease in plasma calcium that increases PTH secretion. This, in turn, mobilizes calcium, phosphate, and hydroxyproline from bone and stimulates the kidney to secrete phosphate. The ability of the kidney to excrete a large quantity of phosphate appears to be important for the deposition of a large quantity of calcium carbonate in the shell. Thus, without the ability of PTH to cause the kidneys to secrete phosphate, the ability to deposit calcium in the shell might be compromised.

In summary, there is general agreement that the avian kidney can secrete phosphate and that infusions of inorganic phosphate or PTE produce net phosphate secretion. Whether PTH actually stimulates net phosphate secretion or inhibits phosphate reabsorption, as we discussed for the reptilian kidney, has not been determined. Thus, the renal handling of phosphate appears to be very similar in birds and reptiles. This similarity is not surprising when the kidneys of these two classes of vertebrates are compared. The kidney of birds is composed of two basic types of nephrons: (1) reptilian nephrons—nephrons which lack a loop of Henle—and (2) mammalian nephrons—nephrons which have a loop of Henle. According to most reports, the reptilian type of nephron is the most numerous (Braun and Dantzler, 1972; Shoemaker, 1972). Whether the capacity of the avian kidney to secrete phosphate occurs in both types of nephrons or only in the reptilian type of nephron is an interesting problem which has not been evaluated.

2.5. Summary of Phosphate Secretion by Nonmammalian Vertebrates

The ability of the kidney to excrete phosphate in excess of the amount filtered across the glomerulus is clearly present in lower vertebrates. In most of these vertebrates, acute elevations in plasma phosphate concentrations consistently produce C_{PO_4}/GFR values greater than 2 and often as great as 15. In reptiles and birds, the infusion of PTH also causes or increases net phosphate secretion. In the lower vertebrates, the ability of the kidney to secrete phosphate is the rule, which suggests that this is important for the homeostatic regulation of phosphate metabolism.

3. IS PHOSPHATE SECRETED BY THE MAMMALIAN KIDNEY?

We wish that we could answer the question "Is phosphate secreted by the (mammalian) kidney?" with either "yes" or "no." Whether the mammalian kidney excretes phosphate in excess of the amount filtered across the glomerulus is still being debated. We believe that the answer to this question will be determined from future investigations rather than from an extensive evaluation of all the studies which suggest net phosphate secretion by the mammalian kidney.

3.1. Use of Renal Clearance Techniques to Assess Phosphate Secretion by the Mammalian Kidney

Three clearance studies performed over the past 47 years are important for understanding our difficulty in stating that the mammalian kidney is capable of secreting phosphate. Pitts (1933) clearly showed that acute increases in plasma phosphate concentration increased urinary phosphate excretion in dogs. The clearance of xylose (C_{xy}) was used to measure GFR, and, except in a few instances, C_{PO_4} was less than C_{xy}. Pitts considered the few urine samples in which C_{PO_4}/C_{xy} was greater than 1 to represent experimental error rather than phosphate secretion. Besides, C_{xy} is known to underestimate GFR; thus, C_{PO_4} was probably consistently less than the true GFR. In a later study, Pitts and Alexander (1944) reexamined this problem in the dog using exogenous creatinine clearance (C_{cr}) to measure GFR. In this study, C_{PO_4}/C_{cr} did not exceed 0.90, even though the plasma phosphate concentration was five to eight times the normal plasma concentration. Handler (1962) attempted to demonstrate net secretion of phosphate in dogs. A number of maneuvers thought to enhance net phosphate secretion were employed. However, C_{PO_4}/C_{in} or C_{PO_4}/C_{cr} was greater than 1.0 in only 8 out of 389 clearance periods in 25 dogs. The highest reported ratio was only 1.13. At plasma phosphate concentrations greater than 15 mM/liter (48 mg/dl), C_{PO_4}/GFR was approximately 0.80. Thus, these investigators did not find evidence for net phosphate secretion by the canine kidney.

Numerous investigators have, however, suggested that the mammalian kidney can secrete phosphate. Thus, in clearance studies in dogs (Ginsburg, 1972), in humans (Webster *et al.*, 1967), and in patients with X-linked hypophosphatemia (Glorieux and Scriver, 1972), C_{PO_4}/C_{in} values greater than 1.0 were reported in 20–50% of the subjects. A finding of a C_{PO_4}/C_{in} greater than 1.0 in a portion of the subjects in an experimental study cannot be considered as proof that net phosphate secretion occurred in these subjects. The problem with such interpretations lies in the variance associated with the measurement of C_{PO_4}/C_{in}. This ratio is based on four measurements (phosphate and inulin concentrations in both plasma and urine). The relative errors of these four measurements are added together when calculating the clearance ratio. A 2–5% error associated with each measurement results in an 8–20% error in the ratio. Thus, ratios considerably greater than 1.0 ($1.08 \rightarrow 1.20$) can be obtained because of random error. Also, it must be considered that the procedures used to elevate phosphate excretion might interfere with the measurements necessary for calculating C_{PO_4}/C_{in}. Indeed, Cook and Simmons (1962) have demonstrated that mannitol, which has often been used in these studies, can interfere with the determination of the phosphate concentration. Such analytical factors make it difficult to conclude that C_{PO_4}/C_{in} values slightly above unity (1.00–1.20) establish the existence of net phosphate secretion.

In many studies, plasma phosphate concentration was considered to equal the phosphate concentration of the glomerular filtrate. However, the plasma phosphate concentration does not give a precise measure of the phosphate concentration of the glomerular filtrate. Grollman (1927) demonstrated that the ultrafiltrate to plasma concentration ratio for phosphate [$(UF/P)_{PO_4}$] was 1.0, except at elevated plasma calcium concentrations where the value of $(UF/P)_{PO_4}$ decreased. Harris *et al.* (1974, 1977) have measured the glomerular fluid to plasma phosphate concentration ratio $[(GF/P)_{PO_4}]$ in Munich–Wistar rats, which have glomeruli accessible to micropuncture. At normal plasma concentrations of phosphate and calcium, these investigators found a $(GF/P)_{PO_4}$ value ranging from 0.79 to 0.98. After the infusion of calcium chloride (plasma calcium increased from 5.7 to 9.2 mEq/liter), $(GF/P)_{PO_4}$ was reduced. Walser (1960) has reported that $(UF/P)_{PO_4}$ in humans can range from 0.81 to 1.00, and Wen (1974) has reported a $(UF/P)_{PO_4}$ value of 1.05 in dogs. Knowing the value of $(GF/P)_{PO_4}$ for each clearance period is essential for determining if C_{PO_4}/C_{in} is indicative of net phosphate secretion.

Such considerations have led Boudry *et al.* (1975) and Tröhler *et al.* (1976) to conclude that net phosphate secretion occurred in rats fed a high-phosphate diet and then given an acute phosphate load. In these studies, C_{PO_4}/C_{in} values of 0.96 ± 0.05 ($n = 6$) and 1.04 ± 0.03 and 1.07 ± 0.01 ($n = 5$) were reported. These investigators either measured the $(UF/P)_{PO_4}$ (0.93 in three rats) or assumed a $(UF/P)_{PO_4}$ slightly less than 1.0. Based on these estimates, both groups of investigators suggested that there was a small but significant net secretion of phosphate. The findings by several investigators of C_{PO_4}/C_{in} values slightly greater than 1.0 have encouraged many others to search for a detectable and possibly significant secretory component for phosphate in the mammalian kidney.

The use of clearance techniques to demonstrate the secretion of phosphate is limited to examining net phosphate secretion. Numerous investigators have had difficulty demonstrating the existence of net phosphate secretion by the mammalian kidney. However, the inability to conclusively demonstrate net phosphate secretion does not negate the existence of a significant secretory component for peritubular-to-luminal flux of phosphate. Several techniques other than steady-state clearance techniques are capable of demonstrating the existence of a peritubular-to-luminal flux of phosphate.

3.2. Evidence of a Peritubular-to-Luminal Flux of Phosphate in the Mammalian Kidney

We have examined whether a detectable peritubular-to-luminal flux of phosphate exists in the kidney of the dog by selectively applying $^{32}PO_4$ to the peritubular compartment and determining if $^{32}PO_4$ entered the tubular fluid. Two approaches were used. In the first (Schneider and McLane, (1977), anesthetized dogs were prepared for micropuncture, and a 2 to 3-cm^2 section of the renal capsule was removed. A small droplet (10 µl) of an isotonic Ringer's bicarbonate solution (pH 7.4) containing $^{32}PO_4$ and [^{3}H]inulin was placed on the exposed surface of the left kidney, and 1-min urine collections were obtained from both kidneys over the next 15 to 20 min. As shown in Fig. 3, the fractional recovery (FR) of [^{3}H]inulin/100 ml/min of GFR was the same for both kidneys, demonstrating that [^{3}H]inulin only entered the nephron by filtration across the glomeruli. The FR of ^{32}PO$_4$/mg/min of urinary phosphate excreted was significantly greater from the left than from the right kidney. If both kidneys excreted recirculating phosphate in a similar fashion, then this difference would demonstrate that some of the ^{32}PO$_4$ applied to the surface of the left kidney entered the tubular lumen directly and appeared in the urine. To demonstrate that recirculating ^{32}PO$_4$ was excreted in a similar fashion by both kidneys, we applied the isotope solution to the surface of a muscle in the neck. Under these circumstances, both the FR of ^{32}PO$_4$/mg/min of urinary phosphate excreted and the FR of [^{3}H]inulin/100 ml/min of GFR were similar from the two kidneys. Thus, we concluded that there was a detectable peritubular-to-luminal flux of phosphate in the dog.

Although a detectable flux of phosphate into the nephron was demonstrated, the magnitude of this flux could not be determined, since the fraction of isotopes that actually entered the peritubular compartment was not known. To obtain an estimate of the fraction of peritubular phosphate which appeared in the urine, ^{32}PO$_4$ and [^{3}H]inulin were directly injected into peritubular vessels on the surface of the kidney (McLane-Vega et al., 1980; Schneider and McLane, 1976). The isotopes, contained in 8–12 nl of an isotonic Ringer's bicarbonate solution (pH 7.4), were injected slowly (0.2–0.5 nl/sec) into a large postglomerular vessel, and 1-min urine collections were obtained from both kidneys. Since the FR of [^{3}H]inulin/100 ml/min of GFR for the injected (0.70 ± 0.09/100 ml/min of GFR) and the noninjected (0.70 ± 0.09/100 ml/min of GFR) kidneys were similar, we concluded that the isotopes had not been injected directly into the tubular lumen. The FR of ^{32}PO$_4$/mg/min of urinary phosphate excreted was significantly greater for the left, injected kidney than for the contralateral, noninjected kidney (Fig. 4). Although there was clearly more ^{32}PO$_4$ in the urine from the injected kidney compared to the control kidney, this difference represented only 0.7 ± 0.2% of the injected isotope. Thus, we concluded that there was a small but detectable flux of phosphate into the nephron of hydropenic dogs.

Although the peritubular-to-luminal flux of phosphate is not a major factor in determining phosphate excretion in hydropenia, it might account for the increase in phosphate excretion accompanying acute volume expansion. To test this hypothesis, we measured the peritubular-to-luminal flux of phosphate in volume-expanded dogs (McLane-Vega et al., 1980; Schneider and McLane, 1976). The fractional clearance of phosphate in these dogs (34.4 ± 5.8%) was twice that of the hydropenic dogs (17.9 ± 2.9%). Following the injection of isotopes into a peritubular capillary,

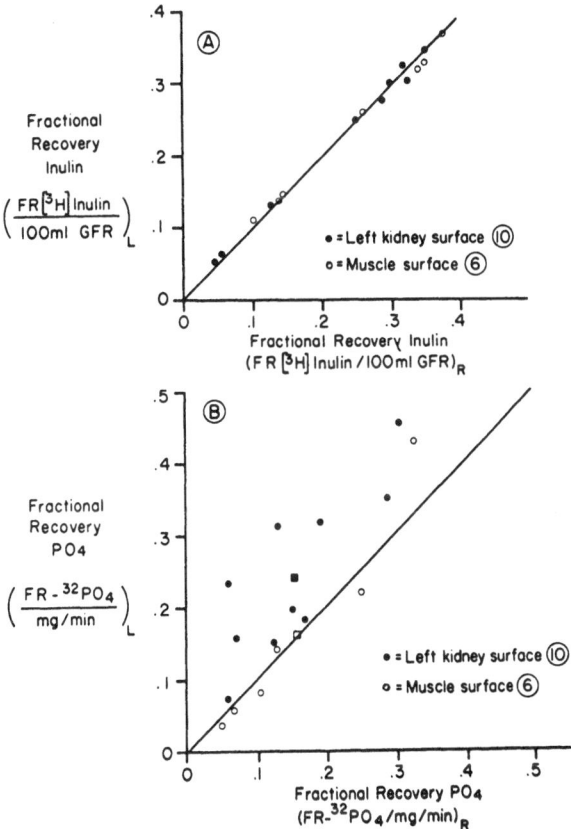

Fig. 3. (A) Fractional recovery of [³H]inulin/100 ml/min of GFR of left kidney (ordinate) as compared to that for right kidney (abscissa). (B) Fractional recovery of phosphate/mg/min of urinary phosphate excretion of the left kidney (ordinate) as compared to that for right kidney (abscissa). Solid circles represent dogs in which isotopes were applied to surface of left kidney. Open circles represents dogs in which isotopes were applied to a muscle in the neck. Solid and open squares represent average values for the respective groups. Circled numbers represent number of animals in each group. (From Schneider and McLane, 1977.)

the FR of [³H]inulin/100 ml/min of GFR for the injected (0.59 ± 0.08/100 ml/min) and the noninjected (0.59 ± 0.08/100 ml/min) kidneys were similar. We concluded from these data that the isotopes had not been injected into a tubule. The FR of ³²PO₄/mg/min of urinary phosphate excretion for the injected kidney (0.0797 ± 0.0088/mg/min) was significantly greater (+0.0101 ± 0.0047/mg/min; $p < 0.05$) than that for the noninjected kidney (0.0696 ± 0.0072/mg/min). This difference, however, represented only 0.31 ± 0.17% of the injected isotope, a value significantly less than that

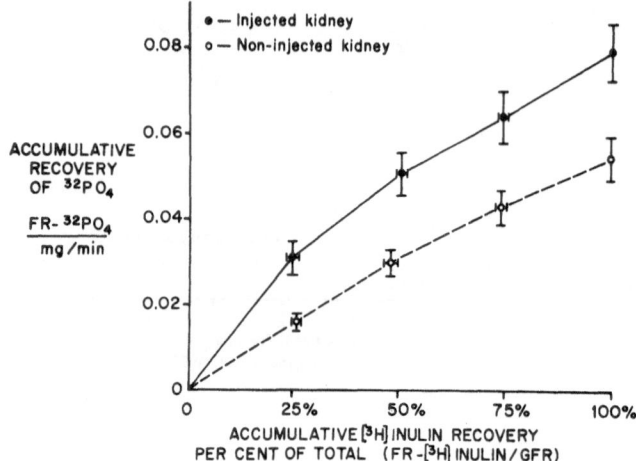

Fig. 4. The urinary excretion of $^{32}PO_4$ following peritubular capillary injection in hydropenic dogs. The accumulative fractional recovery of $^{32}PO_4$ for the injected and noninjected kidneys is plotted as a function of the accumulative recovery of [^3H]inulin (expressed as a percentage of total urinary [^3H]inulin recovery).

found in hydropenic, nonphosphaturic dogs. Thus, we concluded that the phosphaturia accompanying acute extracellular volume expansion was not associated with an increase in the peritubular-to-luminal flux of phosphate. We realize that these results may only reflect events in the superficial nephrons that were perfused. Thus, we have been unable to show an important role for the peritubular-to-luminal flux of phosphate in the dog.

3.2.1. Proximal Tubule as Site of the Peritubular-to-Luminal Flux of Phosphate

In our studies, we could not determine whether the peritubular-to-luminal flux of phosphate occurred along the proximal or distal tubule. Dennis *et al.* (1976, 1977) have measured the bath-to-lumen flux of phosphate in isolated perfused rabbit tubules. These investigators found a small bath-to-lumen flux of phosphate in both the isolated proximal convoluted and proximal straight tubules. This flux was between 7 and 14% of the reabsorptive flux and was not altered by the administration of PTH. These authors concluded that the small bath-to-lumen flux of phosphate probably reflects the passive permeability properties of the tubule rather than a specific secretory pathway.

Several laboratories have attempted to determine if there is a significant peritubular-to-luminal flux of phosphate by using *in vivo* micropuncture or microperfusion techniques. In phosphate-loaded rats, Strickler et al. (1964) did not find any evidence for phosphate secretion by the proximal tubule from measurements of $(TF/P)_{PO_4}$ and inulin concentration ratios $[(TF/P)_{in}]$. Similar results were also reported by others (Boudry et al., 1975; Le Grimellec et al., 1974; Mühlbauer et al., 1977). In contrast, in rats receiving infusions of both phosphate and PTH, Boudry et al. (1975) and Mühlbauer et al. (1977) have reported $(TF/P)_{PO_4}/(TF/P)_{in}$ values above 1.0 for early proximal tubule collections. These authors suggested that phosphate was secreted by the early proximal tubule. However, only in the study by Boudry et al. (1975) was this ratio (1.17 ± 0.06) significantly greater than 1.0. In these experiments, no net secretion of phosphate was found; rather, 30% of the filtered phosphate was reabsorbed by the kidney. It is interesting that the amount of phosphate in early distal tubular fluid and the final urine was the same for phosphate-loaded animals whether or not they received PTH. At least for the superficial nephrons, this reported ability of early proximal tubules to secrete phosphate did not increase the amount of phosphate presented to the superficial distal tubule or the amount of phosphate excreted into the final urine.

Several investigators have used in vivo microperfusion techniques to evaluate the importance of a bidirectional transport process for phosphate along the proximal tubule. Murayama et al. (1972) found that the net reabsorption of phosphate was not significantly different from the luminal-to-peritubular flux of $^{32}PO_4$. If a large peritubular-to-luminal flux of phosphate were present, the luminal-to-peritubular flux of $^{32}PO_4$ should have been significantly greater than the net reabsorption of phosphate. These authors stated that the luminal-to-peritubular flux of $^{32}PO_4$ was 15–20% of the net reabsorption of phosphate; but, because of the variability in their data, this difference was not statistically significant. Boudry et al. (1975) reported that perfusion of proximal tubular segments with a high-specific-activity $^{32}PO_4$ solution was associated with a significant decrease in the specific activity of $^{32}PO_4$ in the collected perfusate. The decrease in specific activity reflects the addition of inorganic phosphate to the perfusion solution, and the authors suggested that this represents a large peritubular-to-luminal flux of phosphate. Greger et al. (1975) pointed out that these authors did not determine if the collected perfusate had been accidentally contaminated. If during the perfusion a fistula between the perfused tubule and either a neighboring tubule or capillary were present, unlabeled phosphate would enter the perfusate and lower its specific activity. While infusing inulin systemically, Greger et al. (1975) perfused proximal tubular segments with an isotonic phosphate and inulin-free solution and measured phosphate and inulin concentrations in the collected perfusate. When the concentration of inulin was undetectable, no measurable concentration of phosphate was found in the perfusate. Only when a significant concentration of inulin was found in the perfusate was there a detectable concentration of phosphate. These data suggest that the decrease in specific activity of phosphate observed by Boudry *et al.* (1975) may have been due, in part, to contamination of the collected perfusate rather than to a large peritubular-to-luminal flux of phosphate. Although Greger *et al.* (1975) failed to find a large peritubular-to-luminal flux of phosphate into the proximal tubule, they noted that a small peritubular-to-luminal flux (an order of magnitude less than the reabsorptive flux) could not be measured by their techniques. Whether the flux of phosphate into the proximal tubule can produce a net secretion of phosphate into the early proximal tubule, as suggested by Boudry *et al.* (1975), has not been verified. Thus, the inability of other investigators to find evidence for anything other than a small peritubular-to-luminal flux of phosphate suggests to us that this flux is best considered to be a small and probably insignificant component of phosphate transport along the proximal tubule.

3.2.2. Distal Nephron Segments as Sites of the Peritubular-to-Luminal Flux of Phosphate

The possibility that there is a secretory component for phosphate transport in the distal part of the nephron has also been of interest. Nicholson (1959) and Nicholson and Shepherd (1959) suggested that phosphate was secreted by the distal nephron of the dog. These authors attempted to selectively damage the distal nephron by a retrograde injection of mercuric chloride via the ureters. A significant reduction in phosphate excretion was observed, which the authors suggested was due to a destruction of a secretory mechanism. Since neither the site(s) nor the nature of the damage caused by the application of mercuric chloride was known, these data do not prove that phosphate was secreted by the distal nephron.

Other investigators have used stop-flow techniques to determine if phosphate was secreted by the distal nephron. Davis *et al.* (1966) reported that the systemic injection of $^{32}PO_4$ during the period of stop-flow resulted in the appearance of $^{32}PO_4$ in the early urine samples, suggesting a secretion of phosphate by the distal tubule. Lambert *et al.* (1964), however, using an identical protocol, could find no evidence for the entrance of phosphate into the distal nephron. The measurement of fluxes into the nephron by the use of renal stop-flow techniques, which elevate intratubular pressures, has been questioned by Lorentz *et al.* (1972). These authors found a marked increase in the "leakiness" of the nephron during elevations in tubular pressure, similar to those obtained in stop-flow experiments. We have recently performed experiments to determine if a detectable secretion of phosphate into the distal nephron occurs at normal intratubular pressures (Schneider and McLane, 1977). After a rapid injection of $^{32}PO_4$ and [^{3}H]inulin into a renal artery of either normal or phosphate-loaded dogs, phosphate never appeared in the urine before inulin. If a significant flux of phosphate into the distal nephron existed, we would have expected $^{32}PO_4$ to appear in the urine before the appearance of [^{3}H]inulin. Thus, at normal intratubular pressures, we could find no evidence for the existence of a detectable peritubular-to-luminal flux of phosphate into the distal part of the nephron.

Boudry et al. (1975) and Mühlbauer et al. (1977) have suggested that the collecting duct may secrete phosphate. This conclusion was based on the observation that in phosphate-loaded rats, the fraction of filtered phosphate leaving the superficial distal tubules was significantly less than the fraction of filtered phosphate excreted into the final urine. These authors felt that this difference probably represented secretion of phosphate but recognized that this difference could also be explained by a heterogeneity of nephron function (i.e., deep nephrons excreting a larger fraction of the filtered phosphate than the superficial nephrons).

Knox et al. (1977) indicated that a heterogeneity of nephron function might account for the apparent secretion of phosphate along the terminal nephron segments of phosphate-loaded rats. These authors observed, as did Boudry et al. (1975), that the fraction of filtered phosphate leaving the superficial distal tubules (51.1 ± 6%) was significantly less than the fraction of filtered phosphate excreted into the final urine (72 ± 6%). They also measured the fraction of filtered phosphate remaining in the deep nephrons by collecting fluid from the thin ascending limbs of Henle's loop, and found that 78 ± 10% of the filtered phosphate was present in these samples. Assuming no reabsorption of phosphate along the ascending limb of Henle's loop, the fraction of filtered phosphate in distal tubules of the deep nephrons would be greater than that in either superficial distal tubules or final urine. These data suggest that a heterogeneity of function between deep and superficial nephrons does exist in the rat and might account for the apparent secretion of phosphate along the terminal nephron segments. However, the data of Knox et al. (1977) do not exclude the possibility of phosphate secretion by the terminal nephron segment.

Two studies utilizing isolated perfused segments of the descending limb of Henle's loop, the thin and thick ascending limbs of Henle's loop (Rocha et al., 1977), and cortical collecting tubules (Dennis et al., 1977) have found that both the bath-to-lumen and the lumen-to-bath fluxes of phosphate are essentially zero. This suggested that the measurements by Knox et al. (1977) reflect the delivery of phosphate to the distal tubules of the deep nephrons. Therefore, we believe that the existence of a significant secretory component for phosphate in the distal part of the nephron has not been satisfactorily established.

4. CONCLUSIONS

The regulation of phosphate balance throughout the vertebrate kingdom is determined in large part by the kidney's ability to adjust the rate at which it excretes phosphate. In lower vertebrates, high rates of phosphate excretion are clearly the results of not only the elimination of phosphate filtered across the glomerulus but also the secretion of phosphate into the nephron. In mammals, a significant secretory component for phosphate has not been established. Although the existence of a small peritubular-to-luminal flux has been established (at least along the proximal nephron), at present, this flux has not been found to be a determinant of urinary phosphate excretion. It appears that the mammalian kidney does not utilize a secretory mechanism in the regulation of phosphate excretion. It is possible, however, that mammals do have a small "remnant" of a phosphate secretory mechanism. However, until several laboratories can consistently demonstrate the importance of phosphate secretion, we believe that renal phosphate excretion by the mammalian kidney is determined by filtration and subsequent reabsorption.

5. REFERENCES

Boudry, J.-F., Troehler, U., Toubabi, M., Fleisch, H., and Bonjour, J.-P.. 1975. Secretion of inorganic phosphate in the rat nephron, *Clin. Sci. Mol. Med.* **48**:475.

Braun, E. J., and Dantzler, W. H., 1972, Function of mammalian-type and reptilian-type nephrons in kidney of desert quail, *Am. J. Physiol.* **222**:617.

Clark, N. B., and Dantzler, W. H., 1972, Renal tubular transport of calcium and phosphate in snakes: Role of parathyroid hormone, *Am. J. Physiol.* **223**:1455.

Clark, N. B., and Wideman, R. F., Jr., 1977, Renal excretion of phosphate and calcium in parathyroidectomized starlings, *Am. J. Physiol.* **233**:F138.

Clark, N. B., Braun, E. J., and Wideman, R. F., Jr., 1976, Parathyroid hormone and renal excretion of phosphate and calcium in normal starlings, *Am. J. Physiol.* **231**:1152.

Clarke, R. W., and Smith, H. W., 1932, Absorption and excretion of water and salts by the elasmobranch fishes. III. The use of xylose as a measure of the glomerular filtrate in *Squalus acanthias*, *J. Cell. Comp. Physiol.* **1**:131.

Cook, B. S., and Simmons, D. H., 1962, Mannitol interference in phosphate determination: Method of correction, *J. Lab. Clin. Med.* **60**:160.

Cortelyou, J. R., 1962, Phosphorus changes in totally parathyroidectomized *Rana pipiens*, *Endocrinology* **70**:618.

Cortelyou, J. R., Quipse, P. A., and McWhinnie, D. J., 1967, Parathyroid extract effects on phosphorus metabolism in *Rana pipiens*, *Gen. Comp. Endocrinol.* **9**:76.

Dantzler, W. H., 1967, Glomerular and tubular effects of arginine vasotocin in water snakes (*Natrix sipedon*), *Am. J. Physiol.* **212**:83.

Davis, B. B., Kedes, L. H., and Field, J. B., 1966, Demonstration of distal tubular flux of phosphorus using modified stop-flow analysis, *Metabolism* 15:482.

Dennis, V. W., Woodhall, P. B., and Robinson, 1976, Characteristics of phosphate transport in isolated proximal tubules, *Am. J. Physiol.* 231:979.

Dennis, V. W., Bello-Reuss, E., and Robinson, R. R., 1977, Response of phosphate transport to parathyroid hormone in segments of rabbit nephron, *Am. J. Physiol.* 233:F29.

Ferguson, R. K., and Wolbach, R. A., 1967, Effects of glucose, phlorizin, and parathyroid extract on renal phosphate transport in chickens, *Am. J. Physiol.* 212:1123.

Ginsburg, J. M., 1972, Effect of glucose and free fatty acid on phosphate transport in dog kidney, *Am. J. Physiol.* 222:1153.

Glorieux, F., and Scriver, C. R., 1972, Loss of a parathyroid hormone-sensitive component of phosphate transport in X-linked hypophosphatemia, *Science* 175:997.

Goldstein, L., and Forster, R. P., 1971, Osmoregulation and urea metabolism in the little skate, *Raja erinacea*, *Am. J. Physiol.* 220:742.

Greger, R. F., Lang, F. C., Knox, F. G., and Lechêne, C. P., 1975, Absence of significant secretory flux of phosphate in the proximal convoluted tubule, *Am. J. Physiol.* 232:F235.

Grollman, A., 1927, The condition of the inorganic phosphorus of the blood with special reference to the calcium concentration, *J. Biol. Chem.* 72:565.

Handler, J. S., 1962, A study of renal phosphate excretion in the dog, *Am. J. Physiol.* 202:787.

Harris, C. A., Baer, P. G., Chiroto, E., and Dirks, J. H., 1974, Composition of mammalian glomerular filtrate, *Am. J. Physiol.* 227:972.

Harris, C. A., Sutton, R. A. L., and Dirks, J. H., 1977, Effects of hypercalcemia on calcium and phosphate ultrafilterability and tubular reabsorption in the rat, *Am. J. Physiol.* 233:F201.

Hernandez, T., and Coulson, R. A., 1957, Inhibition of renal tubular function by cold, *Am. J. Physiol.* 188:485.

Hickman, C. P., Jr., and Trump, B. F., 1969, The kidney, in: *Fish Physiology*, Vol. 1 (W. S. Hoar and D. J. Randall, eds.), pp. 91–239, Academic Press, New York.

Knox, F. G., Haas, J. A., Berndt, T., Marchand, G. R., and Youngberg, S. P., 1977, Phosphate transport in superficial and deep nephrons in phosphate-loaded rats, *Am. J. Physiol.* 233:F150.

Lambert, P. P., Vanderveiken, F., DeKoster, J. P., Kahn, R. J., and DeMyttenaere, M., 1964, Study of phosphate excretion by the stop-flow technique: Effects of parathyroid hormone, *Nephron* 1:103.

Le Grimellec, C., Roinel, N., and Morel, F., 1974, Simultaneous Mg, Ca, P, K, and Cl analysis in rat tubular fluid. IV. During acute phosphate plasma loading, *Pflügers Arch.* 346:189.

Levinsky, N. G., and Davidson, D. G., 1957, Renal action of parathyroid extract in the chicken, *Am. J. Physiol.* 191:530.

Lorentz, W. B., Lassiter, W. E., and Gottschalk, C. W., 1972, Renal tubular permeability during increased intrarenal pressure, *J. Clin. Invest.* 51:484.

Marshall, E. K., and Griffin, A. L., 1933, Excretion of inorganic phosphate by the aglomerular kidney, *Proc. Soc. Exp. Biol. Med.* 31:44.

Martindale, L., 1973, Phosphate excretion in the laying hen (*Gallus domesticus*), *J. Physiol.* 231:439.

McLane-Vega, L. A., Hanson, R. C., and Schneider, E. G., 1980, Peritubular capillary microinjection of PO_4 in hydropenic and acutely volume expanded dogs, *Renal Physiol.*, submitted for publication.

Mühlbauer, R. C., Bonjour, J.-P., and Fleisch, H., 1977, Tubular localization of adaptation to dietary phosphate in rats, *Am. J. Physiol.* 233:F342.

Munz, F. W., and McFarland, W. N., 1964, Regulatory function of a primitive vertebrate kidney, Comp. Biochem. Physiol. 13:381.

Murayama, Y., Morel, F., and Le Grimellec, C., 1972, Phosphate, calcium and magnesium transfers in proximal tubules and loops of Henle, as measured by single nephron microperfusion experiments in the rat, Pflügers Arch. 333:1.

Nicholson, T. F., 1959, The mode and site of the renal action of parathyroid extract in the dog, Can. J. Biochem. Physiol. 37:113.

Nicholson, T. F., and Shepherd, G. W., 1959, The effect of damage to various parts of the renal tubule on the excretion of phosphate by the dog's kidney, Can. J. Biochem. Physiol. 37:103.

Pitts, R. F., 1933, The excretion of urine in the dog. VII. Inorganic phosphate in relation to plasma phosphate level, Am. J. Physiol. 106:1.

Pitts, R. F., and Alexander, R. S., 1944, The renal reabsorption mechanism for inorganic phosphate in normal and acidotic dogs, Am. J. Physiol. 142:648.

Prashad, D. N., and Edwards, N. A., 1973, Phosphate excretion in the laying fowl, Comp. Biochem. Physiol. 46A:131.

Rocha, A. S., Magaldi, J. B., and Kokko, J. P., 1977, Calcium and phosphate transport in isolated segments of rabbit Henle's loop, J. Clin. Invest. 59:975.

Schneider, E. G., and McLane, L. A., 1976, Renal capillary microinjection of $^{32}PO_4$ and ^{3}H-inulin during hydropenia and extracellular volume expansion in the dog, Fed. Proc. Fed. Am. Soc. Exp. Biol. 35:908.

Schneider, E. G., and McLane, L. A., 1977, Evidence for a peritubular-to-luminal flux of phosphate in the dog kidney, Am. J. Physiol. 232:F159.

Shoemaker, V. H., 1972, Osmoregulation and excretion in birds, in: Avian Biology II (D. S. Farner, J. R. King, and K. C. Parkes, eds.), pp. 527–574, Academic Press, New York.

Smith, H. W., 1932, Evolution of fish kidneys, Q. Rev. Biol. 7:1.

Smith, W. W., 1939, The excretion of phosphate in the dogfish, Squalus acanthias, J. Cell. Comp. Physiol. 14:95.

Stolte, H., Galaske, R. G., Eisenbach, G. M., Lechêne, C., Schmidt-Nielsen, B., and Boylan, J. W., 1977, Renal tubular ion transport and collecting duct function in the elasmobranch little skate, Raja erinacea, J. Exp. Zool. 199:403.

Strickler, J. C., Thompson, D. D., Koose, R. M., and Giebisch, G., 1964, Micropuncture study of inorganic phosphate excretion in the rat, J. Clin. Invest. 43:1596.

Trevan, J. W., 1916, The excretion of acid by the kidney, J. Physiol. 50:15.

Tröhler, U., Bonjour, J.-P., and Fleisch, H., 1976, Inorganic phosphate homeostasis: Renal adaptation to the dietary intake in intact and thyroparathyroidectomized rats, J. Clin. Invest. 57:264.

Walker, A. M., and Hudson, C. L., 1937a, The reabsorption of glucose from the renal tubule in amphibia and the action of phlorizin upon it, Am. J. Physiol. 188:130.

Walker, A. M., and Hudson, C. L., 1937b, The role of the tubule in the excretion of inorganic phosphates by the amphibian kidney, Am. J. Physiol. 118:167.

Walser, M., 1960, Protein-binding of inorganic phosphate in plasma of normal subjects and patients with renal disease, J. Clin. Invest. 39:501.

Webster, G. D., Mann, J. B., and Hills, A. G., 1967, The effect of phosphate infusions upon renal phosphate clearance in man: Evidence for tubular phosphate secretion, Metabolism 16:797.

Wen, S. F., 1974, Micropuncture studies of phosphate transport in the proximal tubule of the dog, J. Clin. Invest. 53:143.

Wolbach, R. A., 1970, Phlorizin and renal phosphate secretion in the spiny dogfish, Squalus acanthias, Am. J. Physiol. 219:886.

4

Cellular Mechanisms of Phosphate Transport

FRANKLYN G. KNOX, ANZELM HOPPE,
STEPHEN A. KEMPSON, SUDHIR V. SHAH,
and THOMAS P. DOUSA

1. INTRODUCTION

Transepithelial phosphate transport in the kidney is one to two orders of magnitude more extensive than that in any other organ of the body. Large volumes of glomerular filtrate, 150 liters/day in a normal man, are presented to the renal tubule, from which 80% of the filtered phosphate is reclaimed by this transepithelial phosphate transport system.

Our understanding of the cellular mechanisms of phosphate transport derives from a variety of experimental techniques, including renal clearance, micropuncture, isolated tubule, tissue slice, and biochemical studies on preparations of membranes. Although some of these techniques for the study of phosphate handling in the kidney are extensively covered in other chapters of this book, information from each of these techniques will be collated for the description of our present knowledge on the cellular mechanisms of phosphate transport. It is generally recognized from stop-flow and micropuncture studies that phosphate is reabsorbed predominantly in the proximal tubule. Although there is debate in regard to the existence and significance of phosphate transport in distal segments of the nephron (Knox et al., 1973), this chapter will deal with the cellular mechanisms of phosphate transport only in the proximal tubule because of the predominance of phosphate transport in this segment of the nephron.

In discussing the cellular mechanisms of phosphorus transport, several difficulties and complexities encountered in the analysis of this phe-

79

nomenon should be realized. First, phosphorus is an inorganic ion. Under conditions of physiological pH, it dissociates into at least two different forms (monobasic and dibasic), and the proportion of these two forms can change outside the cell and within the cell depending on small fluctuations in pH.

Another special feature is that phosphorus, unlike other transported ions such as sodium, potassium, or chloride, is incorporated into a multitude of organic compounds, ranging from small ones, such as acyl phosphate, nucleotides, or phospholipids, to huge macromolecules, such as DNA, RNA, or phosphoproteins, Thus, inorganic phosphorus can enter a variety of biosynthetic pathways and be incorporated into nucleotides, mono- and oligosaccharides, and side chains of amino acids through covalent bonds, mostly through esteric bonds, from which it can be released by a variety of hydrolytic enzymes (phosphohydrolases). When inorganic phosphorus enters cells, a fraction can be incorporated into a variety of metabolic pools, and, since in most instances the linkage is a covalent one, phosphorus can reenter the pool of free inorganic phosphorus in the cell only after metabolic cycling. Although net transmembrane and transepithelial phosphorus fluxes can be estimated, the balance of phosphate molecules crossing the cell membrane may depend on the metabolic state of the cell, that is, how much of the phosphorus entering the cell is diverted to metabolism or how much of the phosphorus leaving the cell comes from metabolic pools. Thus, in this aspect as well as the dependence on pH, transport of phosphorus differs from other transported ionic species such as sodium, potassium, chloride, or water.

2. TRANSMEMBRANE MOVEMENT OF PHOSPHATE

2.1. Membrane Composition and Structure

The major cellular components involved in tubular phosphate transport are the membrane lining the lumen of the tubules (sometimes called apical) and the membrane on the peritubular side (sometimes called basolateral, basal, or antiluminal). Therefore, we will review the basic properties of membranes in terms of structural and functional properties in general and with specific attention to membranes of renal cells transporting phosphorus.

Almost half of the mass of the plasma membrane of many cells is composed of complex lipids, and most of the remainder is protein. The amount of carbohydrate present, primarily on the outer surface, is often very small (Bretscher and Raff, 1975; Winzler, 1970), but it is becoming increasingly clear that carbohydrate covalently linked to membrane protein or lipid plays an important role in membrane structure and function (Cook and Stoddart, 1973). Current ideas of membrane structure (Israelachvili, 1977; Singer, 1974) are based primarily on thermodynamic considerations and are centered on the concept of globular protein molecules associated with a lipid bilayer. The proteins are built into the bilayer in an asymmetrical fashion. Some proteins (peripheral) that are associated with the bilayer do not penetrate it, while others (integral) are immersed in the lipid bilayer to varying degrees and are more tightly bound. Some integral membrane proteins, the so-called "transmembrane proteins" (Fig. 1), can span the entire width of the bilayer and project out on either side. The brush-border membrane lining the lumen of the renal proximal tubule contains at least 35–40 distinct protein subunits ranging in size from 10,000 to 360,000 daltons (Neville and Glossmann, 1971). Three glycoprotein subunits account for most of the carbohydrate in the membrane (Glossmann and Neville, 1971). Similar studies on the protein subunit composition of the basolateral membranes of the proximal tubular cell are rare, but there is probably considerably less carbohydrate present than in the luminal membranes (Rostgaard and Thuneberg, 1972).

The luminal membrane of the proximal tubule is characterized by numerous extensions, microvilli, typically arranged in pallisades with axes at a right angle projected into the plane of the tubular lumen surface. This "brush-border" arrangement of the luminal plasma membrane is typical not only for renal proximal tubules but also for some other transporting epithelial cells, such as those lining the small intestine or the bile canaliculi. These three cell types are also quite similar in terms of biochemical composition. However, since the diameter of the lumen of kidney tubules it only 10–30 μm and one kidney contains at least 1,000,000 tubules, the total brush-border surface in the kidney as an organ enormously exceeds the total brush-border surface in the small intestine or

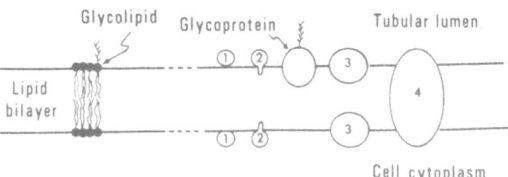

Fig. 1. Hypothetical model of the organization of proteins in the lipid bilayer of the microvillus membrane of the renal brush border. Peripheral (1) and integral (2, 3) proteins are exposed to the cell exterior or interior. Some integral proteins (4) span the bilayer completely. Specific examples of these proteins are (1) actin, α-actinin; (2) γ-glutamyltransferase, leucine aminopeptidase, maltase; and (3, 4) alkaline phosphatase, Mg^{2+}-ATPase, trehalase. Carbohydrate is probably restricted to the external surface of the membrane, in this case, the side facing the lumen of the proximal tubule. References are given in the text.

in the bile canaliculi. The major purpose of the microvilli is probably to increase the total surface available for contact with tubular fluid from which many components are absorbed at high rates.

Microvilli may not only represent passive extensions of the luminal membrane to increase surface area but may also serve as actively moving organelles. Thus, motility of the brush border may be important in transcellular transport by the renal proximal tubule. Rapid movements of the microvilli indicate the presence of a contractile mechanism (Thuneberg and Rostgaard, 1969), and two peripheral proteins associated with the cytoplasmic surface of the microvillus membrane (Fig. 1) may mediate the contractions. One of these proteins is actin, which occurs as filaments arranged in a $1 + 6$ configuration in the core of the microvillus (Rostgaard and Thuneberg, 1972). These filaments are associated with each other and with the membrane through cross-bridges which may be composed of another protein, α-actinin (Booth and Kenny, 1976; Kenny and Booth, 1976). The manner in which such a micromechanical pump might aid overall tubular reabsorption has not been established. It may serve simply to prevent the occurrence of unstirred liquid layers between microvilli or to cause bulk intracellular movement of absorbed solutes. It is interesting to note at this point the report of a system of actin- and myosin-like filaments closely associated with the basal membrane of the proximal tubular cell. It was suggested that this two-filament contractile system may prevent abnormal dilation of the tubule by transient high hydrostatic pressures (Rostgaard *et al.*, 1972).

Microtubules are hollow linear subcellular structures composed of subunits of the heterodimeric globular protein tubulin (Snyder and McIntosh, 1976) and are found in most eucaryotic cells, including those in the renal proximal tubule (Tyson and Bulger, 1973). Much of the interest in microtubules is due to their central role in the control of the structural organization of the cell and in mitosis. In addition to these two roles, microtubules have been shown to play an important role in the action of various hormones, such as vasopressin, on the kidney. It appears that microtubules in the renal cortical cells may be involved in the renal handling of phosphate and its control by parathyroid hormone (PTH). This role is suggested indirectly by observations in the rat that a specific microtubule-disrupting alkaloid, colchicine, perturbs reabsorption of phosphate in the proximal tubule and its regulation by PTH (Dousa *et al.*, 1976). It should be stressed, however, that unlike microfilaments, microtubules are not known with certainty to be directly associated with the luminal or antiluminal membrane, and the exact role of cytoplasmic microtubules in the transport function is still in the realm of speculation. However, it has been shown in several other systems that microtubules may direct or control the structure of the membrane, namely, the movement of the intramembranous particles (Berlin *et al*, 1974; Oliver *et al.*, 1974).

2.2. Phosphate–Membrane Interactions

In consideration of the molecular mechanism by which the phosphate is translocated from the luminal to the peritubular fluid, we will consider certain requirements which are to be satisfied and factors expected to play a role in phosphate transport in the kidney. So far, many of these considerations are based on experiments dealing with phosphate transport in isolated renal tissue or its subfractions.

Inorganic phosphate is a highly polar molecule and will not readily traverse the hydrophobic interior of a biological membrane, although the permeability to phosphate may vary with the phospholipid composition of the membrane, at least as shown in the erythrocyte (Gruber and Deuticke, 1973). Phosphate will cross the membrane much more rapidly via a specific transport system associated with one or more membrane proteins. In general, a prerequisite for the active transport of solutes is binding to a specific protein at a site exterior to the cell. In bacterial cells, the selective transport of carbohydrates, amino acids, and ions, including phosphate, across the plasma membrane is mediated by a class of proteins known as binding proteins (Oxender and Quay, 1976; Simoni, 1972). The various binding proteins may act as the recognition sites for active transport systems. The glucose-binding site in the renal brush-border membrane is closely associated with a protein (Thomas, 1973); likewise, in the erythrocyte membrane, a specific protein fraction may account for the entire glucose transport system (Bloch, 1974; Kasahara and Hinkle, 1976). A role for specific membrane proteins has been demonstrated also in phosphate transport across the inner mitochondrial membrane (Banerjee *et al.*, 1977; Coty and Pederson, 1975; Hadvarg and Kadenbach, 1976) and the erythrocyte membrane (Ho and Guidotti, 1975; Wolosin *et al.*, 1977). It is thus reasonable to expect that one or more membrane proteins are involved in the transport of phosphate across the membrane of the brush border of the renal proximal tubule. The phosphate may have access to a polar pocket in a protein which then traverses the membrane and releases the phosphate on the other side. Alternatively, phosphate may move through a polar channel formed by the tertiary structure of a protein or by the aggregation of two or more protein subunits. In the latter case, the protein(s) involved might span the membrane, and the channel could be opened or closed by minor adjustments in protein configuration triggered by binding of phosphate to the protein at a site exterior to the bilayer. The formation of a transmembrane channel has been suggested (Ho and Guidotti, 1975) to be the mechanism by which the anion transporting protein functions in the erythrocyte membrane. Since active phosphate transport is sodium dependent, as discussed later, the binding site may be held in a conformation favoring phosphate attachment by binding of sodium to a separate adjacent site. A similar proposal has been advanced (Kinne, 1976) as a possible reason for the sodium dependency of the glucose transport system in the renal brush border. Although the major active and rate-limiting step in tubular transport of phosphate is considered to be luminal uptake by the brush-border membrane, phosphate in the proximal tubular cell must cross to the other side of the cell and through the basolateral membranes to reach the peritubular interstitium. The latter process appears to be a sodium-independent passive process, probably facilitated diffusion down a concentration gradient, and may also involve a membrane carrier mechanism.

2.3. Enzymes of the Brush-Border Membrane

Several integral proteins in the brush-border membrane are enzymes, some of which, on the basis of criteria such as their susceptibility to the action of proteases, are more tightly associated with the lipid bilayer than are others (Fig. 1). For example, digestion of isolated membranes with papain releases aminopeptidases, maltase, and γ-glutamyltransferase (Kenny and Booth, 1976) but not alkaline phosphatase (Thomas and Kinne, 1972), trehalase, and Mg^{2+}-ATPase (George and Kenny, 1973). A number of so-called "brush-border localized enzymes" were also found in some other subcellular components or in other tissues. The specificity of their relationship to the brush-border membrane is in the fact that the specific activities of these enzymes are much higher (in many cases, ten times greater) than in the other sites of the cells and that they are organized within the membrane in a specific structured fashion, as suggested and demonstrated by histochemical, light, and electron microscopic investigations. Recall that the brush-border membrane of proximal tubules resembles that of the small-intestinal epithelium and bile canaliculi in terms of ultrastructure and that they are also very similar in terms of specific brush-border enzymes. Therefore, the set of brush-border enzymes found in the renal brush border is very similar, if not identical, to that found in the intestinal and bile canalicular brush-border membranes. A less extensive number of specific enzyme activities was found to be typically associated with the basolateral membranes of the proximal tubular cell. Only the presence of adenylate cyclase, $(Na^+ + K^+)$-ATPase, and Ca^{2+}-ATPase has been repeatedly demonstrated at the present time (Kinne, 1975; Kinne and Schwartz, 1977).

The brush border is the first point at which the constituents of the glomerular filtrate come into contact with the proximal tubule. Although the enzymes of the brush-border membrane are ideally situated for a role in tubular reabsorption, the physiological significance of most of these enzymes remains undetermined to date. A role in amino acid transport has been suggested for γ-glutamyltransferase (Meister and Tate, 1976), but this proposal has been questioned (Wendel *et al.*, 1976). It has been estimated that the potential of the peptidase enzymes for hydrolyzing peptide substrates in the glomerular filtrate greatly exceeds the requirements (Kenny and Booth, 1976). An alternative function in amino acid transport was suggested for these enzymes. A function of trehalose in the renal reabsorption of glucose was proposed (Sacktor, 1968) based on the ATP-dependent synthesis of trehalose from glucose in the membrane, with subsequent hydrolysis of trehalose by trehalase releasing glucose into the cell. There is, however, little evidence that the enzymes involved in trehalose synthesis are present in the brush-border membrane. As mentioned above, a more widely accepted view, of the transmembrane transport of glucose is that a specific carrier is involved. The glucose-binding protein is the only protein in the microvillus membrane for which a specific transport function has been demonstrated. Not all the transport systems in the proximal tubule may be located in the brush-border membrane; for example, $(Na^+ + K^+)$-ATPase and Ca^{2+}-ATPase in the basolateral membrane have been implicated in the active transport of sodium and calcium, respectively (Kinne, 1975).

None of the known enzymes in the brush-border membrane has been specifically implicated in phosphate transport, but alkaline phosphatase deserves consideration. This enzyme is characterized (and defined analytically) by an optimum activity *in vitro* in the pH range 8.2–10.7, but under conditions likely to prevail *in vivo,* alkaline phosphatase has an optimum activity at a physiological pH (Fishman, 1974). In microbiological systems (*Escherichia coli*), the activity of alkaline phosphatase depends on the phosphate concentration in the culture medium. In mammalian tissues, alkaline phosphatase of high specific activity is localized in the brush-border membranes of tissues with important transport functions (kidney, intestine, bile canaliculi, trophoblast), and there is at least some evidence to suggest that the enzyme may be involved in phosphate transport. For example, uptake of phosphate by slices of mouse intestine is proportional to the activity of alkaline phosphatase and ceases when the enzyme activity is blocked by inhibitors of the enzyme such as beryllium or phenylalanine (Moog and Glazier, 1972). Further, the dietary phosphate intake, which markedly modulates renal tubular transport, appears to regulate the activity of the intestinal enzyme (McCuaig and Motzok, 1972). With respect to the kidney, there is no direct evidence that brush-border alkaline phosphatase is involved in phosphate transport, but the first observation which suggested such an association was the finding that alkaline phosphatase activity was specifically increased in kidneys of phosphate-deprived rats (Melani *et al.*, 1967). More recent studies, in which renal cortical alkaline phosphatase activity and phosphate transport were measured in parallel, indicate an apparent reciprocal relationship between phosphate excretion by the kidney and, specifically, membrane-bound alkaline phosphatase activity in the renal cortex (Dousa *et al.*, 1976; Kempson *et al.*, 1977). In thyroparathyroidectomized (TPTX) rats treated with colchicine, renal excretion of phosphate increased and alkaline phosphatase decreased, while another brush-border enzyme, leucine aminopeptidase, was not changed in comparison with controls. In rats placed on a low-phosphate diet, renal phosphate excretion decreased and the specific and total alkaline phosphatase activity markedly increased, but there were no changes in other brush-border enzymes, such as maltase, leucine aminopeptidase, and γ-glutamyltransferase, nor in mitochondrial, lysosomal, or contraluminal membrane enzymes. The specific increase in alkaline phosphatase activity of the luminal brush border was apparent also in histochemical analysis of the renal cortex. Previous work (Melani *et al.*, 1967) also indicated that the increase in alkaline phosphatase in animals on a low-phosphate diet was specific in terms that enzymes of the glycolytic pathway were not influenced by the low-phosphate diet. It has been shown recently that the increase in alkaline phosphatase activity can be prevented by treatment with drugs inhibiting RNA and protein synthesis. In our recent experiments, we examined whether actinomycin D, an inhibitor of RNA synthesis, and cycloheximide, an inhibitor of protein synthesis at the level of translation, influence the enzyme changes and excretory features of renal adaptation to a low-phosphorus diet. Indeed, pretreatment with these two drugs completely or partially blocked the increase in the phosphate reabsorption in response to the low-phosphorus intake and also specifically prevented an increase in renal cortical alkaline phosphatase activity (Shah *et al.*, 1978a,b). Finally, it has been reported that Levamisole, an anthelmintic drug which specifically inhibits alkaline phosphatase, enhanced the fractional excretion of phosphate in dogs (Plante *et al.*, 1977). These findings suggest that alkaline phosphatase may play a role, as yet undetermined, in the transport of phosphate (and possibly of other ions) across the renal brush-border membrane and/or that some other protein component synthesized *de novo* is necessary to increase reabsorption of phosphate.

It is worthwhile to speculate briefly on the molecular mechanism by which alkaline phosphatase may serve in the phosphate transport processes. In the simplest case, alkaline phosphatase, an integral membrane protein, could be the phosphate-transporting protein itself. If it is assumed that phosphate is bound on a specific carrier in the membrane, alkaline phosphatase may be involved in two aspects. It is known that alkaline phosphatase catalyzes not only the hydrolysis of organically bound phosphate but also the transfer of phosphate bound on one organic molecule (donor) to another organic compound (an acceptor molecule) in transesterification reactions, and during such catalysis, a phosphoryl enzyme intermediate is formed (Chen, 1976). Alternatively or additionally, by virtue of its hydrolytic activity, alkaline phosphatase could be involved in the removal of phosphate from the transporting protein (carrier) on the interior of the luminal membrane. A further possibility is that alkaline phosphatase, with its capacity for dephosphorylation, may serve as a regulator of membrane protein phosphorylations. This is based on the general idea that membrane protein phosphorylation, controlled by certain hormones, may be involved in the mechanism of regulation of phosphate transport. That alkaline phosphatase itself may be accessible to hormonal regulation is surmised by its location on a membrane which contains cAMP (cyclic AMP)-binding sites (Insel *et al.*, 1975) and a cAMP-dependent protein kinase (George *et al.*, 1971).

3. CHARACTERISTICS OF PHOSPHATE TRANSPORT

The relationship between phosphate concentrations and transport by the proximal tubule was first described by Pitts (1933) from clearance studies. He characterized the phosphate transport system as a carrier-mediated transport which can be saturated. Several lines of evidence indicate that phosphate is actively (carrier-mediated) rather than passively transported. First, solvent drag as a driving force for phosphate transport can be assumed to be minimal in those experiments where volume reabsorption was held close to zero by the inclusion of an impermeant anion (Lang *et al.*, 1977a). Second, the passive permeability is minimal in comparison to total transport, since there is a negligible passive backflux of phosphate into the tubular lumen, and, as a consequence, the intraluminal concentration of phosphate can reach very low values (Greger *et al.*, 1977). Even in normal physiologic circumstances, with free flow of tubular fluid, the concentration of phosphate in tubular fluid is approximately 60% that of plasma. The free-flow potential is slightly negative in the early proximal tubule and slightly positive, $+1.5$ mV, in later portions of the proximal convoluted tubule, whereas intracellular potentials are markedly negative (Fig. 2). Thus, phosphate must be actively transported against this electrochemical-potential difference. At the luminal cell membrane, two factors oppose the entry of phosphate from the tubular lumen into the cell: the inside negative cell potential and the high intracellular phosphate concentration. At the contraluminal membrane, the transfer of phosphate is favored by the higher intracellular phosphate concentration

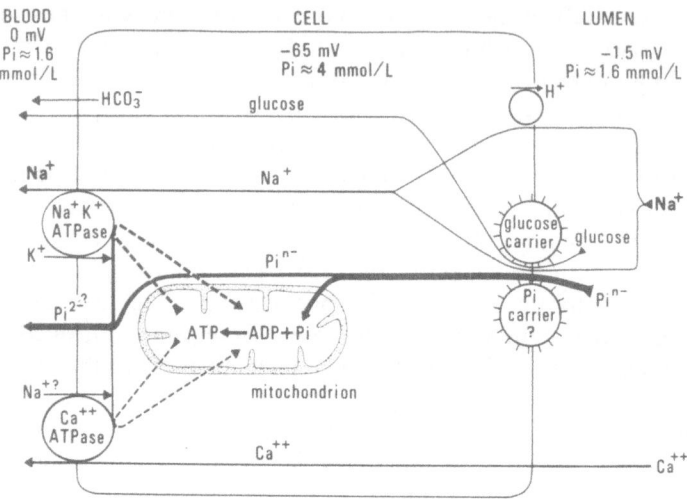

Fig. 2. A saturable sodium-dependent transport mechanism for phosphate located in the luminal membrane. These properties resemble those of the mechanism for glucose transport, and the rates of phosphate and glucose transport are interdependent. Phosphate entry into the cell occurs against both an electrical-potential difference and a small concentration gradient. The driving force for phosphate transport into the cell is sodium entry, which occurs along the electrochemical gradient created by $(Na^+ + K^+)$-ATPase activity in the basolateral membrane. After entry, at least part of the phosphate is transported into mitochondria and serves as a substrate for ATP synthesis. ATP degradation in the basolateral membrane provides locally high concentrations of phosphate, which leaves the cell along the electrochemical gradient. The contralateral transport of phosphate has been shown to occur independently of sodium. The basolateral membranes may be more permeable to HPO_4^{2-} than HPO_4^-. This would explain the effect of changes in cellular pH on phosphate reabsorption (see text). The intracellular concentration of phosphate is taken from Kupfer and Kosovsky (1970).

and the inside negative cell potential. Although transport through two membranes may involve more than one carrier, as long as one step is rate limiting, saturation kinetics may appropriately describe the correlation between transport rate and luminal concentration. In microperfusion experiments, the maximum transport rate of the proximal convoluted tubule was found to be approximately 12 pmol/min/mm (Lang et al., 1977a). Since the first millimeter of proximal tubule is not accessible for microperfusion, these maximum transport rates do not apply to this very early segment. Further, free-flow micropuncture studies would indicate that this segment of the nephron, not accessible to microperfusion, may have a more avid transport rate. Further, transport rates in the late proximal tubule and pars recta have been found to be significant and less than in the proximal convoluted tubule.

An additional characteristic of the phosphate transport system is the affinity for phosphate. The concentration of phosphate at which transport is half maximal is roughly 0.7 mM in the proximal convoluted tubule and 0.2 mM in the late proximal tubule (Lang et al., 1977a). It is noteworthy that the high affinity and limited transport capacity of the late proximal tubule may allow for the low fractional excretions of phosphate in acutely TPTX animals. As plasma phosphate increases this feature may allow for regulation of plasma phosphate concentration even in the absence of PTH.

4. NONHORMONAL FACTORS

4.1. Sodium Dependency of Phosphate Transport

A relationship between sodium and phosphate transport was strongly suggested in clearance experiments in which extracellular fluid volume expansion resulted in a marked natriuresis and phosphaturia in dogs (Agus et al., 1971; Massry et al., 1969; Puschett et al., 1972b; Suki et al., 1969), humans (Steele, 1970), and rats (Frick, 1969, 1972). Although this effect probably involves the release of PTH due to a decreased plasma calcium (Wen, 1974), a close relationship between phosphate and sodium transport in the proximal tubule has been demonstrated independent of the effects of PTH (Schneider et al., 1975). Extracellular fluid volume expansion in TPTX dogs resulted in a blunted phosphaturia as compared with intact dogs, but a relationship between sodium and phosphate excretion was still present (Massry et al., 1969). Similar conclusions have been derived from recollection studies of the proximal tubule in the rat (Beck and Goldberg, 1974; Frick, 1972; Maesaka et al., 1973; Wein, 1974). Many diuretics, such as chlorthiazide, mercurials, furosemide, and ethacrynic acid, cause parallel increases in sodium excretion and phosphaturia in TPTX dogs (Eknoyan et al., 1970). Cardiac glucosides, inhibitors of $(Na^+ + K^+)$-ATPase and sodium transport, increase excretion of both sodium and phosphate (Kupfer and Kosovsky, 1965). In summary, many examples from clearance data suggest a coupling between sodium and phosphate transport. The precise relationship between sodium and phosphate excretion may differ depending upon modulating influences, such as PTH. In addition, it is important to note that segmental differences in sodium and phosphate transport can markedly affect the stoichiometry between these two electrolytes. For example, in sodium depletion, terminal nephron segments markedly reduce the sodium excretion in the urine, and this accordingly alters the relationships between sodium and phosphate as delivered from the proximal tubule.

In micropuncture studies, substitution of sodium by the impermeant cation choline inhibited phosphate transport in the early portions of the proximal convoluted tubule in the rat (Baumann *et al.*, 1975a). Further, in the isolated perfused proximal tubule of the rabbit, ouabain inhibited both sodium and phosphate reabsorption (Dennis *et al.*, 1976). Similarly, in *in vivo* double microperfusion experiments, ouabain inhibited both sodium and phosphate reabsorption when applied to the peritubular microcirculation in the hamster (Ullrich *et al.*, 1977).

In vesicles prepared from the brush border of renal proximal tubules, addition of sodium to the medium markedly enhanced phosphate uptake (Hoffman *et al.*, 1976; Kinne *et al.*, 1977). Further, substitution of sodium by lithium, potassium, rubidium, and cesium or choline resulted in marked decreases in phosphate uptake by the vesicle preparation. The sodium-dependent phosphate uptake by the vesicles occurs against a concentration gradient for phosphate. This sodium-dependent uptake of phosphate was characterized by saturation kinetics qualitatively similar to kinetics observed *in vivo* (Pitts and Alexander, 1944). Arsenate competitively inhibits phosphate uptake by the brush-border vesicles, in agreement with the inhibition of phosphate reabsorption by arsenate reported *in vivo* (Ginsburg and Lotspeich, 1963). Phosphate uptake by the vesicles was enhanced in alkaline medium. Kinne *et al.* (1977) postulate that phosphate transport is electroneutral and is secondary to the active transport of two sodium ions per phosphate ion. This secondary active transport was localized on the brush-border side of the cell and was not found on the antiluminal border of the cell. Hyperpolarization of the brush-border vesicles stimulates phosphate uptake, suggesting that both the potential and chemical gradients for sodium are driving forces for phosphate uptake (Hoffman *et al.*, 1976; Kinne *et al.*, 1977).

This sodium dependency of phosphate transport is not unique to the kidney. Similar relationships, perhaps differing in some specific aspects, have been found in the intestine (Harrison and Harrison, 1963; Taylor, 1974), sea urchin eggs (Chambers, 1963), mammalian nerve fibers (Anner *et al.*, 1973; Straub *et al.*, 1976), fish nerves (Straub *et al.*, 1975), cultured tumor cells (Brown and Lamb, 1975), and squid axon (Caldwell and Lowe, 1970).

In summary, phosphate transport by the brush-border membrane may be characterized as follows: Phosphate transport may be active, secondary to sodium transport, localized in the brush-border membrane but not in the basolateral membrane. The energy requirements for this transport are only indirectly coupled, since the primary energy requirements for the sodium transport are located in the basolateral membrane. Accordingly, the sodium-dependent phosphate uptake in the brush-border membrane utilizes the sodium gradient generated at the basolateral surface of the cell (Fig. 2). Hyperpolarization of vesicles enhances the sodium uptake as well as phosphate uptake, indicating that both the sodium gradient and potential differences serve as driving forces for phosphate transport. The findings of saturation kinetics for phosphate transport and competition with arsenate suggest the existence of a carrier for phosphate in the brush border. Both the concentration gradient for phosphate and potential differences through the antiluminal membrane favor phosphate exit from the cell such that passive phosphate transport through the antiluminal membrane is sufficient to account for phosphate exit. Additionally, this concentration gradient might be enhanced by a local high concentration of phosphate along the cellular site of the basolateral membrane as the result of ATP degradation by the ATPase system. This possibility is emphasized by the finding that radioactivity of intravenously administered [$^{32}PO_4$]sodium hydroxide was recovered in the kidney predominantly in ATP (Kupfer and Kosovsky, 1970).

4.2. Glucose and Phosphate Transport

There are many parallelisms between glucose and phosphate transport in the kidney. For example, glucose and phosphate transport are predominantly, if not exclusively, localized in the proximal tubule. Further, both glucose and phosphate transport are more avid in the early proximal tubule than in later segments of the proximal tubule. Both transport systems are characterized by saturation kinetics, and both transport systems show a sodium dependency. Both systems have been described as carrier-mediated transport systems in the brush-border membrane.

In addition to the similarities of transport mechanisms, competition for transport is suggested by several findings. In clearance and micropuncture experiments, transport of glucose inhibits phosphate reabsorption (Cohen *et al.*, 1956; Ginsburg, 1972; Levitan, 1951). Micropuncture studies in dogs indicate that this effect is specific for glucose and is not secondary to an effect of insulin (DeFronzo *et al.*, 1976). Further, phlorizin inhibits glucose transport, enhances phosphate reabsorption, and reverses glucose-induced phosphaturia (Cohen *et al.*, 1957; Pitts and Alexander, 1944; and Wolbach, 1970). These effects of glucose are shared by other sugars such as fructose and galactose. Phlorizin also inhibits the transport of these sugars in humans and, again, fructose and galactose are also phosphaturic (Fox *et al.*, 1964; Gammeltoft and Kjerulf-Jensen, 1943). The energy supply for glucose and phosphate transport may be shared to some extent, as indicated by the effects of maleate, an inhibitor of succinyl coenzyme A (CoA) transferase, in the kidney. Maleate increases excretion of both phosphate and glucose (Gmaj *et al.*, 1973; Harrison and Harrison, 1954). Further shared mechanisms are suggested by the finding that cardiac glycosides in high doses depress reabsorption of both glucose and phosphate (Czaky *et al.*, 1964; Kupfer and Kosovsky, 1965; Vogel *et al.*, 1965). Since cardiac glycosides also inhibit sodium transport, this provides further evidence linking sodium dependency to both glucose and phosphate transport systems. Phosphate homeostasis also affects transport processes for glucose, as illustrated by the decrease in the Tm for glucose caused by severe phosphate depletion (Gold *et al.*, 1977).

In isolated vesicles from brush borders, glucose, like phosphate, has been shown to be coupled with active sodium transport (Kinne *et al.*, 1977). Similar parallelisms between glucose and phosphate transport have been observed in intestinal preparations as well as in kidney preparations.

In summary, glucose and phosphate transport mechanisms share many common features. These include proximal reabsorption, sodium dependency, competition for transport, and shared characteristics of luminal membrane transport. The sodium gradient and potential differences across the luminal membrane which favor sodium transport may provide a common driving force for glucose, some amino acids, and phosphate transport. There is no direct evidence to indicate that the glucose and phosphate carriers are the same, but both processes may use the same energy source. For example, glucose depolarizes the cell, and this may alter the driving force for phosphate.

4.3. Effect of Acid–Base Balance on Phosphate Transport

There is little question that changes in acid–base balance result in changes in phosphate excretion. The precise relationships are complex, however, and the common denominator has not been elucidated.

Respiratory acidosis. Acute hypercapnia in animals with intact parathyroid glands is associated with an increased excretion of phosphate in the urine (Barker *et al.*, 1957; Brassfield and Behrman, 1941; Denton *et al.*, 1952; Freeman *et al.*, 1957; Gray *et al.*, 1973; Haldane *et al.*, 1924; Levitin *et al.*, 1958; Polak *et al.*, 1961; Schwartz *et al.*, 1965). In TPTX animals, acute hypercapnia also results in increased phosphate excretion (Hoppe and Knox, 1978; Webb *et al.*, 1977).

Respiratory alkalosis. Acute respiratory alkalosis reduces phosphate excretion in humans (Mostellar and Tuttle, 1966) and in TPTX rats (Angielski and Szczepanska-Konkel, 1977) and hamsters (Hoppe and Knox, 1979). Although Malvin and Lotspeich (1956) reported that respiratory alkalosis enhances phosphate excretion, it should be noted that there were no changes in the fractional excretion of phosphate in these studies. In summary, respiratory acidosis is usually associated with a phosphaturia, whereas respiratory alkalosis is associated with an antiphosphaturia.

Acute metabolic acidosis. The production of acute metabolic acidosis, such as that seen following infusion of ammonium chloride, decreases urinary phosphate excretion in TPTX hamsters but then subsequently uncovers the phosphaturic effect of PTH (Knox *et al.*, 1977). In additional studies, metabolic acidosis has been accompanied by phosphaturia in the presence of intact parathyroid glands (Guest, 1942; Haldane *et al.*, 1923; Martin and Jones, 1961; Scott, 1972). It should be noted that a compensatory hypocapnia would be predicted in the presence of acute metabolic acidosis. This feature, noted to affect phosphate excretion, is usually not controlled or evaluated.

Acute metabolic alkalosis. Infusion of sodium bicarbonate has been noted to enhance phosphate excretion in the urine of humans (Mostellar and Tuttle, 1964) and intact (Malvin and Lotspeich, 1956; Mercado *et al.*, 1975) and TPTX (Fulop and Brazeau, 1968) dogs. Puschett and Goldberg reported (1969) that infusion of sodium bicarbonate solution was associated with a greater phosphaturia than infusion of an equivalent volume of sodium chloride, and they suggested that bicarbonate by itself, and not volume expansion, was responsible for the greater phosphaturia. Although both sodium bicarbonate and sodium chloride volume expansion are associated with PTH release, it cannot be ascertained whether the release of PTH was greater in the sodium bicarbonate group. Such might be predicted because of the effects of sodium bicarbonate alkalinization on decreasing ionized calcium concentrations. Mercado *et al.* (1975) reported that in TPTX dogs infused with PTH, sodium chloride or sodium bicarbonate had the same effect on phosphate excretion. No similar studies have been performed in TPTX animals in which equivalent sodium chloride and sodium bicarbonate infusions have been employed. Webb *et al.* (1977) obtained results similar to those of Puschett and Goldberg (1969). Volume expansion with sodium chloride produced a smaller phosphaturia than equivalent expansion of sodium bicarbonate in intact rats. It should be noted that in this case, the rats were normocapnic. The data of Webb *et al.* (1977) indicate that the concentration of calcium in blood is low in the sodium bicarbonate group, again indicating that this greater phosphaturia could be due to enhanced secretion of PTH.

Alkalinization of the urine, such as that following acetazolamide administration or sodium bicarbonate infusion, has been associated with a marked increase in phosphate excretion in intact (Fulop and Brazeau, 1968; Malvin and Lotspeich, 1956) and TPTX (Knox *et al.*, 1976) dogs. From these findings of a correlation between urine alkalinization and inhibition of phosphate reabsorption, it was postulated that the alkaline form of phosphate is less reabsorbable. However, it should be noted that urine alkalinization does not necessarily result in a phosphaturia. For example, as noted above, alkalinization of the urine following lithium administration results in decreased phosphate excretion.

That the acid form of phosphate is reabsorbed predominantly in the proximal tubule can be concluded from recent experiments of Cassola and Malnic (1977). Microperfusion studies of the effect of changes in tubular fluid pH are conflicting. On the one hand, Bank *et al.* (1974) suggest that acid phosphate is predominantly reabsorbed, whereas Baumann *et al.* (1975b) suggest that alkaline phosphate is the predominantly reabsorbed species. Additional studies by Lang *et al.* (1977) suggest that alkaline phosphate is predominantly transported, although the acid form is also transported. In isolated vesicles prepared from brush-border membranes, alkaline phosphate was shown to be preferentially transported over acid phosphate (Hoffman *et al.*, 1976). This finding suggests, for the luminal membrane at least, that alkaline phosphate may be the preferentially transported species. Ullrich (1977) initially reported that phosphate transport is insensitive to ambient pH changes. Recently, however, he has concluded that luminal acidosis and intracellular alkalosis inhibit phosphate transport.

In summary, it is difficult to reconcile changes in acid–base balance in blood, urine, and tubular fluid with a common mechanism. The effect of urinary alkalinization on renal handling of phosphate is discussed in Chapter 8.

An additional important component of acid–base balance is the intracellular compartment. Changes in intracellular pH may play a key role in transepithelial transport of phosphate. Unfortunately, no direct evidence exists to evaluate whether intracellular pH is the common denominator to account for changes in transcellular phosphate transport. However, citrate reabsorption and cellular content may provide an indicator of cellular pH (Adler, 1972b; Adler *et al.*, 1974; Crawford, 1963; Grollman *et al.*, 1961; Ostberg, 1931; Simpson, 1967). The altered citrate metabolism, in turn, is considered to be due to changes in intracellular bicarbonate concentrations. In addition, acute changes in systemic pCO_2 can influence intracellular pH (Adler *et al.*, 1965), whereas changes in systemic bicarbonate concentration and pH do not necessarily reflect changes in cellular pH (Adler *et al.*, 1972a). The metabolic alkalosis in blood which is characteristic of potassium-depleted animals is associated with a cellular acidosis (Alder *et al.*, 1972b; Sanslone and Muntwyler, 1966). Reciprocally, the metabolic acidosis is presumed to accompany an intracellular alkalosis after acute lithium administration (Angielski *et al.*, 1976). Table 1 summarizes the relationship beween phosphate transport and predicted intracellular pH for the kidney. The values presented in Table 1 indicate that changes in phosphate excretion are consistent with the presumed changes in intracellular pH but not with blood, that is, a

Table 1. Acid–Base Status and Phosphate Excretion[a] in TPTX Animals

	FE of PO$_4$	Blood acid–base status	Renal citrate content or excretion	Predicted cell pH	Reference
Lithium administration	↓	Metabolic acidosis	↑	↑	Angielski and Szczpanska-Konkel (1977) Angielski et al. (1976)
Hypocapnia	↓	Respiratory alkalosis	↑	↑	Webb et al. (1977) Hoppe and Knox (1978) Angielski and Szczpanska-Konkel (1977) Adler et al. (1972)
Hypercapnia	↑	Respiratory acidosis	↓	↓	Webb et al. (1977) Hoppe and Knox (1978) Angielski and Szczpanska-Konkel (1977)
K$^+$ depletion[b]	↑	Metabolic alkalosis	↓	↓	Beck and Davis (1975) Adler et al. (1974)

[a] FE, fractional excretion.
[b] In this study, absolute excretion of phosphate in K$^+$-depleted animals is not significantly higher (controls 6.1 ± 2.8 µg/min; K$^+$ depleted, 8.9 ± 2.1 µg/min; $p > 0.05$), but if one corrects for presented filtered load, phosphate excretion in K$^+$-depleted animals is twice as high as in controls.

low excretion of phosphate in intracellular alkalosis and a high excretion of phosphate in intracellular acidosis. We must emphasize, however, that direct measurements of cellular pH with simultaneous measurements of phosphate transport are not available in the literature. Further, the mechanism by which changes in cellular pH might change phosphate transport is also not clear. One of many possibilities is that the basolateral membranes are more permeable to alkaline phosphate, which allows for more avid transcellular transport.

In hypokalemia and severe potassium depletion, intracellular pH of the tubular cells is probably acid (Adler *et al.*, 1974), whereas extracellular pH is clearly alkaline. In a study of potassium-depleted TPTX rats by Beck and Davis (1975), absolute excretion of phosphate was slightly increased, but if these data are expressed in terms of fractional excretion, the values of the latter were twice as high as in control animals. The phosphaturic effect of PTH was still present, but this was significantly reduced in magnitude. Unfortunately, acid–base parameters in blood were not measured in these studies, but it is likely that there was a metabolic alkalosis. In summary, several lines of evidence indicate that phosphate reabsorption is influenced by intracellular pH.

5. HORMONAL REGULATION OF PHOSPHATE AT THE CELLULAR LEVEL

The hormonal regulation of renal phosphate transport is discussed in detail in Chapters 5 and 6. In this section, we would like to consider briefly only the final steps involved in modulating phosphate transport in renal tubules at the cellular level.

At the present stage of our knowledge, it is useful to consider together the effects of hormonal and humoral agents which mediate their affects via cyclic nucleotides. These agents, which are usually polypeptides or biogenic amines, have effects which are rapid in both onset and decline and are mediated by cyclic nucleotides.

Separately, we may consider other possible cellular mechanisms involved in long-term adjustment of phosphate transport.

5.1. Mechanism of Regulation by Cyclic Nucleotides

The only hormone which has been proven to specifically regulate phosphate transport under physiological conditions is PTH (Aurbach and Heath, 1974; Aurbach *et al.*, 1972). In addition, there is considerable evidence that other polypeptides, calcitonin, glucagon, and insulin, in pharmacologic doses or under pathologic circumstances, may also act on renal tubular phosphate transport (Aurbach and Heath, 1974; Aurbach *et al.*, 1972; Butlen and Jard, 1972; DeFronzo *et al.*, 1975, 1976; Dousa, 1976; Dousa and Barnes, 1977; Nizet *et al.*, 1976). Some biogenic amines, such as dopamine (Cuche *et al.*, 1976) and acetylcholine (Schneider *et al.*, 1973), may also be included in this category.

In general, PTH (Aurbach and Heath, 1974; Aurbach *et al.*, 1972; Butler and Jard, 1972; Dousa, 1976; Dousa and Barnes, 1977), calcitonin (Aurbach and Heath, 1974; Aurbach *et al.*, 1972; Cuche *et al.*, 1976; Dousa, 1976; Dousa and Barnes, 1977; Kurokawa *et al.*, 1974), and glucagon (Aurbach and Heath, 1974; Aurbach *et al.*, 1972; Butlen and Jard, 1972; Dousa, 1976; Dousa and Barnes, 1977) are phosphaturic, while insulin (De Fronzo *et al.*, 1975, 1976; Nizet *et al.*, 1976) reduces renal phosphate excretion. All of these agents may act directly or indirectly via cyclic nucleotides (Dousa, 1976). These agents most likely do not enter the cells to exert their effects on phospate transport. It has been shown, or at least it is assumed, that all of these hormones bind on the antiluminal membrane to the specific receptors associated with adenylate cyclase and stimulate, or inhibit, generation of cAMP (DiBella *et al.*, 1974; Kinne, 1975; Marx *et al.*, 1972; Schlatz *et al.*, 1975; Sutcliffe *et al*, 1973; Zull *et al.*, 1977). cAMP generated in response to these hormones then inhibits phosphate transport, resulting in phosphaturia (Aurbach and Heath, 1974; Aurbach *et al.*, 1972). Since, as pointed out earlier, the first point of entry and probably the rate-limiting site of phosphate transport is in the brush border, it is hypothesized that cyclic nucleotides will ultimately act directly or indirectly on brush-border membranes (Kinne, 1975; Murer *et al.*, 1978).

Most of the data regarding the possible role of cyclic nucleotides and protein phosphorylation have been obtained in studies of PTH effects. Perhaps, in a general way, and using a rather great oversimplification, PTH action may be taken as representative of cAMP-mediated inhibition of phosphate transport by other similarly acting agents.

There is considerable evidence that PTH stimulates adenylate cyclase and causes an intracellular accumulation of cAMP (Aurbach and Heath, 1974; Aurbach *et al.*, 1972; Dousa, 1976; Dousa and Barnes, 1977). Exogenous cAMP or its derivative(s) are able to mimic phosphaturic effects of hormones (Bell *et al.*, 1972; Butlen and Jard, 1972; Hamburger *et al.*, 1974; Murer *et al.*, 1978; Rasmussen *et al.*, 1968) in intact animals (Bell *et al.*, 1972; Butlen and Jard, 1972; Rasmussen *et al.*, 1968), in micropuncture studies (Agus *et al.*, 1971), in isolated perfused tubules (Hamburger *et al.*, 1974), in perfused tubules *in situ* (Baumann *et al.*, 1977), and in isolated amphibian membranes (Sellers *et al.*, 1977).

It is generally assumed that, as for other hormones and tissues, cAMP serves as an intracellular mediator in a classical "second-messenger role" (Robison *et al.*, 1971). The intriguing possibility that in the case of renal tubules, cAMP that appears in tubular fluid in response to phosphaturic hormones could also conceivably have a regulatory effect on transport processes, including phosphate transport (Butlen and Jard, 1972; Küntziger *et al.*, 1974), will be considered briefly. In response to PTH, cAMP is increased in both tubular cells and lumen and, primarily by water abstraction, reaches a very high concentration in the distal portion of tubular system and in the final urine (Fig. 3). For example, in the human kidney, high doses of PTH may result in up to a 100-fold increase in the urinary cAMP concentration compared to controls (Aurbach and Heath, 1974; Aurbach *et al.*, 1972). A high-affinity binding site for cAMP has been found in brush-border preparations (Insel *et al.*, 1975). Since under most conditions, brush-border preparations form vesicles with right side out (Kinne and Schwartz, 1976), it can be assumed that the binding is on the luminal surface. Despite this, it has been shown that cAMP added to isolated vesicles from brush borders does not inhibit phosphate transport, but marked inhibition of phosphate transport does occur in vesicles from animals treated with dibutyryl cAMP (Murer *et al.*, 1978). On the other hand, addition of dibutyryl cAMP decreases isotonic phosphate transport in perfused tubules (Baumann *et al.*, 1977; Hamburger *et al.*, 1974).

These findings suggest that cAMP acts directly and on the proximal tubule from the luminal side. Thus, it is quite conceivable that cAMP released into the lumen in the early proximal tubule could act in more distal portions of the nephron (Butlen and Jard, 1972), where its concentration also increases by water abstraction (Fig. 3). As discussed elsewhere, phosphate reabsorption in the distal tubule remains controversial (Knox, 1977).

The mechanism by which a rise in intracellular cAMP produces the ultimate expression of the physiological action of PTH remains unknown (Aurbach and Heath, 1974; Aurbach *et al.*, 1972; Dousa, 1976; Dousa and Barnes, 1977). As proposed by Aurbach *et al.* (1972), the state of phosphorylation of the membrane proteins may be linked to specific functional modifications in membrane permeability and transport; this hypothesis is under investigation. The major components of this protein-phosphorylating system include (1) protein kinase, an enzyme that catalyzes the transesterification of γ-phosphate from ATP to side chains of serine or threonine in polypeptides and that is stimulated by cAMP; (2) a very specific protein substrate that is a component of phosphate transport or a phosphate-transport-regulating system and that is expected to be located in or close to the luminal plasma membrane; and (3) protein phosphatase, which catalyzes the dephosphorylation of proteins (Aurbach *et al.*, 1972; Hosey and Tao, 1977; Kinne *et al.*, 1975).

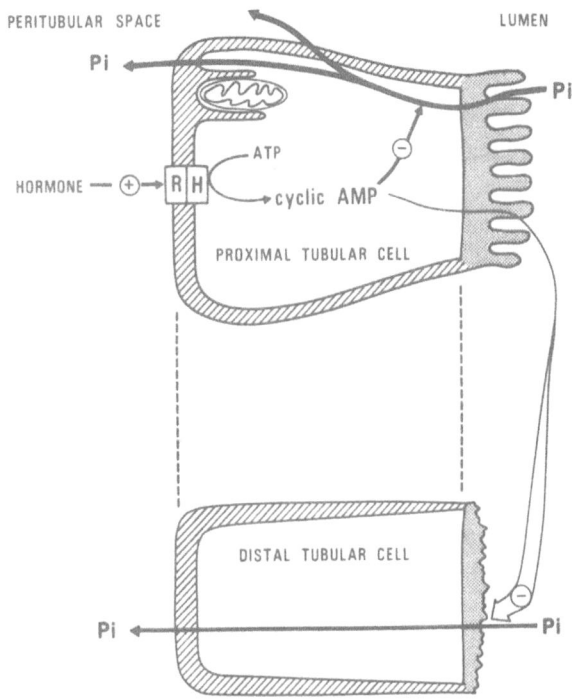

Fig. 3. Mode of cAMP effect on phosphate transport from within the cell (proximal tubular cell) or from the lumen (distal tubular cell). "Distal" means any site along the tubule length distal to the site of cAMP efflux to the lumen under the influence of phosphaturic hormones (e.g., PTH). As the distance from site of efflux increases, cAMP in the lumen becomes progressively more concentrated. H, phosphaturic hormone; R, receptor for the hormone; Pi, inorganic phosphate; ―⊖→, inhibitory action.

The basic elements required for such a reversible mechanism have been found in various preparations from the kidney or renal cortex (Abou-Issa *et al.*, 1974, 1975; Aurbach *et al.*, 1972; DeRubertis and Craven, 1976; Forte *et al.*, 1972, 1975; George *et al.*, 1977; Kim *et al.*, 1977; Kinne *et al.*, 1975; Knox *et al.*, 1977; Sakai *et al.*, 1976; Wombacher *et al.*, 1973). Administration of PTH or calcitonin *in vivo* or addition to tissue slices causes an increase in cAMP and also activation of protein kinase (DeRubertis and Craven, 1976; Knox *et al.*, 1977; Sakai *et al.*, 1976). Studies on isolated cortical tubules also suggest that cAMP-mediated phosphorylations may be involved in the action of PTH (Ausiello *et al.*, 1976).

Although the activation of protein kinase and protein phosphoryla-tions may be an integral part of the kidney's response to PTH, major unresolved questions remain. What is the exact link between activation of protein kinase and inhibition of phosphate transport? What is the nature of the protein(s) involved in phosphorylation by a cAMP-dependent system? Is there an intrinsic membrane protein kinase or a cytosolic protein kinase which is a phosphorylating enzyme?

On the one hand, the presence of cAMP-dependent protein kinase was described in a subfraction of renal cortical membranes containing brush border (Abou-Issa et al., 1975; George et al., 1977; Kinne and Schwartz, 1976; Kinne et al., 1975); this enzyme was activated by addition of cAMP in vitro (George et al., 1977; Kinne et al., 1975), whereas in other reports, renal membrane protein kinase was not activated by cAMP (Abou-Issa et al., 1974; George et al., 1977). Some authors report that membrane protein kinase is rather loosely bound on the membrane and is easily extracted by mild procedures (Abou-Issa et al., 1974; DeRubertis and Craven, 1976; Sakai et al., 1976; Wombacher et al., 1973). Thus, according to one view, cAMP, generated under the influence of PTH at the luminal membrane, activates the brush-border-membrane-bound cAMP-dependent protein kinase. This protein kinase, in turn, would phosphorylate a specific protein involved in the regulation of phosphate transport (Kinne, 1975; Kinne and Schwartz, 1976). However, the majority of cAMP-dependent protein kinase in the cortex is in the cytosol (Abou-Issa et al., 1974; DeRubertis and Craven, 1976; Forte et al., 1972). A second view, which takes that fact into consideration, is that protein involved in phosphate transport may be phosphorylated by the protein kinase that is in the cytosol but in close apposition to the luminal brush border. It should be noted that a protein kinase from cytosol, and which is not sensitive to direct stimulation by cAMP, has been described and extracted from the brush-border fraction (George et al., 1977). It appears that the two alternatives mentioned above (soluble vs. membrane protein kinase) are not necessarily mutually exclusive (Fig. 4). There may even be disadvantages from a regulatory point of view if each of these phosphorylating mechanisms operated alone. If it is assumed (and experimental evidence seems to be in favor to such an assumption) that cAMP is generated in the basolateral membrane (Kinne, 1975; 1972; Schwartz, 1976; Marx et al., 1972; Shlatz et al., 1975), a considerable quantity of cAMP would be bound by regulatory subunits of cytosolic protein kinase, non-protein-kinase-binding proteins (Ueland and Doskeland, 1977), or destroyed by cAMP phosphodiesterase prior to reaching the brush border and the opposite side of the cell. That cAMP can reach the brush border is documented by the finding of increased urinary excretion of cAMP in response to PTH (Aurbach and Heath, 1974; Aurbach et al.., 1972). Therefore, the fine adjustment of such a mechanism (cAMP-sensitive protein kinase that is intrinsic in the brush-border membrane) would be influenced by many cytoplasmic unspecific factors. On the other hand, the access of activated

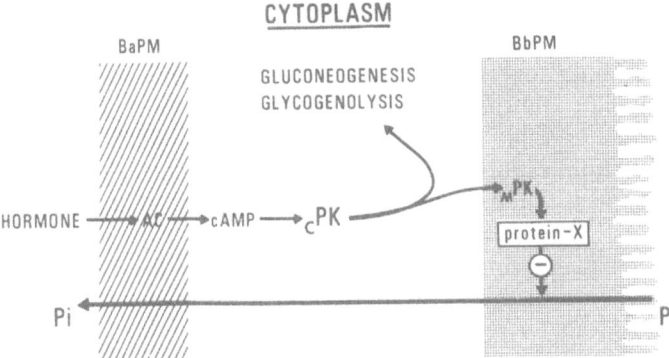

Fig. 4. Hypothetical scheme for the possible role of membrane-bound and soluble protein kinases in regulation of phosphate transport. $_cPK$, cytoplasmic cAMP-dependent protein kinase; $_MPK$, membrane protein kinase within brush border independent of cAMP; protein-X, a protein component involved in control of Pi transport or in phosphate transport itself; AC, adenylate cyclase; Pi, inorganic phosphate; BbPM, brush-border plasma membrane; BaPM, basolateral plasma membrane; —⊖→, inhibitory action.

cytosolic protein kinase to a specific protein substrate intrinsic to the brush border could be hindered by the location of substrate within the infrastructure of the brush-border membrane. Perhaps, just as in the case of activation of glycogen phosphorylase (Soderling and Park, 1974), both soluble and membrane-bound protein kinases may act in sequence and in such a way that cAMP would first activate cAMP-dependent protein kinase in the cytoplasm, which would then activate another specific membrane protein kinase by phosphorylation. The latter membrane-bound protein kinase (activated by cAMP-dependent phosphorylation via action of cytosolic protein kinase) would then finally act on the phosphate-transporting protein or on regulatory protein components of phosphate transport in the brush border (Fig. 4). In addition, the cAMP-dependent protein kinase in cytosol may cause other regulatory adjustments, such as an increase in activity of glycogen phosphorylase (Handler and Orloff, 1963) or stimulation of gluconeogenesis (Nagata and Rasmussen, 1970), which was found to be activated by cAMP in renal cortex. Analogous unresolved questions arise in relation to the other system, such as renal effects of vasopressin (Dousa *et al.*, 1977b; Kinne and Schwartz, 1976).

Another integral enzyme in protein phosphorylation is protein phosphatase, an enzyme that removes phosphate from side chains of amino acids. Protein phosphatase has been found in renal cortex. However, no direct or indirect effects of cyclic nucleotides on protein phosphatase have been reported to date (Abou-Issa *et al.*, 1975; George *et al.*, 1977). It is likely that In cAMP-dependent protein phosphorylation, as in many other systems, the major regulatory point is protein kinase (Hosey and Tao, 1977).

Thus, taken together, the effect of cAMP-mediated hormones on renal phosphate transport through phosphorylation of specific protein(s) appears to be a viable hypothesis. However, the mechanism of specific phosphorylation, especially the nature of the substrate for protein kinase specifically associated with phosphate transport, remains to be elucidated.

Another major component of the membranes are phospholipids, although based on their less strict structural specificity, they are not expected to be a major regulatory component of a highly specialized membrane fraction. In several reports, it was noted that PTH (Beck *et al.*, 1972; Lo *et al.*, 1976) and cAMP (Beck *et al.*, 1972) can increase phospholipid turnover in the kidney and incorporation of phosphate into membrane phospholipids and that cAMP can activate the phosphoinositol kinase (Cunningham, 1968). Although the significance of these observations is uncertain, the possible role of membrane phospholipids should not be completely dismissed from consideration.

Cyclic GMP (cGMP) is another nucleotide which has been found in the kidney (Dousa and Barnes, 1977). In several reports, the effects on cGMP of PTH and other agents influencing renal tubular phosphate handling, such as acetylcholine (Schneider *et al.*, 1973), have been described (Biddulph and Wrean, 1977; Dousa *et al.*, 1977a; Rosenberg and Fogel, 1977; Schneider *et al.*, 1973). It is very difficult to integrate these isolated findings with the concept of cAMP-mediated phosphate regulation. It should be noted that mutual interrelationships between cAMP and cGMP levels are numerous. cAMP was shown to stimulate guanylate cyclase in some systems (Earp *et al.*, 1977) and to stimulate cAMP phosphodiesterase (Chasin and Harris, 1976; Hui *et al.*, 1978) or inhibit it, depending on the type of cAMP phosphodiesterase examined (Chasin and Harris, 1976). Therefore, it is possible that changes in cGMP levels which have been described in response to agents acting on phosphate transport may be secondary to changes in cAMP. Another feature of the cGMP system is its outstanding dependence on calcium (Goldberg and Haddox, 1977). Since PTH, calcitonin, and other agents such as acetylcholine are known to influence calcium transmembrane movement, it is also possible that cGMP changes are basically due to changes in redistribution of calcium elicited by the hormones. These considerations do not exclude the possibility that cGMP may play adirect role in regulation of phosphate transport. However, positive evidence to suggest this is not yet available.

With respect to phosphate transport, the role of calcium as an intracellular mediator is not quite clear. PTH increased intracytoplasmic calcium (Rasmussen, 1972), but an ionophore, which supposedly increased calcium influx, actually decreased phosphaturia (Popovtzer *et al.*, 1977a). Calcium unquestionably serves as a cofactor modulating the biochemical steps involved in regulation of phosphate transport, but it is difficult to make a case for its role as a primary or specific signal.

While a mechanism involving increased cAMP levels and cAMP-dependent phosphorylations applies primarily to phosphaturic agents, another polypeptide, insulin, is antiphosphaturic (DeFronzo *et al.*, 1975, 1976; Nizet, 1976). As in other hormonal systems—basically, those involving intermediate metabolism (Soderling and Park, 1974; Steinberg *et al.*, 1975)—the question arises whether insulin acts through mediation of cyclic nucleotides and phosphorylations in a direction opposite to that of phosphaturic agents. At the present time, there is very little evidence for the involvement of cyclic nucleotides and protein phosphorylation in the antiphosphaturic effect of insulin. Nevertheless, several preliminary observations suggest that insulin opposes the effects of phosphaturic hormones. It was reported that insulin decreased the binding of PTH to renal cortical membranes (Sutcliffe *et al.*, 1973; Zull *et al.*, 1977) and also decreased the activation of adenylate cyclase by PTH (Sutcliffe *et al.*, 1973). Addition of insulin alone to incubated renal cortical slices did not change the concentration of cAMP or cGMP. On the other hand, the effect of PTH of increasing cAMP levels and activating protein kinase, as well as the effect of glucagon of activating a protein kinase, were significantly reduced (Northrup *et al.*, 1979). These observations have been made under very limited experimental conditions but suggest that insulin may act on kidney cortex either through diminishing cAMP accumulation or through other mechanisms antagonizing cellular effects of phosphaturic hormones.

5.2. Other Cellular Mechanisms in Regulation of Phosphate Transport

Besides the phosphaturic and antiphosphaturic agents mentioned above, some other hormones have been shown to influence the renal handling of phosphate, and these cases, cAMP and cAMP-dependent phosphorylation do not seem to be *directly* implicated.

Vitamin D influences the renal handling of phosphate, but the direction of these changes is not clearly established. In some studies, infusion of vitamin D was antiphosphaturic (Popovtzer *et al.*, 1974, 1977b; Puschett *et al.*, 1972a), while in some recent experiments, low doses of vitamin D were phosphaturic in the rat (Bonjour *et al.*, 1977). The mechanism of the direct effect of vitamin D on renal phosphate transport is a matter of speculation at the present time. Since vitamin D is a steroid hormone, it may act directly on the renal tubules as do other steroid hormones, via *de novo* synthesis of a specific protein(s) involved in phosphate transport or its regulation (DeLuca, 1977). Besides such direct action, vitamin D appears to modulate the response of other hormones which act primarily via cAMP and protein phosphorylations. In vitamin-D-deficient animals, adenylate cyclase from renal cortex was less stimulated by PTH *in vitro*, and the renal response to PTH both in terms of increase in urinary cAMP and increase in phosphate excretion was diminished (Forte *et al.*, 1976). The effect of vitamin D and its metabolites on the renal handling of phosphate is discussed in Chapter 7.

A similar modulatory effect on phosphaturic hormone action seems to be exerted by thyroid hormones. In hypothyroid animals, renal cortical adenylate cyclase stimulation by PTH was significantly reduced (Harkcom *et al.*, 1978). Administration of thyroxine caused an increase in the rate of phosphate excretion (Harkcom *et al.*, 1976). However, all of these observations remain to be systematically investigated in depth. The same applies to possible effects of other known hormonal agents on renal phosphate transport, such as steroid sex hormones and glucocorticoids.

Remarkable changes in the rate of renal phosphate transport can occur under circumstances when none of the known hormonal agents is likely to be responsible for such adaptation. The most striking example is the marked increase in renal tubular phosphate reabsorption in response to decreased dietary phosphorus intake (Bonjour *et al.*, 1976; Trohler *et al.*, 1976). While the stimulus for such change is unknown, some observations suggest that the adaptation occurs within the brush border (Murer *et al.*, 1978) and that *de novo* protein synthesis may be involved. It has been shown that brush borders isolated from animals on a low-phosphate diet have a higher capacity for phosphate transport than those from animals with normal phosphate intake (Murer *et al.*, 1979). In recent experiments, we found that inhibitors of protein synthesis prevent the increase in the renal phosphate reabsorption elicited by low-phosphorus diet (Shah *et al.*, 1978a,b). This observation suggests that increased phosphorus transport may be dependent on synthesis of a specific protein which is induced in the course of adaptation to the low phosphorus intake. The effects of dietary phosphate on renal handling of phosphate are discussed in Chapter 9.

6. REFERENCES

Abou-Issa, H., Kratowich, N., and Mendicino, J., 1974, Properties of soluble and bound protein kinase isolated from swine kidney, *Eur. J. Biochem.* **42**:464.

Abou-Issa, H., Mendicino, J., Leibach, F., and Pillion, D., 1975, Phosphorylation and dephosphorylation of renal brush border membranes by protein kinase and phosphoprotein phosphatase, *FEBS Lett.* **50**:121.

Adler, S., Roy, A., and Relman, A. S., 1965, Intracellular acid–base regulation. I. The response of muscle cells to changes in CO_2 tension or extracellular bicarbonate concentration, *J. Clin. Invest.* **44**:8.

Adler, S., Anderson, B., and Zett, B., 1972a, The role of bicarbonate in determining pH heterogeneity in rat diaphragm, *J. Lab. Clin. Med.* **80**:679.

Adler, S., Zett, B., and Anderson, B., 1972b, The effect of acute potassium depletion on muscle cell pH *in vitro, Kidney Int.* **2**:159.

Adler, S., Zett, B., and Anderson, B., 1974, Renal citrate in the potassium deficient rat: Role of potassium and chloride ions, *J. Lab. Clin. Med.* **84**:307.

Agus, Z. S., Puschett, B. J., Senesky, D., and Goldberg, M., 1971, Mode of action of parathyroid hormone and cyclic adenosine 3′,5′-monophosphate on renal tubular phosphate reabsorption in the dog, *J. Clin. Invest.* **50**:617.

Angielski, S., and Szczepanska-Konkel, M., 1977, Restoration of PTH dependent phosphaturia by metabolic (MA), respiratory acidosis (RA) and Diamox (D) in acutely parathyroidectomized (PTX), lithium treated rats, in: *Proceedings of 3rd International Workshop on Phosphate and Other Minerals,* Madrid, Spain.

Angielski, S., Pempkowiak, L., Gmaj, P., Hoppe, A., and Nowicka, C., 1976, The effect of maleate and lithium on renal fuction and metabolism, *in: Renal Metabolism in Relation to Renal Function* (U. Schmidt and U. C. Dubach, eds.), pp. 142–152, Hans Huber, Bern.

Anner, B., Ferrero, J., Jirounek, P., and Straub, R. W., 1973, Na-dependent phosphate-influx into mammalian nerve fibers, *Experientia* **29**:74.

Arruda, J., Richardson, A. L., Wolfson, J. A., Nascimento, L., Rademacher, D. R., and Kurtzman, N. A., 1976, Lithium administration and phosphate excretion, *Am. J. Physiol.* **231**:1140.

Aurbach, G. D., and Heath, D. A., 1974, Parathyroid hormone and calcitonin regulation of renal function, *Kidney Int.* **6**:331.

Aurbach, G. D., Keutmann, H. T., Niall, H. D., Tregear, G. W., O'Riordan, J., Marcus, R., Marx, S. J., and Potts, J. T., Jr., 1972, Structure, synthesis, and mechanism of action of parathyroid hormone, *Recent Prog. Horm. Res.* **28**:353.

Ausiello, D., Handler, J., and Orloff, J., 1976, Effect of parathyroid hormone and cyclic AMP on protein phosphorylation in rabbit kidney cortex, *Biochim. Biophys. Acta* **451**:372.

Banerjee, R. K., Shertzer, H. G., Kanner, B. I., and Racker, E., 1977, Purification and reconstitution of the phosphate transporter from bovine heart mitochondria, *Biochem. Biophys. Res. Commun.* **75**:772.

Bank, N., Aynedjian, H. S., and Weinstein, S. W., 1974, A microperfusion study of phosphate reabsorption by the rat proximal tubule, *J. Clin. Invest.* **54**:1040.

Barker, E. S., Singer, R. B., Elkinton, J. R., and Clark, K. J., 1957, The renal response in man to acute experimental respiratory alkalosis and acidosis, *J. Clin. Invest.* **36**:515.

Baumann, K., de Rouffignac, C., Roinel, N., Rumrich, G., and Ullrich, K. J., 1975a, Renal phosphate transport: Inhomogeneity of local-proximal transport rates and sodium dependence, *Pflügers Arch.* **356**:287.

Baumann, K., Rumrich, G., Papavassiliou, F., and Klöss, S., 1975b, pH dependence of phosphate reabsorption in the proximal tubule of rat kidney, *Pflügers Arch.* **360**:183.

Baumann, K., Chan, Y.-L., Bode, F., and Papavassiliou, F., 1977, Effect of parathyroid hormone and cyclic adenosine 3′,5′-monophosphate on isotonic fluid reabsorption: Polarity of proximal tubular cells, *Kidney Int.* **11**:77.

Beck, L. H., and Goldberg, M., 1974, Mechanism of the blunted phosphaturia in saline-loaded thyroparathyroidectomized dogs, *Kidney Int.* **6:**18, 1974.

Beck, N. P., DeRubertis, F. R., Michelis, M. F., Fusco, R. D., Field, J. B., and Davis, B. B., 1972, Effect of prostaglandin E_1 on certain renal actions of parathyroid hormone, *J. Clin. Invest.* **51:**2352.

Beck, W., and Davis, B. B., 1975, Impaired renal response to parathyroid hormone in potassium depletion, *Am. J. Physiol.* **228:**179.

Bell, N. H., Avery, S., Sinha, T., Clark, C. M., Jr., Allen, D. O., and Johnston, C., Jr., 1972, Effects of dibutyryl cyclic adenosine $3',5'$-monophosphate and parathyroid extract on calcium and phosphorus metabolism in hypoparathyroidism and pseudohypoparathyroidism, *J. Clin. Invest.* **61:**816.

Berlin, R. D., Oliver, J. M., Ukena, T. E., and Yin, H. H., 1974, Control of cell surface topography, *Nature* **247:**45.

Biddulph, D. M., and Wrean, R. W., 1977, Effects of parathyroid hormone on cyclic AMP, cyclic GMP, and efflux of calcium in isolated renal tubules, *J. Cyclic Nucleotide Res.* **3:**129.

Bloch, R., 1974, Human erythrocyte sugar transport. Identification of the essential residues of the sugar carrier by specific modification, *J. Biol. Chem.* **249:**1814.

Bonjour, J.-P., Trohler, U., Mühlbauer, R., and Fleisch, H., 1976, Tubular adaptation of inorganic phosphate (Pi) transport in response to variations in dietary Pi in rats, in: *Renal Metabolism in Relation to Renal Function* (U. Schmidt and U. C. Dubach, eds.), pp. 272–280, Hans Huber. Bern.

Bonjour, J.-P., Preston, C., and Fleisch, H., 1977, Effect of 1,25-dihydroxyvitamin D_3 on the renal handling of Pi in thyroparathyroidectomized rats, *J. Clin. Invest.* **60:**1419.

Booth, A. G., and Kenny, A. J., 1976, A morphometric and biochemical investigation of the vesiculation of kidney microvilli, *J. Cell Sci.* **21:**449.

Brassfield, C. R., and Behrman, V. G., 1941, A correlation of the pH of arterial blood and urine as affected by changes in pulmonary ventilation, *Am. J. Physiol.* **132:**272.

Bretscher, M. S., and Raff, M. C., 1975, Mammalian plasma membranes, *Nature* **258:**43.

Brown, K. D., and Lamb, J. F., 1975, Na-dependent phosphate transport in cultured cells, *J. Physiol.* **251:**58P.

Butlen, D., and Jard, S., 1972, Renal handling of $3',5'$-cyclic AMP in the rat, *Pflügers Arch.* **331:**172.

Caldwell, P. C., and Lowe, A. G., 1970, The influx of phosphate into squid giant axons, *J. Physiol.* **207:**271.

Cassola, A. C., and Malnic, G., 1977, Phosphate transfer and tubular pH during renal stopped flow microperfusion experiments in the rat, *Pflügers Arch.* **367:**249.

Chambers, E. L., 1963, Role of cations in phosphate transport by fertilized sea urchin eggs, *Fed. Proc. Fed. Am. Soc. Exp. Biol.* **22:**331.

Chasin, M., and Harris, D. N., 1976, Inhibitors and activators of cyclic nucleotide phosphodiesterase, *Adv. Cyclic Nucleotide Res.* **7:**225.

Chen, S. T., 1976, Alkaline phosphatase, *Front. Gastrointest. Res.* **2:**109.

Cohen, J. J., Berglund, E., and Lotspeich, W. D., 1956, Renal tubular reabsorption of acetoacetate, inorganic sulfate and inorganic phosphate in the dog as affected by glucose and phlorizin, *Am. J. Physiol.* **184:**91.

Cohen, J. J., Berglund, E., and Lotspeich, W. D., 1957, Interrelations during renal tubular reabsorption in the dog among several anions showing a sensitivity to glucose and phlorizin, *Am. J. Physiol.* **189:**331.

Cook, G. M. W., and Stoddart, R. W., 1973, *Surface Carbohydrates of the Eukaryotic Cell,* Academic Press, New York.

Coty, W. A., and Pederson, P. L., 1975, Phosphate transport in rat liver mitochondria. Membrane components labeled by N-ethylmaleimide during inhibition of transport, *J. Biol. Chem.* **250**:3515.

Crawford, M. A., 1963, The effects of fluoroacetate, malonate and acid–base balance on renal disposal of citrate, *Biochem. J.* **88**:115.

Cuche, J.-L., Marchand, G. R., Greger, R. F., Lang, F. C., and Knox, F. G., 1976, Phosphaturic effect of dopamine in dogs. Possible role of intrarenally produced dopamine in phosphate regulation, *J. Clin. Invest.* **58**:71.

Cunningham, E. B., 1968, The enhancement of phosphoryl transfer by adenosine 3',5'-monophosphate in the presence of a membranous fraction from canine kidney, *Biochim. Biophys. Acta* **165**:574.

Czaky, T. Z., Prachnamboli, K., Eiseman, B., and Ho, P. M., 1964, The effect of digitalis on the renal tubular transport of glucose in normal and heartless dogs, *J. Pharmacol. Exp. Ther.* **150**:275.

DeFronzo, R. A., Cooke, C. R., Anders, R., Fallona, G. R., and Davis, P. J., 1975, The effect of insulin on renal handling of sodium, potassium, calcium, and phosphate in man, *J. Clin. Invest.* **55**:845.

DeFronzo, R. A., Goldberg, N., and Agus, Z. S., 1976, The effects of glucose and insulin on renal electrolyte transport, *J. Clin. Invest.* **58**:83.

DeLuca, H. F., 1977, Vitamin D endocrine system, *Adv. Clin. Chem.* **19**:125.

Dennis, V. W., Woodhall, P. B., and Robinson, R. R., 1976, Characteristics of phosphate transport in isolated proximal tubule, *Am. J. Physiol.* **231**:979.

Denton, D. A., Maxwell, M., McDonald, I. R., Munro, J., and Williams, W., 1952, Renal regulation of the extracellular fluid in acute respiratory acidemia, *Aust. J. Exp. Biol. Med. Sci.* **80**:489.

DeRubertis, F. R., and Craven, P. A., 1976, Hormonal modulation of cyclic adenosine 3',5'-monophosphate-dependent protein kinase activity in rat renal cortex, *J. Clin. Invest.* **57**:1442.

DiBella, F. P., Dousa, T. P., Miller, S. S., and Arnaud, C. D., 1974, Parathyroid hormone receptors of renal cortex: Specific binding of biologically active, ^{125}I-labeled hormone and relationship to adenylate cyclase activation, *Proc. Natl. Acad. Sci. U.S.A.* **71**:723.

Dousa, T. P., 1976, Drugs and other agents affecting the renal adenylate cyclase system, in: *Methods in Pharmacology*, Vol. 4A (M. Martinez-Maldonado, ed.), pp. 293–331, Plenum Press, New York.

Dousa, T. P., and Barnes, L. D., 1977, Cyclic nucleotides in regulation of renal function, in: *Cyclic 3',5'-nucleotides: Mechanism of Action* (H. Cramer and J. Schultz, eds.), pp. 251–262, John Wiley and Sons, London.

Dousa, T. P., Duarte, C. G., and Knox, F. G., 1976, Effect of colchicine on urinary phosphate and regulation by parathyroid hormone, *Am. J. Physiol.* **231**:61.

Dousa, T. P., Barnes, L. D., Ong, S.-H., and Steiner, A. L., 1977a, Immunohistochemical localization of 3',5'-cyclic GMP in rat renal cortex: Effect of parathyroid hormone, *Proc. Natl. Acad. Sci. U.S.A.* **74**:3569.

Dousa, T. P., Barnes, L. D., and Kim, J. K., 1977b, The role of the cyclic AMP-dependent protein phosphorylations and microtubules in the cellular action of vasopressin in mammalian kidney, in: *Neurohypophysis* (A. Moses and L. Share, eds.), pp. 220–235, Karger, New York.

Earp, H. S., Smith, P., Ong, S.-H., and Steiner, A. L., 1977, Regulation of hepatic nuclear guanylate cyclase, *Proc. Natl. Acad. Sci. U.S.A.* **74**:946.

Eisenberg, E., 1965, Effects of serum calcium level and parathyroid extracts on phosphate and calcium excretion in hypoparathyroid patients, *J. Clin. Invest.* **44**:942.

Eknoyan, G., Suki, W. N., and Martinez-Maldonado, M., 1970, Effect of diuretics on urinary excretion of phosphate, calcium and magnesium in thyroparathyroidectomized dogs, *J. Lab. Clin. Med.* **76**:257.

Fishman, W. H., 1974, Perspectives on alkaline phosphatase isoenzymes, *Am. J. Med.* **56**:617.

Forte, L. R., Chao, W.-T. H., Walkenbach, R. J., and Byington, K. H., 1975, Studies of kidney plasma membrane adenosine 3′,5′-monophosphate-dependent protein kinase, *Biochim. Biophys. Acta* **389**:84.

Forte, L. R., Nickols, G. A., and Anast, C. S., 1976, Renal adenylate cyclase and the interrelationship between parathyroid hormone and vitamin D in the regulation of urinary phosphate and adenosine cyclic 3′,5′-monophosphate excretion, *J. Clin. Invest.* **57**:559.

Fox, M., Thier, S., Rosenberg, L., and Segal, S., 1964, Impaired renal tubular function induced by sugar infusion in man, *J. Clin. Endocrinol. Metab.* **24**:1318.

Freeman, S., Jacobsen, A. B., and Williamson, B. J., 1957, acid–base balance and removal of injected calcium from the circulation, *Am. J. Physiol.* **191**:377.

Frick, A., 1969, Mechanism of inorganic phosphate diuresis secondary to saline infusions in the rat, *Pflügers Arch. Gesamte Physiol. Menschen Tiere* **313**:106.

Frick, A., 1972, Proximal tubule reabsorption of inorganic phosphate during saline infusion in the rat, *Am. J. Physiol.* **223**:1034.

Fulop, M., and Brazeau, P., 1968, The phosphaturic effect of sodium bicarbonate and acetazolamide in dog, *J. Clin. Invest.* **47**:988.

Gammeltoft, A., and Kjerulf-Jensen, K., 1943, The mechanism of renal excretion of fructose and galactose in the rabbit, cat, dog and man (with special reference to the phosphorylation theory), *Acta Physiol. Scand.* **6**:368.

George, E. R., Balakir, R. A., Filburn, C. R., and Sacktor, B., 1977, Cyclic adenosine monophosphate-dependent and -independent protein kinase activity of renal brush border membranes, *Arch. Biochem. Biophys.* **180**:429.

George, S. G., and Kenny, A. J., 1973, Studies on the enzymology of purified preparations of brush border from rabbit kidney, *Biochem. J.* **134**:43.

Ginsburg, J. N., 1972, Effect of glucose and free fatty acid on phosphate transport in dog kidney, *Am. J. Physiol.* **222**:1153.

Ginsburg, J. N., and Lotspeich, N. D., 1963, Interrelations of arsenate and phosphate transport in the dog kidney, *Am. J. Physiol.* **205**:707.

Glossmann, H., and Neville, D. M., 1971, Glycoproteins of cell surfaces. A comparative study of three different cell surfaces of the rat, *J. Biol. Chem.* **246**:6339.

Gmaj. P., Hoppe, A., Angielski, S., and Rogulski, J., 1973, Effects of maleate and arsenite on renal reabsorption of sodium and bicarbonate, *Am. J. Physiol.* **225**:90.

Gold, L. W., Massry, S. G., and Friedler, R. M., 1977, Effect of phosphate depletion on renal tubular reabsorption of glucose, *J. Lab. Clin. Med.* **83**:554.

Goldberg, N. D., and Haddox, M. K., 1977, Cyclic GMP metabolism and involvement in biological regulation, *Annu. Rev. Biochem.* **46**:823.

Gray, S. P., Morris, J. E. W., and Brooks, I., 1973, Renal handling of calcium, magnesium, inorganic phosphate and hydrogen ions during prolonged exposure to elevated carbon dioxide concentrations, *Clin. Sci. Mol. Med.* **45**:751.

Greger, R. F., Lang, F. C., Knox, F. G., and Lechêne, C. P., 1977, Absence of significant secretory flux of phosphate in the proximal convoluted tubule, *Am. J. Physiol.* **232**:F235.

Grollman, A. P., Harrison, H. C., and Harrison, H. E., 1961, The renal excretion of citrate, *J. Clin. Invest.* **40**:1290.

Gruber, W., and Deuticke, B., 1973, Comparative aspects of phosphate transfer across mammalian erythrocyte membranes, *J. Membr. Biol.* **13**:19.

Guest, G. M., 1942, Organic phosphates of the blood and mineral metabolism in diabetic acidosis, *Am. J. Dis. Child.* **64**:401.

Hadvarg, P., and Kadenbach, B., 1976, Identification of a membrane protein involved in mitochondrial phosphate transport, *Eur. J. Biochem.* **67**:573.

Haldane, J. B. S., Hill, R., and Luck, J. M., 1923, Calcium chloride acidosis, *J. Physiol. (London)* **57**:301.

Haldane, J. B. S., Wigglesworth, V. B., and Woochon, C. E., 1924, The effect of reaction changes on human inorganic metabolism, *Proc. R. Soc. Med.* **96**:1.

Hamburger, R. J., Lawson, N. L., and Dennis, V. W., 1974, Effect of cyclic adenosine nucleotides on fluid absorption by different segments of proximal tubule, *Am. J. Physiol.* **227**:396.

Handler, J. S., and Orloff, J., 1963, Activation of phosphorylase in toad bladder and mammalian kidney by antidiuretic hormone, *Am. J. Physiol.* **205**:298.

Harkcom, T. M., Hui, Y. S. F., Palumbo, P. J., and Dousa, T. P., 1976, Phosphaturic effect of L-thyroxine (T₄) in hypothyroid rats, *Clin. Res.* **24**:272A.

Harkcom, T. M., Kim, J. K., Palumbo. P. J., Hui, Y. S. F., and Dousa. T. P., 1978, Modulatory effect of thyroid fuction on enzymes of vasopressin-sensitive cyclic AMP system in renal medulla, *Endocrinology* **102**:1475.

Harrison, H. E., and Harrison, H. C., 1954, Experimental production of renal glycosuria, phosphaturia and aminoaciduria by injection of maleic acid, *Science* **120**:606.

Harrison, H. E., and Harrison, H. C., 1963, Sodium, potassium, and interstitial transport of glucose, L-tyrosine, phosphate, calcium, *Am. J. Physiol.* **205**:107.

Ho, M. K., and Guidotti, G., 1975, A membrane protein from human erythrocytes involved in anion exchange, *J. Biol. Chem.* **250**:675.

Hoffman, N., Thees, M., and Kinne, R., 1976, Phosphate transport by isolated renal brush border vesicles, *Pflügers Arch.* **362**:147.

Hoppe, A., and Knox, F. G., 1978, Effect of acute acid–base changes on fractional excretion in TPTX hamsters, *Clin. Res.* **26**:542.

Hosey, M. M., and Tao, M., 1977, Protein kinases and membrane phosphorylation, in: *Current Topics in Membranes and Transport*, Vol. 9 (F. Bronner and A. Kleinzeller, eds.), pp. 233–320, Academic Press, New York.

Hui, Y. S. F., Torres, V. E., Northrup, T. E., and Dousa, T. P., 1978, Differential properties of cyclic nucleotide phosphodiesterases in glomeruli (GL) and tubuli (TB) of rat renal cortex, *Clin. Res.* **26**:41A.

Insel, P., Balakir, R., and Sacktor, B., 1975, The binding of cyclic AMP to renal brush border membranes, *J. Cyclic Nucleotide Res.* **1**:107.

Israelachvili, J. N., 1977, Refinement of the fluid-mosaic model of membrane structure, *Biochim. Biophys. Acta* **469**:221.

Kasahara, M., and Hinkle, P. C., 1976, Reconstitution of D-glucose transport catalysed by a protein fraction from human erythrocytes in sonicated liposomes, *Proc. Natl. Acad. Sci. U.S.A.* **73**:396.

Kempson, S. A., Hui, Y. S. F., Kim, J. K., Knox, F. G., and Dousa, T. P., 1977, Cellular mechanism of renal phosphate handling in rats fed on low phosphate diet, *Clin. Res.* **25**:595A.

Kenny, A. J., and Booth, A. G., 1976, Organization of the kidney proximal-tubule plasma membrane, *Biochem. Soc. Trans.* **4**:1011.

Kim, J. K., Frohnert, P. P., Hui, Y. S. F., Barnes, L. D., Farrow, G. M., and Dousa, T.

P., 1977, Enzymes of cyclic 3',5'-nucleotide metabolism in human renal cortex and renal adenocarcinoma, *Kidney Int.* **12**:172.

Kinne, R., 1975, Polarity of the renal proximal tubular cell, *Med. Clin. North Am.* **59**:615.

Kinne, R., 1976, Properties of the glucose transport system in the renal brush border membrane, *Curr. Top. Membr. Transp.* **8**:209.

Kinne, R., and Schwartz, I. L., 1976, Resolution of the epithelial cell envelope into luminal and contraluminal plasma membranes as a tool for the analysis of transport processes and hormone action, in: *Membranes and Diseases* (L. Bolis, J. F. Hoffman, and A. Leaf, eds.), pp. 331–343, Raven Press, New York.

Kinne, R., and Schwartz, I. L., 1977, Asymmetric distribution of renal epithelial cell membrane function in the action of antidiuretic hormone and parathyroid hormone, in: *Disturbances in Body Fluid Osmolality* (T. E. Andreoli, J. J. Grantham, and F. C. Rector, eds.), pp. 37–55, American Physiological Society, Bethesda.

Kinne, R., Shlatz, L. J., Kinne-Saffran, E., and Schwartz, I. L., 1975, Distribution of membrane-bound cyclic AMP dependent protein kinase in plasma membranes of cells of the kidney cortex, *J. Membr. Biol.* **24**:145.

Kinne, R., Berner, W., Hoffman, N., and Murer, H., 1977, Phosphate transport by isolated renal and intestinal plasma membranes, in: *Phosphate Metabolism* (S. G. Massry and E. Ritz, eds.), pp. 265–277, Plenum Press, New York.

Knox, F. G., 1977, The intrarenal metabolism of phosphate, *Physiologist* **20**:25.

Knox, F. G., Schneider, E. G., Willis, L. R., Strandhoy, J. W., and Ott, C. E., 1973, Site and control of phosphate reabsorption by the kidney, *Kidney Int.* **3**:347.

Knox, F. G., Haas, J. A., and Lechêne, C., 1976, Effect of parathyroid hormone on phosphate reabsorption in the presence of acetazolamide, *Kidney Int.* **10**:216.

Knox, F. G., Preiss, J., Kim, J. K., and Dousa, T. P., 1977, Mechanism of resistance to the phosphaturic effect of the parathyroid hormone in the hamster, *J. Clin. Invest.* **59**:675.

Küntziger, H., Amiel, C., Roinel, N., and Morel, F., 1974, Effects of parathyroidectomy and cyclic AMP on renal transport of phosphate, calcium, and magnesium, *Am. J. Physiol.* **227**:905.

Kupfer, S., and Kosovsky, J. D., 1965, Effect of cardiac glycosides on renal tubular transport of calcium, magnesium, inorganic phosphate and glucose in the dog, *J. Clin. Invest.* **44**:1132.

Kupfer, S., and Kosovsky, J. D., 1970, Renal intracellular phosphate and phosphate excretion: The effect of digoxin and parathyroid hormone, *Mt. Sinai J. Med. N. Y.* **4**:359.

Kurokawa, K., Nagata, N., Sasaki, M., and Nakane, K., 1974, Effects of calcitonin on the concentration of cyclic adenosine 3',5'-monophosphate in rat kidney *in vivo* and *in vitro*, *Endocrinology* **94**:1514.

Lang, F., Greger, R. F., Marchand, G. R., and Knox, F. G., 1977a, Saturation kinetics of phosphate reabsorption in rats, in: *Phosphate Metabolism* (S. G. Massry and E. Ritz, eds.), pp. 153–155, Plenum Press, New York.

Lang, F., Quehenberger, P., Greger, R., Oberleithner, H., and Deetjen, P., 1977b, Effect of luminal pH on renal phosphate reabsorption in intact and thyroparathyroidectomized rats, *Proc. Int. Union Physiol. Sci.* **13**:427.

Levitan, B. A., 1951, Effect in normal man of hyperglycemia and glycosuria on excretion and reabsorption of phosphate, *J. Appl. Physiol.* **4**:225.

Levitin, H., Branscome, W., and Epstein, F. H., 1958, The pathogenesis of hyperchloremia in respiratory acidosis, *J. Clin. Invest.* **37**:1667.

Lo, H., Lehotary, D. C., Katz, D., and Levey, G. S., 1976, Parathyroid hormone-mediated incorporation of ^{32}P-orthophosphate into phosphatidic acid and phosphatidylinositol in renal cortical slices, *Endocr. Res. Commun.* **3**:377.

Maesaka, J. K., Levitt, M. F., and Abramson, R. G., 1973, Effect of saline infusion on phosphate transport in intact and thyroparathyroidectomized rats, *Am. J. Physiol.* **225**:1421.

Malvin, R. L., and Lotspeich, W. D., 1956, Relation between tubular transport of inorganic phosphate and bicarbonate in the dog, *Am. J. Physiol.* **187**:51.

Martin, H. E., and Jones, R., 1961, The effect of ammonium chloride and sodium bicarbonate on the urinary excretion of magnesium, calcium, and phosphate, *Am. Heart J.* **62**:206.

Marx, S. J., Fedak, S. A., and Aurbach, G. D., 1972, Preparation and characterization of a hormone-responsive renal plasma membrane fraction, *J. Biol. Chem.* **247**:6913.

Massry, S. G., Coburn, J. W., and Kleeman, C. R., 1969, The influence of extracellular volume expansion on renal phosphate reabsorption in the dog, *J. Clin. Invest.* **48**:1237.

McCuaig, L. W., and Motzok, I., 1972, Regulation of intestinal alkaline phosphatase by dietary phosphate, *Can. J. Physiol. Pharmacol.* **50**:1152.

Meister, A., and Tate, S. S., 1976, Glutathione and related γ-glutamyl compounds: Biosynthesis and utilization, *Annu. Rev. Biochem.* **45**:559.

Melani, F., Ramponi, G., Farnararo, M., Cocucci, E., and Guerritore, A., 1967, Regulation by phosphate of alkaline phosphatase in the rat kidney, *Biochim. Biophys. Acta* **138**:411.

Mercado, A., Slatopolsky, E., and Klahr, S., 1975, On the mechanisms responsible for the phosphaturia of bicarbonate administration, *J. Clin. Invest.* **56**:1386.

Moog, F., and Glazier, H. S., 1972, Phosphate absorption and alkaline phosphatase activity in the small intestine of the adult mouse and of the chick embryo and hatched chick, *Comp. Biochem. Physiol.* **42A**:321.

Mostellar, M. E., and Tuttle, E. P., 1964, Effect of alkalosis on plasma and urinary excretion of inorganic phosphate in man, *J. Clin. Invest.* **43**:138.

Murer, H., Evers, C., Stoll, R., and Kinne, R., 1978, The effect of parathyroid hormone (PTH) and dietary phosphate on the sodium-dependent phosphate transport system located in the rat renal brush border membrane, in: *Biochemical Nephrology* (W. G. Guder and U. Schmidt, eds.), pp. 455–462, Hans Huber, Bern.

Nagata, N., and Rasmussen, H., 1970, Parathyroid hormone, 3',5'-AMP, Ca^{++}, and renal gluconeogenesis, *Proc. Natl. Acad. Sci. U.S.A.* **65**:368.

Neville, D. M., and Glossmann, H., 1971, Plasma membrane protein subunit composition. A comparative study by discontinuous electrophoresis in sodium dodecyl sulfate, *J. Biol. Chem.* **246**:6335.

Nizet, A., Lefebore, P., Luyckx, A., and Crabbe, J., 1976, Hormonal and nonspecific humoral factors in the interference between sodium, glucose, and phosphate, in: *Renal Metabolism in Relation to Renal Function* (U. Schmidt and U. C. Dubach, eds.), pp. 262–280, Hans Huber, Bern.

Northrup, T. E., Krezowski, P. A., Palumbo, P. J., Kim, J. K., Hui, Y., and Dousa, T. P., 1979, Insulin inhibition of hormone-stimulated protein kinase systems of rat adrenal cortex, *Am. J. Physiol.* **236**:E649.

Oliver, J. M., Ukena, T. E., and Berlin, R. D., 1974, Effects of phagocytosis and colchicine on the distribution of lectin-binding sites on cell surfaces, *Proc. Natl. Acad. Sci. U.S.A.* **71**:394.

Ostberg, O., 1931, Studien über die Zitronen Säureausscheidung der Menschennieren in normalen und pathologischen Zuständen, *Skand. Arch. Physiol.* **62**:81.

Oxender, D. L., and Quay, S. C., 1976, Isolation and characterization of membrane binding proteins, in: *Methods in Membrane Biology*, Vol. 6 (E. D. Korn, ed.), pp. 183–242, Plenum Press, New York.

Pitts, R. F., 1933, The excretion of urine in the dog, *Am. J. Physiol.* **106**:1.

Pitts, R. F., and Alexander, R. S., 1944, The renal reabsorption mechanism for inorganic phosphate in normal and acidotic dogs, *Am. J. Physiol.* **142**:648.

Plante, G., Lehoux, J., and Petitclerc, C., 1977, Increased phosphaturia following inhibition of renal alkaline phosphatase, *Clin. Res.* **25**:444.

Polak, A., Hayie, G. D., Hays, R. M., and Schwartz, W. B., 1961, Effects of chronic hypercapnia on electrolyte and acid–base equilibration. I. Adaptation, *J. Clin. Invest.* **40**:1223.

Popovtzer, M. M., Robinette, J. B., DeLuca, H. F., and Holick, M. F., 1974, The acute effect of 25-hydroxycholecalciferol on renal handling of phosphorus, *J. Clin. Invest.* **53**:913.

Popovtzer, M. M., Robinette, J. B., McDonald, K. M., and Kuruvila, C. K., 1975, Effect of Ca^{++} on renal handling of $PO_4^=$: Evidence for two reabsorptive mechanisms, *Am. J. Physiol.* **229**:901.

Popovtzer, M. M., Flis, R. S., Mehandru, S. K., and Blum, M., 1977a, Effect of divalent cation ionophore (A23187) on renal handling of phosphorus, *Kidney Int.* **12**:164.

Popovtzer, M. M., Blum, M. S., and Flis, R. S., 1977b, Evidence for interference of 25(OH)vitamin D_3 with phosphaturic action of calcitonin, *Am. J. Physiol.* **232**:E515.

Poujeol, P., Chabardès, D., Roinel, N., and de Rouffignac, C., 1976, Influence of extracellular fluid volume expansion on magnesium, calcium and phosphate handling along the rat nephron, *Pflügers Arch.* **365**:203.

Puschett, J. B., and Goldberg, M., 1969, The relationship between the renal handling of phosphate and bicarbonate in man, *J. Lab. Clin. Med.* **73**:956.

Puschett, J. B., Moranz, J., and Kurnick, W. S., 1972a, Evidence for a direct action of cholecalciferol and 25-hydroxycholecalciferol on the renal transport of phosphate, sodium, and calcium, *J. Clin. Invest.* **51**:373.

Puschett, J. B., Agus, Z. S., Senesky, D., and Goldberg, M., 1972b, Effects of saline loading and aortic obstruction on proximal phosphate transport, *Am. J. Physiol.* **223**:851.

Rasmussen, H., 1972, Ionic and hormonal control of calcium homeostasis, *Am. J. Med.* **50**:567.

Rasmussen, H., and Tenenhouse, A., 1970, Parathyroid hormone and calcitonin, in: *Biochemical Actions of Hormones* (F. Litwack, ed.), pp. 365–413, Academic Press, New York.

Rasmussen, H., Pechet, M., and Fast, D., 1968, Effect of dibutyryl cyclic adenosine 3′,5′-monophosphate, theophylline, and other nucleotides upon calcium and phosphate metabolism, *J. Clin. Invest.* **47**:1843.

Robison, G. A., Butcher, R. W., and Sutherland, E. W., 1971, *Cyclic AMP*, Academic Press, New York.

Rosenberg, E. M., and Fogel, A. J., 1977, Role of cyclic 3′,5′-GMP in modulation of cellular uptake of phosphate, *Am. J. Physiol.* **233**:E203.

Rostgaard, J., and Thuneberg, L., 1972, Electron microscopical observations on the brush border of proximal tubule cells of mammalian kidney, *Z. Zellforsch. Mikrosk. Anat.* **132**:473.

Rostgaard, J., Kristensen, B. I., and Nielsen, L. E., 1972, Electron microscopy of filaments in the basal part of rat kidney tubule cells and their *in situ* interaction with heavy meromyosin, *Z. Zellforsch. Microsk. Anat.* **132**:497.

Sacktor, B., 1968, Trehalase and the transport of glucose in the mammalian kidney and intestine, *Proc. Natl. Acad. Sci. U.S.A.* **60**:1007.

Sakai, M., Matushita, S., Nakano, T., Kimura, N., Araki, N., and Nagata, N., 1976, Effects of parathyroid hormone *in vivo* on the protein kinase activity in rat kidney, *Endocrinology* **98**:1443.

Sanslone, W. R., and Muntwyle, E., 1966, Muscle cell pH in relation to chronicity of potassium depletion, *Proc. Soc. Exp. Biol. Med.* **122**:900.

Schneider, E. G., Strandhoy, J. W., Willis, L. R., and Knox, F. G., 1973, Relationship between proximal sodium reabsorption and excretion of calcium, magnesium and phosphate, *Kidney Int.* **4**:369.

Schneider, E. G., Goldsmith, R. S., Arnaud, C. D., and Knox, F. G., 1975, Role of parathyroid hormone in the phosphaturia of extracellular fluid volume expansion, *Kidney Int.* **7**:317.

Schussler, G. C., Verso, M. A., and Nemoto, T., 1972, Phosphaturia in hypercalcemic breast cancer patients, *J. Clin. Endocrinol. Metab.* **35**:497.

Schwartz, W. B., Brackett, W. C., Jr., and Cohen, J. J., 1965, The response of extracellular hydrogen ion concentration to graded degrees of chronic hypercapnia: The physiologic limits of the defense of pH, *J. Clin. Invest.* **44**:291.

Scott, D., 1972, Excretion of phosphorus and acid in the urine of sheep and calves fed either roughage or concentrate diets, *Q. J. Exp. Physiol. Cogn. Med. Sci.* **57**:379.

Sellers, B. B., Hall, J. J., Both, C. W., and Mendoza, S. A., 1977, Active phosphate transport across the urinary bladder of the toad, *Bufo marinus, J. Membr. Biol.* **32**:291.

Shah, S. V., Kempson, S. A., Northrup, T. E., and Dousa, T. P., 1978a, Renal adaptation to low phosphate (P) diet and its blockade by actinomycin D (Act-D), *Clin. Res.* **26**:42.

Shah, S. V., Kempson, S. A., Northrup, T. E., and Dousa, T. P., 1978b, Renal adaptation of rats to low phosphate diet (LPD): Possible role of protein synthesis, *Clin Res.* **26**:476.

Shlatz, L. J., Schwartz, I. L., Kinne-Saffran, E., and Kinne, R., 1975, Distribution of parathyroid hormone-stimulated adenylate cyclase in plasma membranes of cells of the kidney cortex. *J. Membr. Biol.* **24**:131.

Simoni, R. D., 1972, Macromolecular characterization of bacterial transport systems. in: *Membrane Molecular Biology* (C. F. Fox and A. D. Keith. eds.), pp. 289–322, Sinauer Associates, Inc., Stamford, Connecticut.

Simpson, D. P., 1967, Regulation of renal citrate metabolism by bicarbonate ion and pH: Observations in tissue slices and mitochondria, *J. Clin. Invest.* **46**:225.

Singer, S. J., 1974, The molecular organization of membranes, *Annu. Rev. Biochem.* **43**:805.

Snyder, J. A., and McIntosh, J. R., 1976, Biochemistry and physiology of microtubules, *Annu. Rev. Biochem.* **45**:699.

Soderling, T. R., and Park, C. R., 1974, Recent advances in glycogen metabolism, in: *Advances in Cyclic Nucleotide Research,* Vol. 4 (P. Greengard and G. A. Robison, ed.), pp. 283–333, Raven Press, New York.

Steele, T. H., 1970, Increased urinary phosphate excretion following volume expansion in ' normal man, *Metabolism* **19**:129.

Steinberg, D., Mayer, S. E., Khoo, J. C., Miller, E. A., Miller, R. E., Fredholm, B., and Eichner, R., 1975, Hormone regulation of lipase, phosphorylase, glycogen synthase in adipose tissue, in: *Advances in Cyclic Nucleotide Research,* Vol. 5 (G. I. Drummond, eds.), pp. 549–568, Raven Press, New York.

Straub, R. W., Ferrero, J., Jirounek, P., Jones, G. J., and Salamin, A., 1975, Na-dependent transport of orthophosphate in vertebrate non-myelinated nerves at different pH, in: *Proceedings of 6th International Congress of Pharmacology,* Helsinki, Finland, p. 367 (Abstract).

Straub, R. W., Ferrero, J., Jirounek, P., Rouiller. M., and Salamin, A., 1976, Sodium-dependent transport of orthophosphate in nerve fibres, in: *Phosphate Metabolism* (S. G. Massry and E. Ritz, eds.), pp. 333–344, Plenum Press, New York.

Suki, W. N., Martinez-Maldonado, M., Rouse, D., and Terry, A., 1969, Effect of expansion of extracellular fluid volume on renal phosphate handling, *J. Clin. Invest.* **48**:1888.

Sutcliffe, H. S., Martin, T. J., Eisman, J. A., and Pilczyk, R., 1973, Binding of parathyroid hormone to bovine kidney-cortex plasma membranes, *Biochem. J.* **134**:913.

Taylor, A. N., 1974, *In vitro* phosphate transport in chick ileum: Effect of cholecalciferol. calcium, sodium, and metabolic inhibitors. *J. Nutr.* **104**:489.

Thomas, L., 1973, Isolation of N-ethylmaleimide-labelled phlorizin-sensitive D-glucose binding protein of brush border membrane from rat kidney cortex, *Biochim. Biophys. Acta.* **291**:454.

Thomas, L., and Kinne, R., 1972, Studies on the arrangement of aminopeptidase and alkaline phosphatase in the microvilli of isolated brush border of rat kidney, *Biochim. Biophys. Acta.* **255**:114.

Thuneberg, L., and Rostgaard, J., 1969, Motility of microvilli. A film demonstration, *J. Ultrastruct. Res.* **29**:578.

Trohler, U., Bonjour, J.-P., and Fleisch, H., 1976, Inorganic phosphate homeostasis: Renal adaptation to the dietary intake in intact and thyroparathyroidectomized rats, *J. Clin. Invest.* **57**:264.

Tyson, G. E., and Bulger, R. E., 1973, Effect of vinblastine sulfate on the fine structure of proximal tubule cell of rat kidney, *J. Cell Biol.* **59**:349.

Ueland, P. M., and Doskeland, S. O., 1977, An adenosine 3′,5′-monophosphate-adenosine binding protein from mouse liver, *J. Biol. Chem.* **252**:677.

Ullrich, K. J., 1977, Characterization of calcium, phosphate and *para*-aminohippurate transport in the proximal convolution of the mammalian kidney, *Proc. Int. Union Physiol. Sci.* **12**:224.

Ullrich, K. J., Capasso, G., Rumrich, G., Papavassiliou, F., and Klöss, S., 1977, Coupling between proximal tubular transport processes. Studies with ouabain, SITS and HCO_3^- free solutions, *Pflügers Arch.* **368**:245.

Vogel, B., Lauterbach, F., and Kroger, W., 1965, Die Bedeutung des Natriums für die renaler Transporte von Glucose und Para-aminihippursäure, *Pflügers Arch. Gesamte Physiol. Menschen Tiere* **283**:151.

Webb, R. K., Woodhall, P. B., Tisher, C. C., Glaubiger, G., Neelon, F. A., and Robinson, R. R., 1977, Relationship between phosphaturia and acute hypercapnia in the rat, *J. Clin. Invest.* **60**:829.

Wen, S. F., 1974, Micropuncture studies of phosphate transport in the proximal tubule of the dog, *J. Clin. Invest.* **53**:143.

Wendel, A., Hahn, R., and Guder, W. G., 1976, On the role of γ-glutamyltransferase in renal tubular amino acid reabsorption, in: *Renal Metabolism in Relation to Renal Function* (U. Schmidt and U. C. Dubach, eds.), pp. 426–436, Hans Huber, Bern.

Winzler, R. J., 1970, Carbohydrates in cell surfaces, *Int. Rev. Cytol.* **29**:77.

Wolbach, R. A., 1970, Phlorizin and renal phosphate secretion in the spiny dog fish, *Squalus acanthias, Am. J. Physiol.* **219**:886.

Wolosin, J. M., Ginsburg, H., and Cabantchik, Z. I., 1977, Functional characterization of anion transport system isolated from human erythrocyte membranes, *J. Biol. Chem.* **252**:2419.

Wombacher, H., Reuter-Smerdka, A., and Korber, F., 1973, Cyclic adenosine 3′,5′-monophosphate dependent kinases in rat kidney, *FEBS Lett.* **30**:313.

Zull, J. E., Malbon, C. C., and Chuang, J., 1977, Binding of tritiated bovine parathyroid hormone to plasma membranes from bovine kidney cortex, *J. Biol. Chem.* **252**:1071.

5

The Effects of Parathyroid Hormone on Renal Phosphate Handling

KAI LAU, STANLEY GOLDFARB, and
MARTIN GOLDBERG

1. INTRODUCTION

Parathyroid hormone (PTH) has been known to produce phosphaturia in a variety of species (Agus *et al.*, 1971; Amiel *et al.*, 1970; Bell *et al.*, 1972). This response is most strikingly demonstrated in individuals with primary hyperparathyroidism, in whom excess phosphaturia and hypophosphatemia correlate closely with measured elevations in serum PTH levels (Aurbach and Heath, 1974). On the other hand, the role of PTH in the regulation of phosphate (PO_4) homeostasis in normal subjects has been more difficult to ascertain. For example, studies from several laboratories have revealed that a variety of agents may influence the urinary excretion of PO_4 in the absence of PTH including extracellular fluid volume expansion (Amiel *et al.*, 1970), diuretics (Fulop and Brazeau, 1968), the level of dietary PO_4 intake (Steele, 1976), insulin (DeFronzo *et al.*, 1976), mild hyperglycemia (DeFronzo *et al.*, 1976), phlorizin infusion (Nussbaum *et al.*, 1978), and changes in systemic pH (Fulop and Brazeau, 1968; Puschett and Goldberg, 1969).

These observations suggest that PO_4 transport at either the tubular or whole-kidney level may be affected by a number of agents other than PTH. However, careful analysis of each of these experimental maneuvers reveals that the endogenous level of PTH (or that achieved by exogenous infusions) profoundly influences the magnitude of response to these agents. Thus, changes in plasma PTH levels probably exert the most important influence over day-to-day PO_4 homeostasis. In this chapter, the

115

evidence for this conclusion will be reviewed, as will the data which indicate that PTH has an effect on PO_4 transport in the various segments of the nephron. We shall also discuss the interaction of PTH and various hormonal and nonhormonal phosphaturic agents, as well as the mechanism of action of PTH on the kidney.

2. THE EFFECT OF PTH IN VARIOUS SEGMENTS OF THE NEPHRON

2.1. Proximal Convoluted Tubule

A major focus of the study of the phosphaturic action of PTH has been to investigate the various nephron segments which may be affected by the hormone. Initial studies utilizing the technique of micropuncture (Strickler et al., 1964) suggested that the proximal convoluted tubule was a critical, if not the only, site of action of PTH on the nephron. Since that time, a number of free-flow micropuncture studies (Agus et al., 1971; de Rouffignac et al., 1973; Frick, 1972) in a variety of species have confirmed the clear-cut effect of PTH in reducing proximal tubular PO_4 reabsorption.

This effect of PTH has also been analyzed by ablation of the parathyroid glands (PTX) to acutely or chronically remove the influence of PTH. Under these circumstances, the proximal tubular reabsorption of PO_4 is markedly enhanced, often by 25% of initial levels (Beck and Goldberg, 1973, 1974; Frick, 1972). These studies of PTX animals have also revealed other characteristics of proximal tubular PO_4 transport. Whereas in intact animals, PO_4 transport closely parallels fluid reabsorption—tubular fluid (TF) to ultrafilterable (UF) PO_4 ratio $[(TF/UF)_{PO_4}]$ remains constant at a range between 0.6 and 0.95, indicating proportionate PO_4 and water transport along the nephron—in acute PTX, the ratio falls progressively along the nephron (Fig. 1).

Thus, PTH, even at physiologic, nonstimulated levels, exerts an important influence on proximal tubular PO_4 reabsorption. In its absence, a specific PTH-sensitive component of this PO_4 reabsorptive system is unmasked. While the inhibitory effects of PTH on proximal tubular PO_4 transport have been confirmed in microinjection studies utilizing radioactive tracers (Brunette et al., 1973; Staum et al., 1972) as well as by the techniques of microperfusion and droplet analysis (Ullrich, 1977), it should be noted that recent studies of this phenomenon occurring in the isolated perfused rabbit tubule have revealed conflicting data (Dennis et al., 1976). In the latter experiments, PTH was without effect on net PO_4 efflux from this segment. However, species differences may underly this negative response, since recent data suggest that the rabbit may not re-

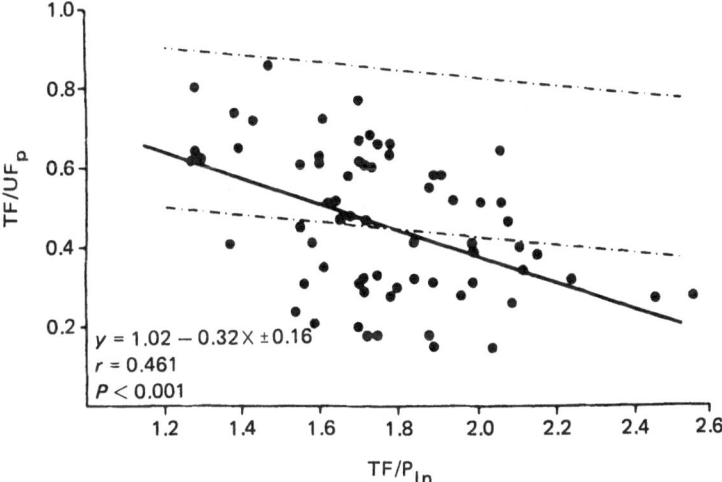

Fig. 1. Correlation of tubular fluid/ultrafiltrate PO_4 ratio [(TF/UF)$_P$] with tubular fluid/ plasma inulin ratio [(TF/P)$_{In}$] in the proximal tubule of acutely thyroparathyroidectomized (TPTX) dogs. The solid line is the calculated regression. The broken lines enclose the 95% confidence band for (TF/UF)$_P$ vs. (TF/P)$_{In}$ in intact dogs. (From Beck and Goldberg, 1974.)

spond to pharmacologic infusions of PTH with a phosphaturia (Berndt *et al.*, 1978).

2.2. Pars Recta—Loop of Henle

Amiel and co-workers (1970) first demonstrated apparent PO_4 transport beyond the late proximal tubule. In acutely PTX rats, while 34% of filtered PO_4 was delivered from the last portions of the accessible surface convolutions of the proximal tubule, only 11% of filtered PO_4 was found at the earliest puncture sites in the superficial distal convoluted tubules. These observations were later confirmed in intact (Knox *et al.*, 1974) and PTX rats (Colindres *et al.*, 1976) as well as in psammomys (de Rouffignac *et al.*, 1973). In addition, a number of studies which examined tubular PO_4 handling in acutely PTX animals found that an increment in delivery of PO_4 out of the proximal tubule produced by extracellular volume expansion (saline) or carbonic anhydrase inhibition (acetazolamide) did not result in a rise in urinary PO_4 excretion (Beck and Goldberg, 1973, 1974; Frick, 1972; Maesaka *et al.*, 1973). These data indirectly suggested that PO_4 was reabsorbed somewhere in the nephron beyond the accessible proximal convoluted tubule. Moreover, since these maneuvers produce a phosphaturia of a similar degree to the increment in the delivered load of PO$_4$ from the proximal tubule in the presence of intact parathyroid glands, it is apparent that these "distal" nephron sites may be responsive to the inhibitory effects of PTH.

A series of recent experiments suggests that the segment of the nephron between the late proximal tubule and early distal tubule which is inaccessible to micropuncture, the pars recta, may be the tubular locus of PO$_4$ reabsorption. First, studies of the isolated perfused rabbit tubule by Dennis *et al.* (1976) have shown that while the pars recta has a fairly low rate of PO$_4$ reabsorption (approximately 30% of that found in the pars convoluta), it is nonetheless a potential site of substantial PO$_4$ reabsorption. Moreover, this segment was responsive to PTH inhibition, as the PO$_4$ efflux rate fell from 2.64 ± 0.41 to 1.91 ± 0.2 pmol/mm/min. While the previously noted caveat against direct extrapolation from data derived from this preparation to whole-kidney characteristics in other species must be invoked, the results do suggest the potential role for this system in PTH-mediated PO$_4$ transport.

Further evidence for pars recta PO$_4$ transport, albeit indirect, derives from two separate experimental studies. First, the stationary microperfusion studies of Lang *et al.* (1977a) show PO$_4$ efflux from perfusate instilled in the pars recta and descending limb of the loop of Henle. Second, data from the isolated perfused rabbit loop of Henle show this nephron segment to be virtually impermeable to PO$_4$ (Rocha *et al.*, 1977), suggesting that the site of PO$_4$ transport in the microperfusion studies was likely to be the pars recta. A synthesis of these data would suggest that the only nephron segment between the late accessible proximal convoluted tubule and the early distal convoluted tubule which is capable of PO$_4$ reabsorption and PTH inhibition is the pars recta. However, it should be emphasized that 25% of the late proximal convoluted tubule and 20% of the early distal convoluted tubule are not accessible to micropuncture and may therefore represent the transport sites for PO$_4$ inferred from the free-flow micropuncture studies described above.

Thus, it would appear that a component of PTH action is due to inhibition of PO$_4$ transport in the nephron segments between the late proximal tubule and early distal convoluted tubule. This site is likely to be, at least in part, the pars recta of the proximal tubule, but these conclusions are tentative and await a great deal of confirmatory experimental data.

2.3. Distal Convoluted Tubule and Terminal Nephron

Several studies have recently documented an important role of the distal convoluted tubule as well as the terminal nephron (cortical collecting tubule and medullary collecting duct) in tubular PO$_4$ reabsorption and the phosphaturic effects of PTH. Recent micropuncture studies reported in preliminary form by Chiu *et al.* (1974), Colindres *et al.* (1976), Lau *et al.* (1977), and Lechêne *et al.* (1978) have shown that between 5 and 15% of the filtered load of PO_4 can be reabsorbed along the superficial distal convoluted tubule, and this transport system may be inhibited by PTH (Colindres *et al.*, 1976). While these data are in apparent conflict with earlier microinjection studies which were unable to show any PO_4 transport or PTH effect in the distal portions of the nephron (Brunette *et al.*, 1973; Staum *et al.*, 1972), the microinjection technique has recently been refined utilizing extremely slow injection rates to more closely approximate *in vivo* conditions, and PO_4 transport along the distal nephron has been demonstrated (Poujeol *et al.*, 1977).

While distal convoluted tubular transport of PO_4 may represent an important component of renal PO_4 handling, the regulation of final urinary PO_4 excretion apparently resides in the terminal nephron. This conclusion derives from the number of studies which show a large difference between the amount of PO_4 delivered from the late distal convoluted tubule and that which appears in the final urine (Amiel *et al.*, 1970; Carone, 1964; Chiu *et al.*, 1974). This difference is magnified in PTX animals, implying a PTH-inhibitable system.

It should be pointed out that some controversy surrounds the conclusion that the terminal nephron regulates final urinary PO_4 excretion. Since the entire population of renal tubules contributes to the final urine while only a very small number of surface tubules are sampled in micropuncture experiments, it has been postulated that heterogeneity between nephrons could be a factor in apparent terminal nephron reabsorption. This controversy has been the subject of a recent extensive review (Knox *et al.*, 1977b). The data forwarded by Knox *et al.* (1977a) for PO_4-loaded animals, in which more PO_4 was found in the hairpin turn of the loop of Henle of juxtamedullary nephrons than in superficial distal convoluted tubules, lend support to the concept of nephron heterogeneity for PO_4 transport. Juxtamedullary nephrons might reabsorb more or less PO_4 than superficial nephrons and contribute a component of tubular fluid to the medullary collecting duct that is different in PO_4 content from that of superficial tubules. Thus, a difference between urinary and distal tubular fluid PO_4 could represent medullary collecting duct and cortical collecting tubule reabsorption or merely the mixing of the deep-nephron tubular fluid with that of the superficial nephrons.

This issue remains unresolved, since it has not been possible to quantify the total amount of urinary PO_4 derived from the filtrate of these two nephron populations. However, recent preliminary data by Bengele *et al.* (1978) using the technique of microcatheterization of the medullary collecting duct have shown that in PTX animals, PO_4 content falls with distance along this nephron structure. Intact animals show no such effect, again suggesting the importance of PTH action in modulating terminal-nephron PO_4 reabsorption.

In summary, PTH leads to phosphaturia through inhibition of PO_4 transport at all nephron sites shown to be capable of PO_4 reabsorption. While the precise locus of PO_4 transport beyond the sites accessible to micropuncture study remain controversial, it is likely that PTH acts to reduce PO_4 transport in the collecting duct system.

3. MODE OF ACTION OF PTH

In the evaluation of the phosphaturic action of PTH, a distinction must be made between the effects of the withdrawal of PTH by PTX and the response to the exogenous administration of PTH, since both of these techniques have been utilized in the study of PTH action. In the PTX preparation, the acute removal of PTH stimulates PO_4 reabsorption along the entire nephron and lowers urinary PO_4 excretion to extremely low levels. Thus, removal of PTH unmasks a continually suppressed PO_4 reabsorptive system. Moreover, at least in nephron segments beyond the proximal convoluted tubule, this increased capacity for PO_4 reabsorption may prevent any alteration in proximal tubular PO_4 transport from being manifested in the final urine. In contrast, the acute infusion of PTH in supraphysiologic or pharmacologic amounts produces direct inhibition of PO_4 reabsorption in all nephron segments which are capable of PO_4 transport and leads to a marked rise in PO_4 excretion.

The renal response to the withdrawal of PTH through changes in renal tubular PO_4 handling may be most clearly seen in the blunted phosphaturia of saline loading in PTX animals. Saline expansion in either intact or PTX dogs results in a large increment in the delivered load of PO_4 from the proximal tubule (Fig. 2). Yet, whereas in intact animals virtually all of this incremental load reaches the final urine, in PTX dogs there is a markedly reduced phosphaturia (Beck and Goldberg, 1974). Similar results are seen during acetazolamide infusion (Beck and Goldberg, 1973). Experiments in which PTH levels are maintained constant by exogenous infusion and saline expansion is superimposed demonstrate that the entire saline-produced increment in the delivered load of PO_4 from the proximal tubule appears in the final urine (Goldfarb et al., 1978). These data suggest that even physiologic, nonstimulated levels of PTH exert an important influence over tubular PO_4 handling.

These results suggest the following pattern of renal PO_4 handling. Whole-kidney PO_4 reabsorption may be viewed as the sum of PO_4 reabsorption in the proximal tubule and in nephron segments beyond the proximal tubule. In fact, experiments using PO_4 infusions have shown that the

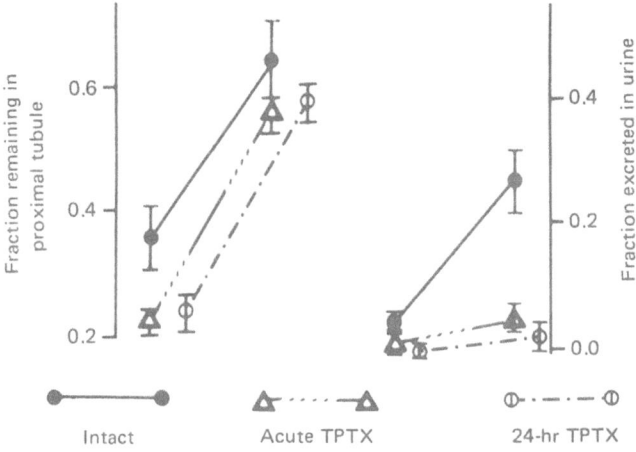

Fig. 2. Effect of saline infusion on the fraction of filtered PO_4 remaining in the late proximal tubule (on the left) and on fractional PO_4 excretion in the urine (on the right) in intact, acutely TPTX, and 24-hr TPTX dogs. Lines connect mean values before and after saline. (From Beck and Goldberg, 1974.)

classical Tm_{PO_4} which exists for the whole kidney is derived from a proximal tubular Tm and a distal-nephron Tm (Goldfarb et al., 1975). The proximal system is sensitive to PTH, its second messenger, cyclic AMP (cAMP) (Goldfarb et al., 1978), and a variety of other agents, including extracellular fluid volume expansion (Colindres et al., 1976; Frick, 1972), carbonic anhydrase inhibition (Beck and Goldberg, 1973; Knox et al., 1976), mild hypercalcemia (Goldfarb et al., 1978), hyperglycemia (De-Fronzo et al., 1976), and metolazone (Fernandez and Puschett, 1973). These agents may act to primarily reduce sodium transport, which is known to be closely linked to proximal tubular PO_4 reabsorption (Agus et al., 1971; Dennis et al., 1976). However, in the nephron segments beyond the proximal tubule, it may be shown that reduction of sodium transport does not influence PO_4 reabsorption (Chiu et al., 1974; Goldfarb et al., 1975). Only PTH (or cAMP) may reduce the large PO_4 reabsorptive capacity of this "distal" nephron system and allow the increment in distal-nephron PO_4 delivery produced by these proximal-tubular-active agents to appear in the final urine. It should be noted that the effect of the withdrawal of PTH may also be demonstrated on the proximal convoluted tubule. There, PTX leads to avid PO_4 reabsorption and a reduction in the delivered load of PO_4 from approximately 50% of filtered PO_4 to 25% of filtered PO_4. This effect occurs without a measurable change in fluid or sodium reabsorption. Thus, studies in the acutely PTX animal demonstrate the effects of PTH in masking a potent PO_4 reabsorptive system which resides both in and beyond the late proximal convoluted tubule.

The direct effects of PTH may be seen when supraphysiologic or pharmacologic levels of the hormone are achieved by exogenous infusion (Agus *et al.*, 1971; Eisenberg, 1965; Goldfarb *et al.*, 1975) or by the production of acute hypocalcemia (Cuche *et al.*, 1976). In this circumstance, PO_4 transport has been reported to be reduced in the proximal tubule (Agus *et al.*, 1971), the pars recta (Dennis *et al.*, 1977), the distal convoluted tubule (Colindres *et al.*, 1976), and the collecting duct (Bengele *et al.*, 1978). The effect in the proximal tubule can be shown to be additive to the inhibition of PO_4 transport produced by extracellular volume expansion (Wen, 1974) or carbonic anhydrase inhibition (Knox *et al.*, 1976). The net effect of these actions is a pronounced rise in urinary PO_4 excretion during the production of acutely elevated levels of PTH.

In summary, the effects of PTH on PO_4 handling may be divided into the response to the withdrawal of PTH, which reduces PO_4 reabsorption at tubular sites within and beyond the late proximal convoluted tubule and allows increments in delivered loads of PO_4 from the proximal tubule to appear in the final urine, and the direct effects of PTH. The latter refers to the acute inhibition of PO_4 reabsorption at all nephron sites of potential PO_4 transport by exogenous or endogenous increments in plasma PTH levels and results in a marked phosphaturia.

4. MECHANISM OF THE PHOSPHATURIC EFFECT OF PTH

PTH may inhibit PO_4 reabsorption by virtue of a number of discrete actions. First, PTH-induced adenyl cyclase stimulation may lead to a change in some aspect of membrane or cellular function which results in a specific reduction in net PO_4 reabsorption. In applying such an hypothesis, Rasmussen and colleagues propose that the rise in cAMP content of cells may act to increase the intracellular concentration of calcium and PO_4 (Rasmussen *et al.*, 1968). If this were to occur, the transmembrane gradient for inorganic PO_4 would rise and could lead to reduced transepithelial PO_4 transport. This hypothesis awaits the development of sensitive techniques for the measurement of intracellular inorganic PO_4.

Second, the effect on PO_4 transport may be produced as a secondary phenomenon. In this formulation, stimulation of cAMP production leads to a reduction in sodium transport, which, in turn, leads to a fall in PO_4 reabsorption (Agus *et al.*, 1971). Lorentz (1974, 1976) has forwarded an interesting hypothesis relating to this formulation, in which the action of PTH, at least in the proximal convoluted tubule, leads to a nonspecific increase in proximal tubular permeability. Thus, effects of PTH (and cAMP) on fluid and PO_4 as well as sodium and calcium transport could be related to increased back diffusion through the lateral intercellular spaces (Lorentz, 1976). This hypothesis needs to be tested in other systems, however, and to be confirmed by other investigators. It apparently does not explain the observation that during marked extracellular volume expansion with saline, PTH has an additive, specific effect of inhibiting PO_4 reabsorption in the dog (Wen, 1974).

Third, a rise in cAMP levels could somehow lead to alkalinization of the proximal tubular fluid, either through an effect on the enzyme carbonic anhydrase or through another system. The change in tubular fluid could markedly alter the ionic form of PO_4 and thereby influence its capacity to penetrate epithelial membranes.

While none of these potential mechanisms is mutually exclusive, the cAMP system appears to be invariably involved in PTH-induced phosphaturia. We will now examine the experimental evidence for and against each of these hypotheses as well as the data which support the central role for cAMP activation.

4.1. Role of Adenyl Cyclase–cAMP System

There is a great deal of evidence indicating that the phosphaturic action of PTH is mediated via the adenyl cyclase–cAMP system. The sequence of biochemical events has been reviewed recently (Aurbach and Heath, 1974): PTH interacts with specific receptors on the contraluminal membrane (Melson et al., 1970), resulting in activation of adenyl cyclase, which, in turn, produces an increase in intracellular concentration of cAMP (Chase and Aurbach, 1967, 1968; Melson et al., 1970; Russell et al., 1968; Streeto, 1969). The cyclic nucleotide stimulates a protein kinase on the luminal membrane (Kinne et al., 1975; Shlatz et al., 1975), leading to phosphorylation of luminal membrane proteins (Kinne et al., 1975; Shlatz et al., 1975). A fraction of the cAMP generated in the cell is added to the tubular fluid and escapes inactivation by phosphodiesterase to 5'-AMP, resulting in a rapid and sustained increase in urinary excretion of cAMP (Buttlen and Jard, 1972; Chase and Aurbach, 1967; Kaminsky et al., 1970).

Evidence supporting the role of cAMP in mediating the effects of PTH is compelling. First, PTH administration selectively stimulates renal cortical adenyl cyclase in the rat (Chase and Aurbach, 1968), hamster (Knox et al., 1977c), and rabbit (Streeto, 1969), leading to an increase in renal tissue cAMP concentration within minutes (Chase and Aurbach, 1967). A rise in urinary cAMP excretion follows PTH administration (Chase and Aurbach, 1967; Chase et al., 1969; Knox et al., 1977c) and precedes the phosphaturic effect of the hormone, whether the hormone is given exogenously (Chase and Aurbach, 1967) or its endogenous secretion is stimulated (Mercado et al., 1975). It can be shown that urinary cAMP is derived almost exclusively from the kidney under the stimulation of PTH, since plasma cAMP minimally rises (Kaminsky et al., 1970). This cAMP-stimulating action of PTH can be further localized in the cortical tubules, unlike an effect of antidiuretic hormone (ADH) on medullary structures (Marx et al., 1972).

Second, PTH-sensitive adenyl cyclase activity has been systemically studied along the entire rabbit nephron. It was found in the pars convoluta and pars recta of the proximal tubule, the cortical portion of the thick ascending limb, and the granular segments of the distal convoluted tubule and cortical collecting tubule (Chabardès et al., 1975) (Fig. 3). In general, PTH has little or no effect on the adenyl cyclase activity within the renal medulla (Streeto, 1969). Except for the loop of Henle, all of these nephron segments correspond to the known sites of action of PTH on PO_4 reabsorption. However, it should be remembered that, while consistent with the concept of cAMP as the cellular mediator of PTH action, the presence of adenyl cyclase should not necessarily be equated specifically with its phosphaturic effect. For example, the enzyme may be involved in known actions of PTH other than phosphaturia, namely, effects on fluid (Agus et al., 1971, 1973; Goldfarb et al., 1978; Hamburger et al., 1976), bicarbonate (Bank and Aynedjian, 1976; Bank et al., 1974; Dennis, 1976; Knox et al., 1976; Rector et al., 1965), and divalent cation transport (Agus et al., 1973; Burnatowska et al., 1977; Sutton et al., 1976).

Third, exogenous cAMP and/or dibutyryl cAMP administration mimics many, if not all, of the physiological actions of PTH, such as inhibition of proximal tubular reabsorption of fluid (Agus et al., 1971; Amiel et al., 1970, 1976; Baumann et al., 1977; Gill et al., 1971; Goldfarb et al., 1975; Hamburger et al., 1974; Küntziger et al., 1974), bicarbonate (Bank and Aynedjian, 1976; Puschett and Zuabach, 1976), and PO_4 (Agus et al., 1973; Arruda et al., 1976; Burnatowska et al., 1977; Dennis et al., 1977; Gill and Casper, 1971; Küntziger et al., 1974). Qualitatively and quantitatively similar effects on "distal" PO_4 reabsorption are also shared by cAMP and dibutyryl cAMP on the one hand and PTH on the other hand (Amiel et al., 1976; Goldfarb et al., 1975; Küntziger et al., 1974). Indeed, enhancement of calcium and magnesium reabsorption by PTH has been shown to be mediated by cAMP in the hamster (Burnatowska et al., 1977).

Fourth, a crucial role for cAMP is evident by the abolition of the phosphaturic effect of PTH if either cAMP generation or its action is inhibited. According to the proposed concept, the phosphaturic action of PTH can be blocked at at least two different steps in the previously outlined sequence. Interference with or inhibition of the activation of adenyl cyclase will prevent generation of cAMP, as seen under a variety of phys-

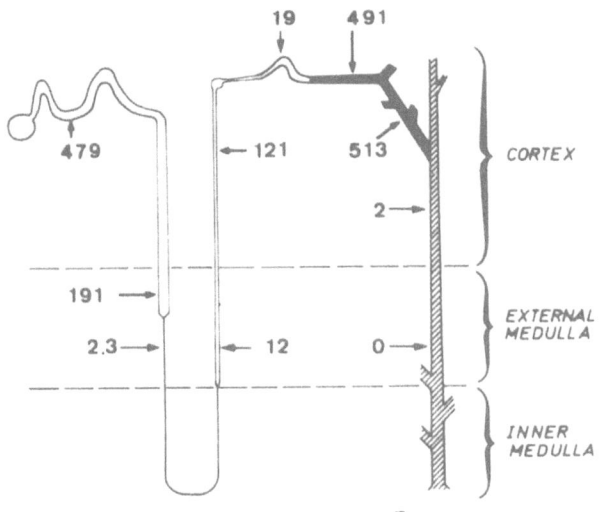

PTH (1U/ml) - Δ cAMP formed (10^{15} mol/mm /30 min.)

Fig. 3. Mean values for PTH-sensitive adenyl cyclase activity in ten portions of the rabbit nephron. The data correspond to the increase in cAMP generation (stimulated minus control) in response to PTH. Starting from the glomerulus, the values indicated correspond to the following segments: proximal convoluted tubule, pars recta, thin descending limb, medullary ascending limb, cortical ascending limb, distal convoluted tubule (granular), distal convoluted tubule (bright), cortical collecting tubule (granular), cortical collecting tubule (light), and medullary collecting tubule. (From Chabardès et al., 1975.)

iological and pathophysiological states—hypercalcemia (Beck et al., 1974; Popovtzer et al., 1977), hypomagnesemia (Slatopolsky et al., 1977), acute metabolic acidosis (Beck et al., 1975b), and clinically in type I pseudohypoparathyroidism (Chase et al., 1969; Sinha et al., 1977). Little or no phosphaturia ensues following PTH administration in these conditions. As predicted by this concept, bypassing the cAMP step with exogenous dibutyryl cAMP can overcome the block due to increased serum calcium (Amiel et al., 1976) or to metabolic acidosis (Beck et al., 1975b). Interference with the cellular action of cAMP could also blunt the phosphaturic effect of PTH, such as that seen after lithium pretreatment in dogs (Arruda et al., 1976). Arruda et al. (1976) observed that prior treatment with lithium for several days interfered with the phosphaturic action of cAMP given either exogenously or endogenously stimulated in response to PTH infusion. This observation has a clinical correlate in those cases of magnesium deficiency associated with nephrocalcinosis (Curiel et al., 1977) and in type II pseudohypoparathyroidism (Drezner et al., 1973). In these clinical disorders, cAMP excretion was appropriate in response to PTH, but no phosphaturia ensued. Thus, in these conditions, the abnormality could lie in the expression of cAMP action at the cellular level rather than in PTH-induced cAMP generation. There are also experimental correlates in hamsters (Knox *et al.*, 1977c) and chronic PO_4 depletion (Steele, 1976). The latter is resistant to PTH due to a failure to respond to either endogenously produced cAMP or exogenously adminstered dibutyryl cAMP (Harter *et al.*, 1974).

The fifth line of evidence that the adenyl cyclase–cAMP system mediates the phosphaturic effect of PTH is derived from recent micropuncture experiments using the shrinking-split-droplet method in combination with simultaneous perfusion of blood capillaries (Baumann *et al.*, 1977). The results of these studies indicate that PTH inhibits isotonic fluid reabsorption in renal proximal tubules preferentially and more effectively when applied from the contraluminal cell side, the site of adenyl cyclase localization (Marx *et al.*, 1972). Furthermore, the data indicate that cAMP inhibits fluid reabsorption with greater potency when applied from the luminal cell side, the sites of specific cAMP binding (Insel *et al.*, 1975) and cAMP-dependent protein kinase activity (Kinne *et al.*, 1975, Shlatz *et al.*, 1975). Confirmation of *in vitro* biochemical studies by these *in vivo* observations indicates the functional polarity of the proximal tubular cells in regard to PTH action. These results further support the concept of cAMP as the cellular mediator of these effects. These same studies demonstrated not only that both cAMP and PTH inhibit fluid transport but also that maximal effective doses of the two agents are not additive (Baumann *et al.*, 1977). At comparable concentrations (10^{-4} M), this effect on fluid transport was shared by dibutyryl cAMP and N^6-butyryl cAMP but not by the other nucleotides tested (deoxy-cAMP, 5'-AMP, cGMP, dibutyryl cGMP), further emphasizing the specificity of cAMP and its functional similarity with PTH.

Thus, several lines of evidence support the contention that PTH influences PO_4 transport as well as that of other species by elaborating cAMP within the renal tubular cell. The mechanism whereby increased cAMP leads to changes in PO_4 reabsorption remains unclear. As noted above, one hypothesis asserts that the tubular effects of PTH are primarily expressed by changes in sodium transport with secondary alterations in PO_4 reabsorption. A second declares that PTH affects changes in PO_4 transport by altering tubular fluid pH. We will consider these postulates in the following sections.

4.2. Role of Inhibition of Sodium Reabsorption—Sodium-Dependent Phosphate Transport Hypothesis

Supraphysiological doses of PTH cause a reduction in proximal tubular sodium and fluid reabsorption by approximately 20–30% (Agus *et al.*, 1973; Bank and Aynedjian, 1976; Hamburger *et al.*, 1976; Knox *et al.*, 1974, 1976; Wen, 1974). Since PO_4 reabsorption is closely linked to sodium and fluid transport along the proximal tubule under a variety of physiological and pharmacological maneuvers (Agus *et al.*, 1971, 1973; Beck and Goldberg, 1973, 1974; Goldfarb *et al.*, 1978; Knox and Lechêne, 1975; Maesaka *et al.*, 1973; Puschett *et al.*, 1972; Schneider *et al.*, 1975; Wen, 1974), it was earlier thought that the proximal tubular inhibition of PO_4 reabsorption by PTH might be mediated via a primary inhibition of sodium transport. Since both extracellular fluid volume expansion and PTH infusion may lead to an increase in the permeability of the proximal tubule to a variety of ions, the view that PTH may primarily act on sodium transport is further strengthened (Lorentz, 1976). As opposed to the PO_4 exit across the contraluminal cell border, which may be passive and sodium independent, entry across the brush-border membrane into the epithelial cell is apparently active and coupled with sodium entry. Recent studies with isolated brush-border-membrane vesicles suggest that PTH may decrease the maximum rate of sodium-dependent PO_4 transport by 30–50% (Ullrich, 1977).

On the other hand, there are a number of observations which indicate that the parallelism between sodium and PO_4 transport is not absolute and that dissociation in their transport may occur throughout the entire nephron, particularly under the influence of PTH. In thyroparathyroidectomized (TPTX) dogs, PTH augments the inhibition of proximal PO_4 reabsorption due to saline expansion (Wen, 1974) despite no further inhibition of fluid reabsorption, suggesting a discrete effect of PTH on PO_4 reabsorption. This dissociation of PO_4 and sodium transport is also seen in acetazolamide-treated TPTX dogs with maximal inhibition of carbonic anhydrase, since administration of PTH induces an additional effect on proximal PO_4 rejection and final urine excretion but does not alter sodium transport (Knox *et al.*, 1976). These data indicate an effect unrelated to sodium and/or bicarbonate reabsorption.

Studies utilizing other techniques also suggest that PTH may independently influence the transport of sodium and PO_4. Thus, microperfusion studies of isolated rabbit proximal tubules indicate that PTH decreases fluid (Hamburger *et al.*, 1976) but not PO_4 (Dennis *et al.*, 1977) efflux (reabsorption) in the pars convoluta, whereas it decreases PO_4 (Dennis *et al.*, 1977) but not fluid (Hamburger *et al.*, 1976) efflux in the pars recta. Furthermore, in the pars convoluta, no correlation was found between fluid efflux and PO_4 efflux (Dennis *et al.*, 1976).

Micropuncture studies also suggest the dissociation of PO_4 and sodium transport in the distal nephron. Following maneuvers which reduce the transport of sodium and PO_4 in the proximal tubule of the PTX animal, there is virtually complete reabsorption of all of the increased distal delivery of PO_4 but reabsorption of only part of the increased load of sodium (Beck and Goldberg, 1973, 1974; Knox *et al.*, 1976; Maesaka *et al.*, 1973; Wen, 1974). Conversely, when PTH is present or exogenously administered, almost all of the increased sodium delivered out of the proximal tubule due to inhibition of proximal tubular reabsorption by PTH is reabsorbed in the distal nephron (Agus *et al.*, 1971, 1973; Wen, 1974). This complete dissociation in the distal nephron would argue against inhibition of sodium transport as an important mediator of inhibition of PO_4 reabsorption at that tubular site.

Thus, while PTH has an important action of inhibiting proximal tubular sodium reabsorption as well as that of PO_4, a variety of experimental techniques and maneuvers suggest that the alteration in sodium transport is not the sole mechanism of action for the inhibition of PO_4 reabsorption. Although this effect may be contributory to the increased PO_4 delivery to the distal nephron, the latter site represents a locus where PO_4 and sodium transport are clearly dissociated.

4.3. Role of Tubular Fluid Alkalinization

Several workers have forwarded the hypothesis that alterations in tubular fluid pH may influence the reabsorption of PO_4. These views have arisen from both theoretical considerations as well as the direct observations of the potent phosphaturic effect of bicarbonate infusions. Since acute PTH infusions are known to alkalinize the urine in a manner similar to bicarbonate administration, it has been proposed that a component of the phosphaturic action of PTH may be mediated through this effect on tubular fluid pH.

As described elsewhere in this book (Chapter 8), a rise in tubular fluid pH, by converting the ionic PO_4 from the monovalent to the divalent form, could theoretically reduce PO_4 transport, since more highly charged species generally cross cell membranes at a reduced rate. If PTH were to alkalinize tubular fluid, it could conceivably reduce PO_4 transport primarily through this effect. Several observations support the hypothesis that tubular fluid alkalinization mediates the phosphaturic effect of PTH.

First, at the whole-kidney level, PTH administration leads to bicarbonaturia (Arruda *et al.*, 1977; Crumb *et al.*, 1974; Diaz-Buxo *et al.*, 1975; Knox *et al.*, 1976) and/or decreased bicarbonate reabsorption (Diaz-Buxo *et al.*, 1975; Karlinsky *et al.*, 1974), as has been repeatedly observed since the initial demonstration of this phenomenon by Ellsworth and Nicholson (1935). These effects are independent of volume status (Fulop and Brazeau, 1968) and can be produced by cAMP (Karlinsky *et al.*, 1974). This response closely mimics the renal response to acetazolamide, since this diuretic leads to reduced proximal tubular reabsorption of fluid (Beck and Goldberg, 1973; Dennis, 1976; Knox *et al.*, 1976; Wen, 1974) and PO_4

(Beck and Goldberg, 1973; Dennis, 1976; Wen, 1974) and leads to striking phosphaturia in humans (Puschett and Goldberg, 1969) and dogs (Crumb et al., 1974; Fulop and Brazeau, 1968). In fact, it has been proposed that PTH is an inhibitor of carbonic anhydrase activity in the kidney and that this effect explains its renal actions (Beck et al., 1975a). This hypothesis is further strengthened by observations of the isolated perfused proximal tubule in which the effects of PTH in inhibiting fluid transport were critically dependent on the presence of bicarbonate in the perfusion fluid. The removal of bicarbonate or the addition of acetazolamide completely blocks this effect of PTH, implying that PTH acted through inhibition of bicarbonate reabsorption.

Thus, the bicarbonaturic effect of PTH at the whole-kidney level, the inhibition of proximal tubular HCO_3^- transport, and the similarity (perhaps even in mechanism of action) between PTH and acetazolamide all suggest the possibility that alkalinization of tubular fluid might play a crucial role in the phosphaturic effect of PTH. On the other hand, a number of different studies and experimental techniques argue against this interpretation.

First, PTH does not consistently produce a bicarbonaturia despite a clear-cut phosphaturic response (Bank and Aynedjian, 1976; Puschett and Zuabach, 1976). This observation appears to be explained by distal-nephron reabsorption of any increment in delivered load of bicarbonate out of the proximal tubule produced by PTH administration (Bank and Aynedjian, 1976; Puschett and Zuabach, 1976). If this is the case, then proximal tubular fluid alkalinization might still occur and thereby increase distal-nephron PO_4 delivery and PO_4 excretion in the final urine. Thus, an absent bicarbonaturia would not completely rule out this hypothesis.

Second, the contention that PTH may inhibit carbonic anhydrase activity has not been confirmed (Garg, 1975). Apparently, the dosage of PTH used in the in vitro studies was high enough to produce nonspecific effects (Garg, 1975). Thus, PTH action and acetazolamide action may not be identical. This conclusion is further supported by the studies of Knox et al. (1976), who found that superimposition of PTH on maximal doses of acetazolamide results in increased phosphaturia without additional bicarbonaturia. Importantly, micropuncture studies of these combined infusions revealed a dissociation of the inhibitory effects of PTH on PO_4 transport in the proximal tubule from any further effect on fluid transport. Thus, at least a component of the phosphaturic effect of PTH is independent of inhibition of carbonic anhydrase activity. Moreover, any inference that inhibition of carbonic anhydrase activity leads to a rise in proximal tubular fluid pH may be erroneous, because an acidic disequilibrium pH may actually result from the inhibition of carbonic anhydrase in the proximal tubule (Rector et al., 1965).

A third line of argument against the tubular fluid alkalinization theory as mediating the effects of PTH comes from direct studies of *in situ* PO_4 transport in high- and low-pH perfusates (Baumann *et al.*, 1975b; Lang *et al.*, 1977b). In these studies, tubular fluid alkalinization resulted in *enhanced* PO_4 reabsorption. Moreover, direct inhibition of H^+ ion secretion by 4-acetamido-4'-isothiocyano-2,2'-disalfonic stilbene (SITS) had no effect on PO_4 reabsorption in the proximal tubule of chronically PTX rats (Ullrich, 1977).

In light of these conflicting and often equivocal experimental data, it must be concluded that the hypothesis of tubular fluid alkalinization has yet to be proven by more definitive studies. Direct measurement of PO_4 transport at various levels of tubular fluid pH and of tubular fluid pH at various lengths from the glomerulus and at various doses of PTH would be useful in testing this hypothesis.

In summary, therefore, the bulk of the evidence discussed above would favor the adenyl cyclase–cAMP system as the prime mediator of the phosphaturic action of PTH. While an inhibition of either sodium or bicarbonate reabsorption may explain some component of the reduction in PO_4 reabsorption seen after PTH administration, concrete and unequivocal evidence that these effects mediate the response to increased cAMP production and thereby lead to phosphaturia is not available at present.

ACKNOWLEDGMENTS. This work was supported by a research grant from the National Heart and Lung Institute (HL-00340), by the Veterans Administration, and by a training grant from the National Institute of Arthritis, Metabolic and Digestive Diseases (1 T32 AM-07006). Stanley Goldfarb is a Research and Education Associate of the Veterans Administration. We would like to thank Toni Snock and Kathy Bressler for their secretarial assistance. We would also like to thank Drs. Chabardès, Imbert, and Morel for their permission to use an illustration from their previous work (Chabardès *et al.*, 1975).

5. REFERENCES

Agus, Z. S., Puschett, J. B., Senesky, D., and Goldberg, M., 1971, Mode of action of parathyroid hormone and cyclic adenosine 3',5'-monophosphate on renal tubular phosphate reabsorption in the dog, *J. Clin. Invest.* **50:**617.
Agus, Z. S., Gardner, L. B., Beck. L. H., and Goldberg, M., 1973, Effect of parathyroid hormone on renal tubular reabsorption of calcium, sodium and phosphate, *Am. J. Physiol.* **224:**1143.
Amiel, C., Küntziger, H. E., and Richet, G., 1970, Micropuncture study of handling of

phosphate by proximal and distal nephron in normal and parathyroidectomized rat. Evidence for distal reabsorption, *Pflügers. Arch.* **317**:93.

Amiel, C., Küntziger, H. E., Conette, S., Corioeur, C., and Bergamioux, N., 1976, Evidence for a parathyroid hormone-independent calcium modulation of phosphate transport along the nephron, *J. Clin. Invest.* **57**:256.

Arruda, J. A. L., Richardson, J. M., Wolfson, J. A., Nascimento, L., Rademacher, D. A., and Kurtzman, N. A., 1976, Lithium administration and phosphate excretion, *Am. J. Physiol.* **231**:1140.

Arruda, J. A. L., Nascimento, L., Westenfelder, C., and Kurtzman, N. A., 1977, Effect of parathyroid hormone on urinary acidification, *Am. J. Physiol.* **232**:429.

Aurbach, G. D., and Heath, D. A., 1974, Parathyroid hormone and calcitonin regulation of renal function, *Kidney Int.* **6**:331.

Bank, N., and Aynedjian, H. S., 1976, A micropuncture study of the effect of parathyroid hormone in renal bicarbonate reabsorption, *J. Clin. Invest.* **58**:336.

Bank, N., Aynedjian, S., and Weinstein, S. W., 1974, A microperfusion study of phosphate reabsorption by the rat proximal renal tubule, *J. Clin. Invest.* **54**:1040.

Baumann, K., de Rouffignac, C., Roinel, N., Rumrich, G., and Ullrich, K. J., 1975a, Renal phosphate transport: Inhomogeneity of local-proximal transport rates and sodium dependence, *Pflügers Arch.* **356**:287.

Baumann, K., Rumrich, G., Papavassiliou, F., and Kloss, S., 1975b, pH dependence of phosphate reabsorption in the proximal tubule of rat kidney, *Pflügers Arch.* **360**:183.

Baumann, K., Chan, Y.-L., Bode, F., and Papavassiliou, F., 1977, Effect of parathyroid hormone and cyclic adenosine 3',5'-monophosphate on isotonic fluid reabsorption: Polarity of proximal tubular cells, *Kidney Int.* **11**:77.

Beck, L. H., and Goldberg, M., 1973, Effects of acetazolamide and parathyroidectomy on renal transport of sodium, calcium and phosphate, *Am. J. Physiol.* **224**:1136.

Beck, L. H., and Goldberg, M., 1974, Mechanism of the blunted phosphaturia in saline-loaded thyroparathyroidectomized dogs, *Kidney Int.* **6**:18.

Beck, N., Singhi, H., Reed, S. W., and Davis, B. B., 1974, Direct inhibitory effect of hypercalcemia on renal actions of parathyroid hormone, *J. Clin. Invest.* **53**:712.

Beck, N., Kim, K. S., Wolak, M., and Davis, B. B., 1975a, Inhibition of carbonic anhydrase by parathyroid hormone and cyclic AMP in rat renal cortex *in vitro, J. Clin. Invest.* **55**:149.

Beck, N., Kim, H. P., and Kim, K. S., 1975b, Effect of metabolic acidosis on renal action of parathyroid hormone, *Am. J. Physiol.* **228**:1483.

Bell, N. H., Avery, S., Sinha, T., Clark, C. M., Jr., Allen, D. O., and Johnston, C., Jr., 1972, Effects of dibutyryl cyclic adenosine 3',5'-monophosphate and parathyroid extract on calcium and phosphorus metabolism in hypoparathyroidism and pseudohypoparathyroidism, *J. Clin. Invest.* **51**:816.

Bengele, H. H., Lechêne, C., and Alexander, E. A., 1978, Phosphate (P) transport along the medullary collecting duct (MCD), *Clin. Res.* **26**:456A.

Berndt, R., Marchand, G., Sell, T., Haas, J., Dousa, T., and Knox, F., 1978, The effects of parathyroid hormone (PTH) and calcitonin (CT) on electrolyte and cyclic AMP (cAMP) excretion in the rabbit, *Fed. Proc. Fed. Am. Soc. Exp. Biol.* **37**:728.

Brunette, M. G., Taleb, L., and Carrière, S., 1973, Effect of parathyroid hormone on phosphate reabsorption along the nephron of the rat, *Am. J. Physiol.* **225**:1076.

Burnatowska, M. A., Harris, C. A., Sutton, R. A. L., and Dirks, J. H., 1977, Effects of PTH and cAMP on renal handling of calcium, magnesium and phosphate in the hamster, *Am. J. Physiol.* **233**:F514.

Buttlen, D., and Jard, S., 1972, Renal Handling of 3',5'-cAMP in the rat. The possible role of luminal 3',5' cyclic AMP in the tubular reabsorption of phosphate, *Pflügers Arch.* **331**:172.

Carone, F. F., 1964, Micropuncture study of renal phosphate excretion and action of parathyroid hormone, *Clin. Res.* 12:249.

Chabardès, D., Imbert, M., and Morel, F., 1975, Localization of PTH action sites along the rabbit nephron, in: *Phosphate Metabolism in Kidney and Bone, International Workshop* (L. V. Avioli, P. Bordier, H. Fleisch, S. Massry, and E. Slatopolsky, eds.), pp. 123–132, Nouvelle Imprimerie, Paris.

Chase, L. R., and Aurbach, G. D., 1967, Parathyroid function and the renal excretion of 3',5' adenylic acid, *Proc. Natl. Acad. Sci. U.S.A.* 58:518.

Chase, L. R., and Aurbach, G. D., 1968, Renal adenyl cyclase. Anatomically separate sites for parathyroid hormone and vasopressin, *Science* 159:545.

Chase, L. R., Melson, G. L., and Aurbach, G. D., 1969, Pseudohypoparathyroidism, defective excretion of 3',5'-AMP in response to parathyroid hormone, *J. Clin. Invest.* 48:1832.

Chiu, P. J. S., Agus, Z. S., and Goldberg, M., 1974, Effect of thyroparathyroidectomy (TPTX) on renal phosphate transport in the rat, *Clin. Res.* 22:520A.

Colindres, R. E., Pastoriza-Munoz, E., Lassiter, W. E., and Lechêne, C., 1976, Effect of extracellular volume expansion (V Exp) on phosphate (P) reabsorption along the nephron in thyroparathyroidectomized (TPTX) rats, in: *Proceedings of the 9th Annual Meeting of the American Society of Nephrology*, Washington, D.C., p. 2.

Crumb, C. K., Martinez-Maldonado, M. Eknoyan, M., and Suki, W. N., 1974, Effects of volume expansion, purified parathyroid extract and calcium on renal bicarbonate absorption in the dog, *J. Clin. Invest.* 54:1287.

Cuche, J.-L., Oh, G. E., Marchand, G. R., and Knox, F. G., 1976, Lack of effect of hypocalcemia on renal phosphate handling, *J. Lab. Clin. Med.* 88:271.

Curiel, M. D., Palomo, F. R., Castrillo, J. M., and Rapado, A., 1977, The effect of PTE infusion in hypomagnesemic states, in: *Proceedings of the 3rd International Workshop on Phosphate and Other Minerals*, Madrid, Spain, p. 19.

DeFronzo, R. A., Goldberg, M., and Agus, Z. S., 1976, The effects of glucose and insulin on renal electrolyte transport, *J. Clin. Invest.* 58:83.

Dennis, V. W., 1976, Influence of bicarbonate on parathyroid hormone-induced change in fluid absorption by the proximal tubule, *Kidney Int.* 10:373.

Dennis, V. W., Woodhall, P. B., and Robinson, R. R., 1976, Characteristics of phosphate transport in isolated proximal tubule, *Am. J. Physiol.* 231:979.

Dennis, V. W., Bello-Reuss, E., and Robinson, R. R., 1977, Response of phosphate transport to parathyroid hormone in segments of rabbit nephron, *Am. J. Physiol.* 233:F29.

de Rouffignac, C., Morel, F., Niss, N., and Roinel, N., 1973, Micropuncture study of water and electrolyte movements along the loop of Henle in psammomys with special reference to magnesium, calcium and phosphorus, *Pflügers Arch.* 344:309.

Diaz-Buxo, J. A., Oh, C. E., Cuche, J. L., Marchand, G. R., Wilson, D. M., and Knox, F. G., 1975, Effects of extracellular fluid volume contraction and expansion on the bicarbonaturia of parathyroid hormone, *Kidney Int.* 8:105.

Drezner, M., Neelon, F. A., and Lebovitz, H. E., 1973, Pseudohypoparathyroidism type II: A possible defect in the reception of the cyclic AMP signal, *N. Engl. J. Med.* 289:1056.

Eisenberg, E., 1965, Effects of serum calcium levels and parathyroid extracts on phophsate and calcium excretion in hypoparathyroid patients, *J. Clin. Invest.* 44:942.

Ellsworth, R., and Nicholson, W. M., 1935, Further observations upon the changes in the electrolytes of the urine following the injection of parathyroid extract, *J. Clin. Invest.* 14:823.

Fernandez, P. D., and Puschett, J. B., 1973, Proximal tubular actions of metolazone and chlorothiazide, *Am. J. Physiol.* 225:954.

Frick, A., 1972, Proximal tubule reabsorption of inorganic phosphate during saline infusion in the rat, *Am. J. Physiol.* **223:**1034.

Fulop, M., and Brazeau, P., 1968, The phosphaturic effect of sodium bicarbonate and acetazolamide in dogs, *J. Clin. Invest.* **47:**983.

Garg, L. C., 1975, Effect of parathyroid hormone and adenosine-3',5' monophosphate on renal carbonic anhydrase, *Biochem. Pharmacol.* **24:**437.

Gill, J. R., Jr., and Casper, A. G. T., 1971, Renal effects of adenosine 3',5'-monophosphate and dibutyryl adenosine 3',5'-cyclic monophosphate, *J. Clin. Invest.* **50:**1231.

Goldfarb, S., Beck, L. H., Agus, Z. S., and Goldberg, M., 1975, Tubular sites of action of dibutyryl cyclic AMP on renal phosphate reabsorption, in: *Phosphate Metabolism in Kidney and Bone, International Workshop* (L. V. Avioli, P. Bordier, H. Fleisch, S. Massry, and E. Slatopolsky, eds.), pp. 135–144, Nouvelle Imprimerie, Paris.

Goldfarb, S., Bosanac, P., Goldberg, M., and Agus, Z. S., 1978, Effects of calcium on renal tubular phosphate reabsorption, *Am. J. Physiol.* **234:**F22.

Hamburger, R. J., Lawson, N. L., and Dennis, V. W., 1974, Effects of cyclic adenosine nucleotides on fluid absorption by different segments of proximal tubule, *Am. J. Physiol.* **227:**396.

Hamburger, R. J., Lawson, N. L. and Schwartz, J. H., 1976, Response to parathyroid hormone in define segments of proximal tubule, *Am. J. Physiol.* **230:**286.

Harter, H. R., Mercado, A. M., Rutherford, W. E., Rodriguez, H., Slatopolsky, E., and Klahr, S., 1974, Effects of phosphate depletion and parathyroid hormone on renal glucose reabsorption, *Am. J. Physiol.* **227:**1422.

Insel, P., Balakir, R., and Sacktor, B., 1975, The binding of cyclic AMP to renal brush border membranes, *J. Cyclic Nucleotide Res.* **1:**107.

Kaminsky, N. I., Broadus, A. E., Hardman, J. G., Jones, D. L., Jr., Ball, J. H., Sutherland, E. W., and Liddle, G. W., 1970, Effects of parathyroid hormone on plasma and urinary adenosine 3'5'-monophosphate in man, *J. Clin. Invest.* **49:**2387.

Karlinsky, M. L., Sager, D. S., and Kurtzman, N. A., 1974, Effect of parathormone and cyclic adenosine monophosphate on renal bicarbonate reabsorption, *Am. J. Physiol.* **227:1226.**

Kinne, R., Shlatz, L. J., Kinne-Saffnan, E., and Schwartz, I. L., 1975, Distribution of membrane-bound cyclic AMP-dependent protein kinase in plasma membranes of cells of the kidney cortex, *J. Membr. Biol.* **24:**145.

Knox, F. G., and Lechêne, C., 1975, Distal site of action of parathyroid hormone on phosphate reabsorption, *Am. J. Physiol.* **229:**1556.

Knox, F. G., Schneider, E. G., Willis, L. R., Straudhoy, J. W., Oh, C. E., Cuche, J.-L., Goldsmith, R. S., and Arnaud, C. D., 1974, Proximal tubular reabsorption after hyperoncotic albumin infusion, *J. Clin. Invest.* **53:**501.

Knox, F. G., Haas, J. A., and Lechêne, C. P., 1976, Effect of parathyroid hormone on phosphate reabsorption in the presence of acetazolamide, *Kidney Int.* **10:**216.

Knox, F. G., Haas, J. A., Berndt, T., Marchand, G. R., and Youngberg, S. P., 1977a, Phosphate transport in superficial and deep nephrons in phosphate-loaded rats, *Am. J. Physiol.* **233:**F150.

Knox, F. G., Oswald, H., Marchand, G. R., Spielman, W. S., Haas, J. A., Berndt, T., and Youngberg, S. P., 1977b, Phosphate transport along the nephron, *Am. J. Physiol.* **233:**F261.

Knox, F. G., Preiss, J., Kim, J. K., and Dousa, T. P., 1977c, Mechanisms of resistance of the phosphaturic effect of parathyroid hormone in the hamster, *J. Clin. Invest.* **59:**675.

Küntziger, H., Amiel, C., Roinel, N., and Morel, F., 1974, Effects of parathyroidectomy and cyclic AMP on renal transport of phosphate, calcium, and magnesium, *Am. J. Physiol.* **227:**905.

Lang, F., Greger, R., Marchand, G. R., and Knox, F. G., 1977a, Stationary microperfusion study of phosphate reabsorption in proximal and distal nephron segements, *Pflügers Arch.* **368**:45.

Lang, F., Oberleithner, H., Greger, R., and Deetjen, P., 1977b, Role of blood pH for phosphate reabsorption during phosphate loading in thyroparathyroidectomized rats, in: *Proceedings of the 3rd International Workshop on Phosphate and Other Minerals,* Madrid, Spain, p. 10.

Lau, K., Agus, Z. S., Goldberg, M., and Goldfarb, S., 1977, Chronic phosphate depletion: Changes in segmental calcium and phosphate reabsorption, in: *Proceedings of 10th Annual Meeting of the American Society of Nephrology,* Washington, D.C., p. 6.

Lechêne, C., Colindres, R. E., and Knox, F. G., 1978, Electron probe microanalysis of the renal effect of parathyroid hormone, in: *Endocrinology of Calcium Metabolism* (D. H. Copp and P. V. Talmage, eds.), p. 230, Excerpta Medica, Amsterdam.

Lorentz, W. B., Jr., 1974, The effect of cyclic AMP and dibutyryl cyclic AMP on the permeability characteristics of the renal tubule, *J. Clin. Invest.* **53**:1250.

Lorentz, W. B., Jr., 1976, Effect of parathyroid hormone on renal tubular permeability, *Am. J. Physiol.* **231**:1401.

Maesaka, J. K., Levitt, M. F., and Abramson, R. G., 1973, Effect of saline infusion on phosphate transport in intact and thyroparathyroidectomized rats, *Am. J. Physiol.* **225**:1421.

Marx, S. J., Fedak, S. A., and Aurbach, G. D., 1972, Preparation and characterization of a hormone responsive renal plasma membrane fraction, *J. Biol. Chem.* **247**:6913.

Melson, G. L., Chase, L. R., and Aurbach, G. D., 1970, Parathyroid hormone sensitive adenyl cyclase in isolated renal tubules, *Endocrinology* **86**:511.

Mercado, A., Slatopolsky, E., and Klahr, S., 1975, On the mechanisms responsible for the phosphaturia of bicarbonate administration, *J. Clin. Invest.* **56**:1386.

Nussbaum, P., Lau, K., DeFronzo, R., Agus, Z. S., Goldberg, M., and Goldfarb, S., 1978, Interactions of insulin, phlorizin, and PTH on renal tubular phosphate transport, *Clin. Res.* **26**:472a.

Popovtzer, M. M., Flis, R. S., Mahandru, S. S., and Blum, M., 1977, Effect of the divalent cation Ionophore (A23187) on renal handling of phosphorus. *Kidney Int.* **12**:164.

Poujeol, P., Coman, B., Toriway, C., and de Rouffignac, C., 1977, Phosphate reabsorption in rat nephron terminal segments, *Pflügers Arch.* **371**:39.

Puschett, J. B., and Goldberg, M., 1969, The relationship between the renal handling of phosphate and bicarbonate in man, *J. Lab. Clin. Med.* **73**:956.

Puschett, J. B., and Zuabach, P., 1976, Acute effects of parathyroid hormone on proximal bicarbonate transport in the dog, *Kidney Int.* **9**:501.

Puschett, J. B., Agus, Z. S., Senesky, D., and Goldberg, M., 1972, Effects of saline loading and aortic obstruction on proximal phosphate transport, *Am. J. Physiol.* **223**:851.

Rasmussen, H., Pechet, M., and Fast, D., 1968, Effect of dibutyryl cyclic adenosine 3',5'-monophosphate, theophylline and other nucleotides upon calcium and phosphate metabolism, *J. Clin. Invest.* **47**:1843.

Rector, F. C., Jr., Carter, N. W., and Seldin, D. W., 1965, The mechanism of bicarbonate reabsorption in the proximal and distal tubules of the kidney, *J. Clin. Invest.* **44**:278.

Rocha, A. S., Magaldi, J. B., and Kokko, J. P., 1977, Calcium and phosphate transport in isolated segments of rabbit Henle's loop, *J. Clin. Invest.* **59**:975.

Russell, R. G. G., Casey, P. A., and Fleisch, H., 1968, Stimulation of phosphate excretion by the renal arterial infusion of 3',5'-AMP: A possible mechanism of action of parathyroid hormone, *Calcif. Tissue Res. (Suppl.)* **2**:54.

Schneider, E. G., Goldsmith, R. S., Arnaud, C. D., and Knox, F. G., 1975, Role of parathyroid hormone in the phosphaturia of extracellular fluid volume expansion, *Kidney Int.* **7**:317.

Shlatz, L. J., Schwartz, I. L., Kinne-Saffran, E., and Kinne, R., 1975, Distribution of parathyroid hormone-stimulated adenylate cyclase in plasma membranes of cells of the kidney cortex, *J. Membr. Biol.* **24**:131.

Sinha, T. K., Allen, D. O., Queener, S. F., and Bell, N. H., 1977, Effects of acetazolamide in the renal excretion of phosphate in hypoparathyroidism and pseudohypoparathyroidism, *J. Lab. Clin. Med.* **89**:1188.

Slatopolsky, E., Lewis, J., Martin, K., and Klahr, S., 1977, On the hypophosphatemia of magnesium depletion in the rat, in: *Proceedings of the 10th Annual Meeting of the American Society of Nephrology*, Washington, D.C., p. 8.

Staum, B. B., Hamburger, R. J., and Goldberg, M., 1972, Tracer microinjection study of renal tubular phosphate reabsorption in the rat, *J. Clin. Invest.* **51**:2271.

Steele, T. H., 1976, Renal resistance to parathyroid hormone during phosphorus deprivation, *J. Clin. Invest.* **58**:1461.

Streeto, J. M., 1969, Renal cortical adenyl cyclase effect of parathyroid hormone and calcium, *Metabolism* **18**:968.

Strickler, J. C., Thompson, D. D., Koose, R. M., and Giebisch, F., 1964, Micropuncture study of inorganic phosphate excretion in the rat, *J. Clin. Invest.* **43**:1596.

Sutton, R. A. L., Wong, N. L. M., and Dirks, J. H., 1976, Effects of parathyroid hormone on sodium and calcium transport in the dog nephron, *Clin. Sci.* **51**:345.

Ullrich, K. J., 1977, Mechanisms of cellular and subcellular transport of phosphate, in: *Proceedings of the 3rd International Workshop on Phosphate*, Madrid, Spain, p. 3.

Wen, S. F., 1974, Micropuncture studies of phosphate transport in the proximal tubule of the dog, *J. Clin. Invest.* **53**:143.

Effects of Hormones Other than Parathyroid Hormones on Renal Handling of Phosphate

EBERHARD RITZ, WILHELM KREUSSER, and
JÜRGEN BOMMER

1. INTRODUCTION

Hormones other than PTH or the vitamin D sterols have definite effects on renal handling of Pi. Although phosphaturic or antiphosphaturic actions of such hormones, for example, insulin, have been known for decades (Allen *et al.*, 1925), this area has been investigated in much less detail than have the effects of PTH. The problem is further complicated by the numerous interactions among the various hormones and by their effects on variables which are known to influence tubular transport of Pi, for example, net intestinal absorption of Pi, extracellular fluid volume, acid–base state, and tubular handling of Na. The nephronal sites of action and the molecular mechanisms by which net tubular transport of Pi is affected are not known for most of the hormones discussed below. This field awaits careful and comprehensive study in the future. It also remains

Abbreviations used in this chapter: ACTH, adrenocorticotrophic hormone; ADH, antidiuretic hormone (= vasopressin); C_{in}, inulin clearance; C_{Pi}, phosphate clearance; CT, calcitonin; DOCA, deoxycorticosterone acetate; GFR, glomerular filtration rate; GH, (human) growth hormone; iPTH, immunoreactive parathyroid hormone; P_i, inorganic phosphate; PEI, phosphate excretion index; PTH, parathyroid hormone; PTX, parathyroidectomy; RPF, renal plasma flow; T_3, triiodothyronine; T_4, thyroxine; TF/P, concentration ratio of tubular fluid to plasma; Tm_{Pi}/GFR, tubular maximal reabsorption capacity for Pi per unit glomerular filtration rate; TPTX, thyroparathyroidectomy; TRP, fractional tubular reabsorption of Pi.

to be clarified whether the effects on renal handling of Pi are due to direct actions of the hormones on the kidney or to their effects on extrarenal organs.

2. GROWTH HORMONE (GH)

2.1. The Effects of GH on Serum Pi Levels

It has long been recognized that fasting serum Pi is higher in patients with acromegaly (Reifenstein *et al.*, 1946). In these patients, there is a good correlation between circulating GH and serum Pi levels, so that serum Pi is a clinically useful index for the activity of the disease. Such hyperphosphatemia is reversible with therapy or after administration of ergocryptine (Belforte *et al.*, 1977).

Whereas serum Pi does not change, or rises only slightly, after short-term administration of GH in humans (Corvilain and Abramow, 1962; Henneman *et al.*, 1960), a significant rise in serum Pi is observed after long-term administration of GH to hypophysectomized or pituitary-intact individuals (Corvilain and Abramow, 1962). This hyperphosphatemic response is also elicited by reduced tetra-*S*-carbamidomethyl-GH (Connors *et al.*, 1973). This finding indicates that the hormonal effect of GH with respect to serum and urinary Pi is not dependent upon the presence of intact disulfide bridges which are the prerequisite for the immunoreactivity of GH.

In experimental animals, GH exhibits a biphasic effect on serum Pi, that is, an initial decrease which is followed by a later increase (Durand *et al.*, 1976). The early fall in serum Pi in the presence of diminished urinary excretion of Pi has been related to an insulin-like effect of GH which would lead to sequestration of Pi in the intracellular space. A logarithmic dose–response relationship exists for the hyperphosphatemic effect of GH. The rise in serum Pi is dependent upon a permissive effect of thyroxine.

It has not been clarified to what extent variations in serum Pi with age depend upon GH. Fasting serum Pi is higher in babies (Todd *et al.*, 1939) and in children (Bullock, 1930), and it falls to normal adult levels after puberty (Thalassinos *et al.*, 1970). High serum Pi levels in children were thought to be related to increased GH levels (Greenwood *et al.*, 1964). However, plasma GH levels respond to numerous physiological stimuli and are highly variable. In more recent studies, the difference in plasma GH levels between children and adults was not striking (Boucher, 1972). In addition, in pituitary dwarfs, serum Pi levels are still higher than in adult control patients (Corvilain and Abramow, 1972); therefore, the difference in serum Pi levels between children and adults cannot be due entirely to the difference in plasma GH concentration.

There is a tendency for serum Pi levels to rise again in advanced age (Keating et al., 1969). However, as shown by Morgan (1973), the rise in serum Pi occurs only in women and takes place after the age of menopause. Aitken et al. (1973a) also found significantly higher serum Pi levels after the menopause. In addition, a significant direct correlation was found between serum Pi and plasma GH levels. It was suggested that the postmenopausal relative hyperphosphatemia was consistent with increased GH activity. In contrast, in men, serum Pi continues to fall gradually throughout life.

The effect of GH on growth is mediated by somatomedin(s) (Van den Brande, 1975) which are synthesized predominantly in the liver and to a lesser extent in the kidney and other tissues. There is at least one report that serum Pi levels are normal or inadequately low for age (New et al., 1972) in "Laron dwarfs" (hereditary somatomedin deficiency; Laron et al., 1968). If confirmed, this finding would be compatible with the notion that the effect of GH on serum Pi (and possibly on renal handling of Pi) is mediated by somatomedin(s). This interesting question requires further study.

2.2. Extrarenal Effects of GH on Pi Metabolism

After administration of GH, Pi balance becomes positive both in humans and in experimental animals (Beck et al., 1957; Ikkos et al., 1959). Pi retention is due to the anabolic effect of GH and is accompanied by increased net intestinal absorption of Pi (Henneman et al., 1960). GH stimulates bone growth and bone remodeling, but the effect on net bone balance is variable (Rasmussen and Bordier, 1974).

2.3. Effects of Gh on Renal Handling of Pi

GH is a renotropic hormone (Gershberg, 1960). This is illustrated by the prompt increase in endogenous creatinine clearance upon administration of GH to normal individuals or patients with hypopituitarism. In dogs, GH raises GFR, RPF, tubular maximal secretion of para-amino-hippurate (Tm_{PAH}) (Davis, 1954; White, 1949), and tubular maximal reabsorption of sulfate (Tm_{SO_4}) (Gershberg and Gash, 1956).

The effects of GH on tubular handling of Pi can be clearly dissociated from such renotropic effects. Administration of GH causes an acute fall in urinary Pi excretion both in humans (Corvilain and Abramow, 1962) and in experimental animals such as dogs (Corvilain and Abramow, 1964) or rats (Durand *et al.*, 1976). The hypophosphaturic response to GH occurs within three hours (Durand *et al.*, 1976). The rise in serum Pi without a concomitant rise in urinary Pi suggests that the phenomenon is of renal origin. Cattaneo *et al.* (1964) studied five patients with acromegaly and found a parallel rise in GFR and Tm_{Pi}; this finding would indicate that Tm_{Pi}/GFR is unchanged in patients with GH oversecretion. In contrast, Corvilain and Abramow (1962) and Bijvoet (1976) found an increase in Tm_{Pi}/GFR after long-term administration of human GH to normal individuals (Table 1) or patients with hypopituitarism and after long-term administration of bovine GH to dogs. In addition, the elevation in Tm_{Pi}/GFR was found to be higher in active acromegalics than in adult control patients and successfully treated acromegalic patients (Corvilain and Abramow, 1972). These findings would indicate that GH raises the intrinsic reabsorptive capacity of the tubule for Pi independent of the hormone's effect on renal hemodynamics and the associated rise in filtered load of Pi. The effects of GH on the kidney appear to be reversible, since both GFR and Tm_{Pi}/GFR are normalized after successful treatment (Corvilain and Abramow, 1972).

There are marked interspecies differences with respect to responsiveness to foreign species of GH. In humans, a growth response can only be elicited by administering GH of human origin (Ikkos *et al.*, 1959) or of simian origin (Beck *et al.*, 1957), but systematic studies in humans on the renal response to GH of various species have not been performed.

Table 1. Effects of Human GH on Renal Function and Plasma Phosphorus Level[a,b]

Age (yr)	Fasting plasma (mg/100 ml)		GFR (ml/min)		$(Tm_{Pi}/GFR) \times 100$ (mg/100 ml)	
	A	B	A	B	A	B
26	2.77	4.01	51	63	2.92	4.05
44	3.35	3.01	114	151	2.83	3.51
26	3.31	3.51	136	151	3.20	3.26
29	2.81	3.00	121	133	2.71	3.44
33	2.13	2.89	116	144	2.52	3.18
28	2.78	2.93	91	114	2.02	4.03
36	2.89	2.83	77	93	2.18	2.54
33	2.74	3.31	102	115	2.59	3.34
26	3.65	3.97	131	157	3.45	3.33
27	2.80	3.39	137	132	3.10	3.55
	$p < 0.05$		$p < 0.001$		$p < 0.01$	

[a] After Corvilain and Abramow (1962).
[b] Abbreviations: A, control values; B, values after human GH administration.

Tm$_{Pi}$/GFR is also high in children as compared with normal adults (Corvilain and Abramow, 1972). However, Tm$_{Pi}$/GFR is also higher in pituitary dwarfs than in normal adults, so that it appears unlikely that the comparatively potent Pi transport system in children is entirely due to endogenous GH.

Data from micropuncture experiments demonstrate enhanced proximal tubular Na reabsorption in GH-treated rats (Simone and Solomon, 1970), although such antinatriuretic action was not confirmed by Rabkin *et al.* (1975); but no data are available on the site of action of GH on Pi reabsorption.

2.4. Factors Related to the Effects of GH on Tubular Transport of Pi

The effect of GH on tubular reabsorption of Pi is not necessarily a direct one. Receptors for GH have not been demonstrated in renal tissue, and there is no evidence that GH affects generation of cyclic AMP (cAMP) or gluconeogenesis in isolated proximal tubules (Guder, 1976).

GH was reported to cause a pronounced retention of Na, resulting in an expansion of the extracellular fluid space in humans (Ikkos *et al.*, 1959) and in rats (Batts *et al.*, 1954). The presence of the adrenal cortex does not seem to play a determinant role in Na retention (Ikkos *et al.*, 1959). However, using apparently purer preparations, Rabkin *et al.* (1975) were unable to observe such Na retention. Furthermore, volume expansion in itself would decrease rather than increase net tubular reabsorption of Pi.

A dose-dependent increase in urinary Ca is frequently observed after administration of GH to humans (Beck *et al.*, 1957) and animals. An increase in net intestinal absorption of Ca was demonstrated with the balance technique (Henneman *et al.*, 1960), and this finding was confirmed using radioisotope techniques. The increase in net intestinal absorption of Ca is sometimes insufficient to account for the rise in urinary Ca, and an additional effect of GH on net bone resorption has also been postulated (Fraser and Harrison, 1960). Although an increase in serum Ca after administration of GH to experimental animals has not been observed, ultrastructural evidence of suppressed parathyroid gland activity has been described, at least by some authors (Altenähr and Kampf, 1976). On the other hand, Rasmussen (1968) proposed that retention of Pi and increased Ca excretion should lead to a tendency to hypocalcemia; this, in turn, should induce compensatory oversecretion of PTH. However, in view of the experiments of Corvilain and Abramow (1964), it appears unlikely that GH affects net tubular Pi reabsorption by inhibiting the secretion of PTH or by preventing a peripheral action of PTH. These authors demonstrated a rise in Tm_{Pi}/GFR in TPTX dogs. In addition, they showed that GH does not modify the action of PTH on the renal tubule, since Tm_{Pi}/GFR was lowered by PTH both before and after GH administration.

There is some controversy over whether insulin, which affects tubular transport of Pi (see below), is released by GH (Stuart-Mason, 1972). In addition, GH appears to directly affect renal tubular glucose transport; $Tm_{glucose}$ falls after hypophysectomy in dogs and is restored by GH (Wesson, 1969), and $Tm_{glucose}$ is high in acromegalic persons (Gershberg, 1960). There are well-known interactions between tubular transport of glucose and tubular transport of Pi (Wesson, 1969).

Finally, recent evidence presented by McIntyre (1978) suggests that administration of GH elevates circulating levels of 1,25-dihydroxyvitamin D, the active metabolite of vitamin D. This substance could influence tubular transport of Pi; this is discussed in Chapter 7.

3. VASOPRESSIN (ANTIDIURETIC HORMONE; ADH)

3.1. Effects of ADH on Serum Pi Levels

Patients with diabetes insipidus do not commonly exhibit abnormal serum Pi concentrations. In addition, administration of physiological doses of ADH does not consistently affect serum Pi levels.

In acute experiments, supraphysiological doses of ADH cause a consistent increase in serum Pi levels (Arruda *et al.*, 1977, 1978). Since such an increase in serum Pi after ADH administration occurs in the presence of increased urinary Pi excretion, the extra-Pi must originate from tissue pools. The increase in serum Pi is independent of the parathyroid status and occurs both in parathyroid-intact and in PTX animals. Experiments of Heidenreich *et al.* (1964) point to a metabolic effect of ADH, since this hormone increased hepatic glycogenolysis with a concomitant decrease in hepatic glycogen content and an increase in serum glucose and lactate. This would lead to increased delivery of Pi to the extracellular space.

3.2. Effects of ADH on Renal Handling of Pi

Although the antidiuretic effect of ADH has been established for a long time, the natriuretic and phosphaturic properties of ADH have been investigated only recently (Arruda *et al.*, 1977, 1978; Eisinger *et al.*, 1970a,b; Kurtzman *et al.*, 1975; Martinez-Maldonado *et al.*, 1971; Wen, 1974).

The natriuretic response is rapid in onset, of brief duration, and similar in potency to that seen after the administration of either ethacrynic acid or furosemide (Brooks and Pickford, 1958; Chan and Sawyer, 1962; Humphreys *et al.*, 1970; Martinez-Maldonado *et al.*, 1971). Diuresis associated with ADH is characterized by an increase in Na, K, Cl, and P excretion, as well as by a marked increase in urinary volume. The diuretic effect of ADH is not contingent upon the presence of preexisting water diuresis, since it is also seen in antidiuretic animals; it is not dependent upon a rise in systemic blood pressure, since it is observed even in animals in which the rise of blood pressure is prevented by administration of nitroprusside; furthermore, the diuretic effect of ADH does not require a change in GFR or RPF (Kurtzman *et al.*, 1975; Wen, 1974).

Eisinger *et al.* (1970a,b) found that the administration of ADH to humans produced phosphaturia when the control levels of Pi excretion were low, while in individuals with high basal urinary Pi, ADH was without effect. The phosphaturic action of ADH was subsequently confirmed by Martinez-Maldonado *et al.* (1971), Wen (1974), Kurtzman *et al.* (1975), and Arruda *et al.* (1977, 1978). Martinez-Maldonado *et al.* (1971) observed a significant rise in Pi excretion and Pi clearance upon injection of ADH into the renal artery of dogs undergoing hypotonic saline diuresis.

There is no complete unanimity as to the site in the nephron where ADH inhibits tubular reabsorption of Pi. In a recollection micropuncture study, Wen (1974) observed no change in TF/P for inulin [$TF/P)_{in}$] in the proximal tubule of TPTX dogs that had been given pressor doses of ADH (Table 2). But, at the same time, ADH caused natriuresis, and it was concluded that natriuresis resulted from inhibition of Na reabsorption in the distal nephron. In contrast, TF/P for ultrafilterable Pi increased consistently in the proximal tubule, irrespective of changes in blood pressure. The dissociation of Na and Pi transport in the proximal tubule led Wen to conclude that ADH inhibits Pi transport in the proximal tubule and Na reabsorption in the distal tubule.

Kurtzman *et al.* (1975) demonstrated that the maximal rate of bicarbonate and glucose reabsorption was not depressed by infusion of ADH, while fractional Pi excretion was markedly increased. The absence of an effect of ADH on reabsorption of glucose or bicarbonate indicates that if there is a proximal effect of this agent, it is a limited one, affecting only tubular reabsorption of Pi. These authors assumed that the diuretic action of ADH was due to an inhibitory effect on Na reabsorption at a point in the nephron distal to the proximal tubule.

The mechanisms through which ADH inhibits the tubular reabsorption of Pi are not as yet elucidated. Buckalew and Nelson (1974) had found suggestive evidence for an extrarenal natriuretic factor after ADH administration. Such a factor may be responsible for the phosphaturia. How-

Table 2. Proximal Tubular Micropuncture Data[a-c]

Dogs[d]	Experimental phase	MBP (mm Hg)	GFR (ml/min)	$(TF/P)_{in}$	$(TF/UF)_{PO_4}$	$(TF/UF)_{PO_4}/(TF/P)_{in}$
5(24)	Control	127 ± 4	33.9 ± 4.5	1.69 ± 0.05	0.70 ± 0.07	0.42 ± 0.04
	Vasopressin	147 ± 6[e]	44.2 ± 6.9[b]	1.53 ± 0.08[e]	0.89 ± 0.09[f]	0.62 ± 0.08[f]
6(29)	Control	130 ± 8	34.3 ± 4.4	1.60 ± 0.10	0.61 ± 0.05	0.39 ± 0.04
	Vasopressin	127 ± 8	35.7 ± 5.0	1.60 ± 0.13	0.80 ± 0.04[e]	0.52 ± 0.04[e]

[a] Wen (1974).
[b] Values are mean ± SEM.
[c] Abbreviations: MBP, mean blood pressure; $(TF/UF)_{PO_4}$, TF/P for ultrafilterable phosphate.
[d] Numbers in parentheses denote tubular fluid samples.
[e] $p < 0.05$.
[f] $p < 0.01$.

ever, such systemic effects appear unlikely in view of the experiments of Martinez-Maldonado *et al.* (1971), who observed an ipsilateral rise in Pi clearance after injection of ADH into the renal artery of dogs.

A phosphaturic response similar to the one seen with ADH was observed after infusing cAMP into the renal artery (Martinez-Maldonado *et al.*, 1971). It was concluded that the phosphaturia following the administration of ADH resulted from inhibition of Na reabsorption in response to increased intracellular formation of cAMP. Senft *et al.* (1968) observed a rise of cAMP in the renal cortex of rats who had been dehydrated for four to five days, and ADH, like PTH, was found to stimulate cortical adenyl cyclase *in vitro* (Aurbach, 1976). However, Morel *et al.* (1976) failed to observe any stimulation of adenyl cyclase in the pars convoluta and the pars recta of isolated proximal tubules. ADH-sensitive adenyl cyclase has been clearly demonstrated, however, in the glomerulus (Ichikawa and Brenner, 1977) and in the renal medulla (Dousa and Valtin, 1976).

In conclusion, ADH at supraphysiological dose levels directly inhibits renal tubular reabsorption of Pi by mechanisms independent of changes in systemic blood pressure, renal hemodynamics, or PTH secretion. Some evidence points to an action of ADH on Pi reabsorption in the proximal tubule, and such action may be mediated by an adenyl cyclase system. The nephron segment(s) where ADH inhibits Pi transport is not as yet determined.

4. THYROID HORMONES (THYROXINE AND TRIIODOTHYRONINE)

4.1. Effects of Thyroid Hormones on Serum Pi Levels

Patients with hyperthyroidism are known to have higher serum Pi levels than euthyroid patients (Adams *et al.*, 1967; Aub *et al.*, 1929; Clerkin *et al.*, 1964; Malamos *et al.*, 1969; Morgan, 1973; Mosekilde *et al.*, 1977; Parsons and Anderson, 1964). Bijvoet and Majoor (1965) found a positive correlation between Tm_{Pi}/GFR and the level of protein-bound iodine. We have found a positive correlation between serum Pi concentrations and serum T_4 levels (Fig. 1). The elevation in serum Pi levels is reversible, since serum Pi levels fall after treatment of thyrotoxicosis (Parsons and Anderson, 1964).

In contrast, in patients with hypothyroidism, serum Pi levels are lower than in normal individuals (Malamos *et al.*, 1969), and serum Pi levels rise after therapy with thyroid extract (Albright *et al.*, 1931; Breitbarth, 1940).

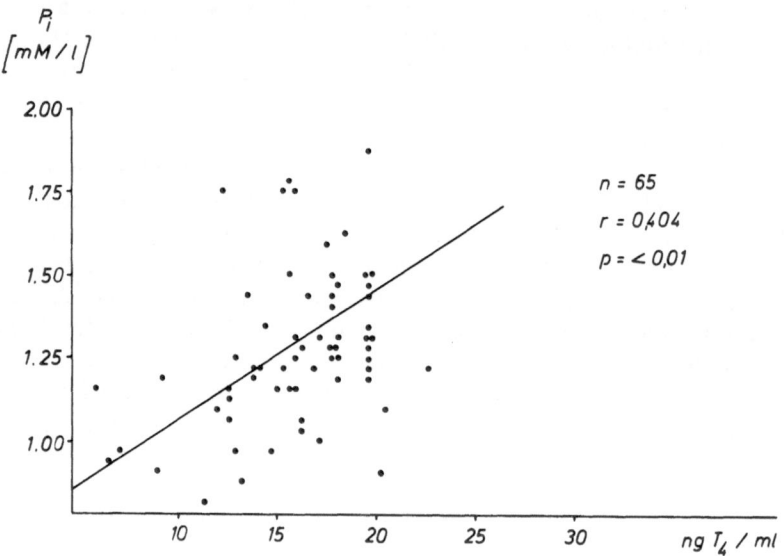

Fig. 1. Correlation between serum Pi and serum T_4 levels in hyperthyroid patients.

Administration of thyroid extract raises serum Pi in normal humans (thyrotoxicosis factitia) and animals. The same effect on serum Pi is seen after administration of T_4 or T_3. Beisel *et al.* (1958) observed an increase in serum Pi after administration of T_3 to dogs, and Perault-Staub and Staub (1972) and Bommer *et al.* (1979) found a rise in mean serum Pi after chronic administration of T_4 to rats.

4.2. Extrarenal Effects of Thyroid Hormones on Pi Metabolism

In the steady state, a change in serum Pi may be due either to changes in the amount of Pi entering the extracellular fluid space or to changes in the renal threshold for Pi. There is good evidence that thyroid hormones influence both extrarenal Pi metabolism and renal handling of Pi.

Pfleger *et al.* (1958) claimed that treatment with T_4 increased radiophosphate influx into intestine; however, Noble and Matty (1967), using the everted-gut-sac technique in rats, found that treatment with T_4 decreased Pi transfer out of the duodenum and had no effect of Pi transport in the lower part of the small intestine. Net intestinal absorption of Pi in humans with thyrotoxicosis, as observed in balance studies, was either increased (Albright *et al.*, 1931; Schittenhelm and Eisler, 1928) or unchanged (Jones *et al.*, 1966). Bommer *et al.* (1979) reported an increase in net intestinal Pi absorption in rats treated with T_4. The increase in net intestinal Pi absorption contrasts with the consistent decrease in net intestinal Ca absorption. Impaired intestinal Ca transport was observed both in humans (Schittenhelm and Eisler, 1928; Singhelakis *et al.*, 1974) and in experimental animals (Friedland *et al.*, 1965; Noble and Matty, 1967).

Thyroid hormones clearly act on bone, independent of PTH, as demonstrated by the observations of Meunier *et al.* (1972) and Bordier *et al.* (1967) in thyrotoxic humans and in animals with experimental thyrotoxicosis (Bommer *et al.*, 1973). Bone mass decreases, as demonstrated by reduced cortical width and increased cortical porosity. These alterations can all be documented by microradioscopy (Meema and Schatz, 1970) and by photon-absorption techniques (Grehn *et al.*, 1973). Fasting urinary Ca excretion (Nordin, 1976) and urinary hydroxyproline (Kivirikko *et al.*, 1965) are elevated. These findings point to increased net bone resorption.

4.3. Effects of Thyroid Hormones on Renal Handling of Pi

Daily urinary Pi excretion is higher in patients with thyrotoxicosis on a self-selected diet than in normal individuals (Aub *et al.*, 1929; Malamos *et al.*, 1969; Robertson, 1942). In addition, urinary Pi excretion rates in the fasting state are elevated in animals with experimental thyrotoxicosis as compared to pair-fed control animals (Bommer and Ritz, 1974). Acute administration of T_3 results in a rapid phosphaturic response (Beisel *et al.*, 1958). In contrast, following acute administration of T_4, no change in urinary Pi is seen for several hours; however, after a lag time of up to 48 hours, an increase in urinary Pi was observed by Albright *et al.* (1931) in humans and by Bommer *et al.* (1979) in rats.

Thyroid hormones increase both GFR and RPF (Katz *et al.*, 1975). Since both GFR and serum Pi are elevated, it follows that the filtered load of Pi is high in thyrotoxic patients (Parsons and Anderson, 1964) and in animals with experimental thyrotoxicosis (Bommer and Ritz, 1974; Bommer *et al.*, 1976).

Several investigators found diminshed fractional Pi excretion (Adams *et al.*, 1967; Bortz *et al.*, 1961; Harden *et al.*, 1964) and a low (Harden *et al.*, 1964) or normal (Nordin and Fraser, 1960) PEI in patients with thyrotoxicosis. However, since both parameters are sensitive to changes in Pi load (Bijvoet, 1976), this finding in itself does not prove a change in the intrinsic capacity of the tubule to reabsorb Pi. However, an elevated Tm_{Pi}/GFR in thyrotoxic patients was reported (Bijvoet, 1969; Bijvoet and Majoor, 1965; Malamos *et al.*, 1969; Parsons and Anderson, 1964). Gellissen and Brodelh (1965) found diminished Tm_{Pi} in newborns with congenital athyreosis and in increase in Tm_{Pi} upon therapy.

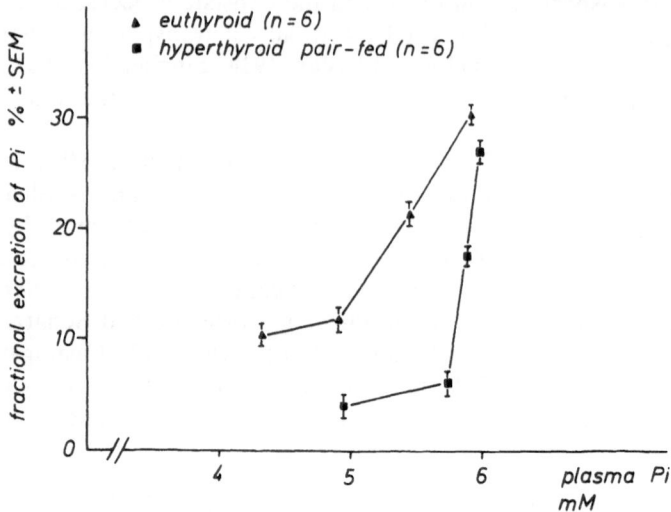

Fig. 2. Effect of Pi infusion on fractional excretion of Pi in hyperthyroid PTX rats. (From Bommer et al., 1979.)

Other authors concluded that T_3 diminishes tubular capacity to reabsorb Pi (Beisel et al., 1958); however, these authors measured TRP under conditions of changing GFR and serum Pi, and conclusions about tubular reabsorptive capacity are therefore potentially subject to error.

In experimental animals, increased tubular reabsorption of Pi could be demonstrated after administration of T_4 (Bommer and Ritz, 1974; Bommer et al., 1976, 1979); that is, at different serum Pi concentrations, the rate of tubular reabsorption of Pi was higher in thyrotoxic animals than in controls, when serum Pi concentrations were raised by infusion of Pi as shown in Fig. 2. Conversely, tubular reabsorption of Pi is apparently reduced in hypothyroid animals (Bommer et al., 1976).

4.4. Factors Related to the Effects of Thyroid Hormones on Renal Handling of Pi

In thyrotoxicosis, many factors are altered which are known to affect renal tubular transport of Pi. Pi reabsorption is decreased by extracellular volume expansion (Frick, 1968; Massry et al., 1969), and extracellular fluid space is reduced in experimental thyrotoxicosis (Bommer et al., 1976). However, increased tubular reabsorption of Pi in animals with experimental thyrotoxicosis is maintained under conditions of volume expansion (Bommer et al., 1979), as shown in Fig. 3.

Vitamin D metabolism is altered in thyrotoxicosis, as indicated by low circulating 25-hydroxyvitamin D_3 levels in thyrotoxic patients (Velentzas *et al.*, 1977); no information is available on 1,25-dihydroxyvitamin D_3 levels. It is conceivable that alterations in vitamin D metabolism might contribute to the change in tubular Pi transport, since 1,25-dihyroxyvitamin D (Bonjour *et al.*, 1977), and possibly other vitamin D metabolites (see Chapter 7), may affect tubular Pi transport.

Plasma GH levels, as measured by radioimmunoassay, were reported to be high in thyrotoxic patients (Braumann *et al.*, 1973), and GH levels rise during administration of T_4 to hypothyroid rats (Kikuyama *et al.*, 1974; Wilkins *et al.*, 1974). However, even after hypophysectomy, experimental thyrotoxicosis caused an increase in serum Pi (Bommer *et al.*, 1979). Although tubular transport of Pi was not directly measured in these experiments, the effect of T_4 on tubular transport of Pi does not appear to be mediated by changes in GH (or other hypophyseal hormones).

There is no reliable information available on serum CT levels in thyrotoxic patients. We found that administration of T_4 caused a marked increase in serum Pi even in TPTX animals. Therefore, the effect of T_4 does not seem to be dependent upon changes in CT secretion.

Adaptation to dietary intake of Pi appears to be a major determinant of tubular reabsorptive capacity for Pi (Tröhler *et al.*, 1976). However, in the experimental study of Bommer *et al.* (1979), the effect of T_4 on Pi reabsorption was observed under conditions of pair-feeding, so that mechanisms other than dietary adaptation must be involved. Alterations in urinary acid excretion do not appear to play a role. T_4 does not have any known effect on renal acid excretion (Zinsman and Boccino, 1968), and

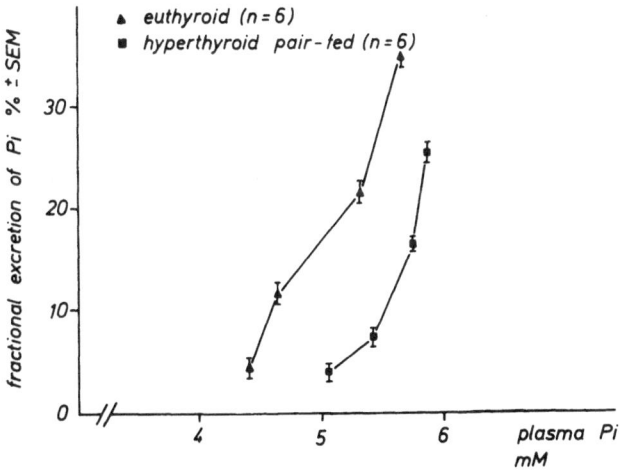

Fig. 3. Effect of Pi infusion on fractional excretion of Pi in hyperthyroid PTX rats with extracellular volume expansion. (From Bommer *et al.*, 1979.)

normal urinary excretion of titratable acid and ammonium excretion were found in hyperthyroid patients both under basal conditions and after loading with ammonium chloride (Katz *et al.*, 1975; Zinsman and Boccino, 1968).

Various authors have proposed that the rise in serum Pi levels in hyperthyroid patients results from suppression of PTH secretion (Adams *et al.*, 1967; Harden *et al.*, 1964; Krane, 1971; Nordin, 1973; Raisz, 1972). The following sequence of events was postulated: T_4 stimulates net bone resorption and thus increases ionized serum Ca levels; this, in turn, suppresses PTH secretion and, consequently, increases tubular reabsorption of Pi. According to these authors, hyperphosphatemia would ensue as a result of suppressed parathyroid activity. This concept finds some support in the clinical observation that hypercalcemia does occur in patients with thyrotoxicosis (Frizel *et al.*, 1967). There is much confusion in the literature with regard to iPTH levels in thyrotoxic patients; increased (Bommer *et al.*, 1975; Burman *et al.*, 1976), normal, and decreased (Bouillon and de Moor, 1974) levels have been reported. Such differences may be related to immunoheterogeneity of PTH. We found that concomitant measurements with carboxyterminal and aminoterminal antibodies gave widely different results.

The effect of T_4 on tubular reabsorption of Pi is not, at least not exclusively, dependent upon a circulating PTH, since increased serum Pi and elevated tubular reabsorption of Pi at a given serum Pi could be demonstrated even in PTX rats after chronic administration of T_4. In addition, the change in tubular transport of Pi was not paralleled by changes in urinary excretion of cAMP. To the extent that urinary cAMP excretion reflects intracellular events in tubular cells, no evidence for the participation of an adenyl cyclase system is found in these studies (Bommer *et al.*, 1979). Although changes in urinary cAMP excretion have been reported in hyperthyroid patients (Carter and Heath, 1977; Tucci and Kopp, 1976), no definite conclusions can be drawn from such findings, since urinary cAMP excretion may also be affected by catecholamines (Bommer *et al.*, 1976).

In conclusion, the study of Bommer *et al.* (1979) documents that T_4 influences the intrinsic tubular capacity for Pi reabsorption by mechanisms independent of adaptation to dietary Pi intake, PTH, GH, CT, and changes in extracellular fluid space. The effect of T_4 on net tubular transport of Pi may involve either one or a combination of the following factors: changes in a critical Pi compartment of tubular cells, as postulated for the increased tubular reabsorption of Pi in the Pi depletion syndrome (Steele and DeLuca, 1976); changes in transepithelial Na transport, to which Pi transport is secondarily linked (Ullrich, 1977); or alterations in vitamin D metabolism. Studies by Ismail-Beigi and Edelman (1971) showed an increase in Na,K-stimulated ATPase under the influence of T_4 in various tissues, and such an increase was also demonstrated in the kidney (Katz and Lindheimer, 1973). Therefore, a primary effect of T_4 on Na–Pi cotransport appears possible.

5. CALCITONIN (CT)

5.1. Effects of CT on Serum Pi Levels

No consistent alterations of serum Pi levels are known in patients with CT oversecretion secondary to medullary thyroid carcinoma (Melvin and Tashjian, 1968) or in patients without endogenous CT, that is, thyroidectomized patients (Mazzuoli et al., 1967). Administration of supraphysiological doses of porcine or salmon CT to patients with Paget's disease (Bijvoet and Jansen, 1967; Haddad et al., 1970; Hamilton, 1970) or those with hypercalcemia (Zilva and Nicholson, 1973) lowered serum Pi levels, although not consistently. Administration of crude CT extracts (Hirsch et al., 1973), porcine and bovine CT (Kenny and Heiskell, 1965), or salmon CT (Roycroft and Talmage, 1973) to rats produces a fall in serum Pi levels. Such a fall in serum Pi is not only independent of PTH, since it occurs also in PTX animals (Roycroft and Talmage, 1973; Talmage and Anderson, 1974), but is also independent of renal loss of Pi, since it occurs also in nephrectomized animals (Anderson and Talmage, 1973; Talmage and Anderson, 1974). Hypophosphatemia in response to the administration of various CT preparations has also been observed in rats (Sørensen and Hindberg, 1972), in sheep (Barlet, 1972), and in kittens (Indech and Jowsey, 1971). In humans, hypophosphatemia is not commonly observed (Ardaillou et al., 1967b; Juan et al., 1976) unless there is an underlying condition of high bone turnover, for example, Paget's disease (Bijvoet et al., 1968).

CT lowers serum Ca, (Foster et al., 1966) and this hypocalcemic effect has been related to the known inhibitory effect of the hormone on bone resorption (Queener and Bell, 1975), although an additional effect of CT on movement of Ca from the extracellular space to soft tissues has been demonstrated by Yamaguchi et al. (1975) in a study using high doses of porcine CT in TPTX rats. It has been suggested that the hypophosphatemic effect of this hormone is due to similar mechanisms. However, the hypophosphatemic and hypocalcemic effects of CT can be dissociated with the use of ethane-1-hydroxy-1,1-diphosphonic acid (EHDP), as demonstrated by Talmage and Anderson (1974). The hypophosphatemic effect of CT appears to be due to multiple factors and could be related to the following events: inhibition of the movement of Pi from bone to extracellular fluid, increased movement of Pi from the extracellular fluid space to soft tissues, and augmented urinary excretion of Pi (Talmage *et al.*, 1972). Convincing arguments have been advanced that CT lowers serum Pi primarily by augmenting its exit from the circulation rather than by inhibiting its release from bone, as originally believed (Talmage *et al.*, 1972). This effect of CT on serum Pi is not feedback controlled, since Pi infusion failed to increase circulating levels of CT (Talmage *et al.*, 1972).

5.2. Extrarenal Effects of CT on Pi Metabolism

In normal persons and in patients with hypoparathyroidism, net intestinal absorption of Pi was significantly diminished upon administration of high doses of synthetic salmon CT (Juan *et al.*, 1976).

The effect of CT on bone mineral turnover has been reviewed recently (Queener and Bell, 1975). CT primarily inhibits bone resorption, and this effect can also be demonstrated *in vitro* (Friedman and Raisz, 1965).

Crude CT, injected subcutaneously into rats, failed to consistently alter the Pi content of kidney, small intestine, submaxillary salivary glands, and lens in the study of Kenny and Heiskell (1965). However, Meyer and Meyer (1975) observed an increase in liver Pi upon administration of CT to rats. Such a rise in liver Pi occurred despite the fall in serum Pi, and indirect evidence pointed against intracellular sequestration of Pi as high-energy Pi esters. In contrast, CT prevented the rise in Pi content of the kidney which normally occurred in thyroidectomized lambs when supplemented with T_4 (Barlet, 1972).

5.3. Renal Effects of CT

No consistent effects of CT on renal hemodynamics have been reported in rats (Gekle, 1972) and in humans (Haas *et al.*, 1971), although such an effect has been reported in dogs (Charbon and Pieper, 1970).

In rats, an increase in urinary Pi excretion has been noted after administration of crude bovine or hog thyroid extract (Kenny and Heiskell, 1965) and after administration of porcine, human, and salmon CT (Aldred *et al.*, 1970a,b); Milhaud and Mouhktar, 1966; Milhaud *et al.*, 1966; Robinson *et al.*, 1966; Sørensen and Hindberg, 1972; Williams *et al.*, 1972). A similar effect has been found in sheep (Barlet *et al.*, 1971), pigs (Russell and Fleisch, 1968), cows (Barlet *et al.*, 1971), and rabbits (Salako *et al.*, 1971). The dog is remarkable in that CT is without effect on phosphaturia, at least after PTX (Clark and Kenny, 1969; Pak *et al.*, 1970; Puschett *et al.*, 1974; Russell and Fleisch, 1968). Although CT in itself was not phosphaturic in this species, it has been claimed that CT inhibited the antiphosphaturic action of 25-hydroxyvitamin D_3 in moderately volume-expanded dogs (Puschett et al., 1974). In addition, in the pig, only very large doses of CT provoked phosphaturia, and no consistent effect was obtained after PTX (Clark and Kenny, 1969; Russell and Fleisch, 1968). In humans, a clear-cut phosphaturic effect of porcine, bovine, human, and salmon CT has been documented in a large number of studies (Cochran et al., 1970; Courvoisier et al., 1970; Haas and Dambacher, 1968; Langer et al., 1971; Martin and Melick, 1969; Milhaud et al., 1970; Paillard et al., 1972; Sørensen and Hindberg, 1972); the phosphaturic response occurs after acute administration of CT and is sustained during long-term administration of the hormone (Bijvoet and Froeling, 1973).

In the past, it was doubted whether the phosphaturic response after administration of CT was a specific hormonal effect. This action of the hormone has been ascribed to impurities in the preparations (Ziegler et al., 1967), and the variable change of Pi excretion with different CT preparations has been attributed to variations in the Mg/Ca ratio of the solvent (Pechet et al., 1967). However, phosphaturia has been elicited with the use of synthetic CT preparations in humans and other species, as described above. The phosphaturic effect of CT has also been ascribed to an increase in the secretion of PTH in response to the hypocalcemia induced by CT, but the phosphaturia occurred in hypoparathyroid humans (Haas et al.., 1971; Paillard et al., 1972; Sørensen and Hindberg, 1972) and in TPTX animals (Milhaud et al., 1966; Robinson et al., 1966). Rasmussen et al. (1967) suggested that the phosphaturic response to CT is a nonspecific effect to hypocalcemia, since similar phosphaturia was observed following injection of sufficient ethylene(bis)oxyethylene-nitrilotetraacetate (EGTA) to produce an idential fall in plasma ionized Ca. However, phosphaturia was observed even in subjects in whom the hypocalcemic effect was negligible because of low bone turnover (Ardaillou et al., 1976b), and it was also observed when the hypocalcemic effect of CT was prevented by infusion of Ca (Paillard et al., 1972).

In view of these findings, a direct renal effect of CT can no longer be doubted. Since phosphaturia occurs without significant changes in GFR and at unchanged or falling serum PI concentrations, it has been concluded that such phosphaturia is due to a tubular action of CT (Ardaillou, 1975; Paillard et al., 1972).

Le Grimellec and Lechêne (1970) reported data suggesting that the increase in endogenous CT secretion following Ca infusion into the thyroid artery increased the proximal tubular reabsorption of Pi. However, the micropuncture study of Gekle (1972) showed a decrease in proximal tubular $(TF/P)_{Pi}$ without a change in GFR, and the author concluded that CT decreased proximal tubular reabsorption of Pi. However, $(TF/P)_{in}$ was

not determined, and it remains undecided whether CT specifically interferes with a Pi transport system or whether its effect is secondary to an
action on net reabsorption of fluid and other electrolytes.

5.4. Factors Related to the Effects of CT on Renal Handling of Pi

The available data do not answer the question whether the effect of
CT on phosphaturia is due to direct interaction between CT and a Pi
transport system or whether it is secondary to changes in renal handling
of Na or other electrolytes induced by CT; irrespective of this consideration, however, there is now clear evidence for the presence of CT
receptors on renal cells, as revealed by high-affinity binding of radiolabeled CT (Marx and Aurbach, 1975; Marx *et al.*, 1972; Queener and Bell,
1975; Sraer and Ardaillou, 1973). There is also evidence for CT-stimulated
adenyl cyclase in renal tissue (Chabardès *et al.*, 1976; Dousa, 1974; Loreau *et al.*, 1975; Marx and Aurbach, 1975; Marx *et al.*, 1972; Melson *et
al.*, 1970; Murad *et al.*, 1970). However, phosphaturia and natriuresis
have been shown in humans, dogs, and cows in which CT receptors and
CT-activated adenyl cyclase could not be demonstrated (Dousa, 1974;
Marx and Aurbach, 1975). It remains undecided whether the inability to
demonstrate CT receptors and CT-activated adenyl cyclase is related to
the insensitivity of existing methods or whether this finding points to some
actions of CT by mechanisms other than adenyl cyclase.

After administration of CT to rats, Kurokawa *et al.* (1974) observed
an increase of urinary cAMP *in vivo* and *in vitro* which preceded the
phosphaturic response. In addition, the effect of CT on renal cAMP was
not additive to the effect of PTH (Kurokawa *et al.*, 1974; Loreau *et al.*,
1975). However, other authors (Heersche *et al.*, 1974; Marx *et al.*, 1972)
could not confirm these findings. In humans, Ardaillou (1975) observed
an increase in serum cAMP and in urinary excretion of cAMP secondary
to a rise in filtered cAMP, but no change was found in the nephrogenous
portion of urinary and renal venous cAMP, although a marked natriuretic
effect was observed. The author concluded that CT affected renal ex-
traction of extrarenal cAMP, presumably of osseous origin, by enhancing
cAMP uptake at the peritubular site. This observation would be compatible with the notion that CT acts through mechanisms other than
cAMP.

Several authors who studied the effects of CT on various systems
reported some actions which were apparently unrelated to the adenyl
cyclase system. In an Ussing chamber, preparation under short-circuit
conditions, a marked effect of CT on secretion of Cl or water and inhibiton
of Na resorption was observed without any detectable change in tissue

cAMP (Walling *et al.*, 1977). The authors speculated that in this system, CT might act by mechanisms other than adenyl cyclase, although their method may not have detected small increases of cAMP in some critical subcellular compartment. Effects of CT unrelated to adenyl cyclase have also been demonstrated by Dreyfus *et al.* (1976) in the gut, where CT in supraphysiological doses antagonized contractile responses to acetylcholine and the cholinergic response to electrical field stimulation. This action of CT has been ascribed to interaction with muscarinic receptors. An effect of CT on the energy charge of renal cells has been reported by Ogata *et al.* (1975), but the mechanisms of this action are poorly defined. *In vitro*, CT has important effects on renal subcellular content of Ca and P (Borle, 1975), and it has been concluded that CT stimulates cellular uptake of Ca and inhibits efflux of Ca from the cells (Borle, 1969), although Kenny and Heiskell (1965) had found a decrease in renal Ca content after administration of CT *in vivo*. An effect of synthetic CT on Ca uptake by mitochondria has been demonstrated (Borle, 1975), but it is unknown whether this polypeptide can directly interact with intracellular membranes *in vivo*. On the basis of radiokinetic studies with renal cell cultures, Borle concluded that CT depresses the Ca efflux from the cell (Borle, 1969, 1975; Harrell *et al.*, 1973), whereas other authors concluded that CT stimulates Ca efflux from the cell (Copp, 1973; Rasmussen, 1971; Rasmussen *et al.*, 1971). It is unknown whether the effects of CT on the ionic composition of the cytosols are mediated exclusively by the adenyl cyclase system.

A coordinate occurrence of high-affinity binding of radiolabeled salmon CT and CT-activated adenyl cyclase was observed by Marx and Aurbach (1975); in addition, parallel loss of the binding and of the hormonal sensitivity of the enzyme was observed after Lubrol treatment (Marx and Aurbach, 1975; Loreau *et al.*, 1977). A parallel decrease in the number of receptor sites for CT and CT-activated adenyl cyclase was observed in an interesting experimental model by Loreau *et al.* (1977). High-affinity binding sites were distributed in fractions in which the specific activity of hormone-sensitive adenyl cyclase was greatest. CT binding and activation of adenyl cyclase occurred at similar hormone concentrations, and the relative potencies of CT analogues were similar whether measured by competition for high-affinity binding sites or by their effects on adenyl cyclase. There was a close parallelism between biological potency and affinity to the receptor for different CTs, in the following order: salmon CT > porcine CT > ovine CT > bovine CT > human Ct. In PTX rats, CT binding to renal receptors was found to be the result of an increased number of receptor sites with no change in affinity. Such a finding is compatible with a feedback mechanism controlling the synthesis of receptor sites according to the level of plasma

CT, similar to the regulatory role of insulin or glucagon on the number of their respective receptors on plasma membranes.

Experiments of Marx *et al.* (1972) and Kurokawa *et al.* (1974) had established that CT-sensitive adenyl cyclase in the kidney was confined to renal cortex and outer medulla. Microdissection studies (Chabardès *et al.*, 1976; Morel *et al.*, 1978) established that CT-dependent adenyl cyclase activity in the rabbit nephron was present in three segments, namely, the medullary and cortical portions of the thick ascending limb of the loop and the bright portion of the distal convoluted tubule (Fig. 4). The sensitivity of these segments was high, since half-maximal stimulation corresponded to CT concentrations ranging between 0.07 and 0.1 nM. The stimulation factor (up to 30-fold) was high enough to account for the stimulation ratio in whole-kidney-cortex homogenates, and the authors concluded that it was not necessary to postulate an action of CT on adenyl cyclase in the proximal tubule which they found to be unresponsive to CT along its entire length. This finding is surprising in view of the demonstrated action of CT on proximal tubular reabsorption, as suggested

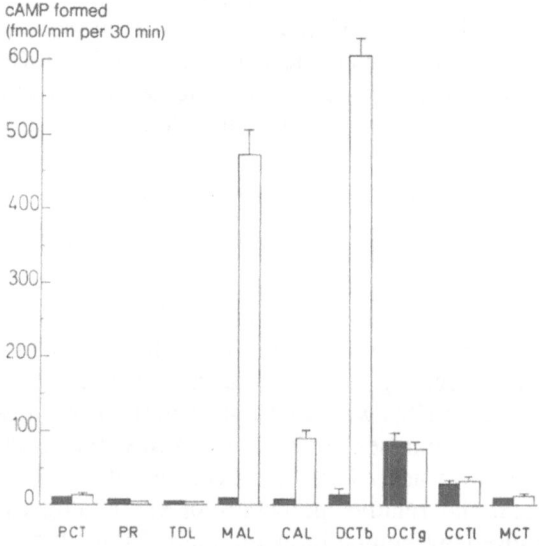

Fig. 4. Distribution of CT-dependent adenyl cyclase activity along the rabbit kidney tubule. PCT, Proximal convoluted tubule; PR, pars recta of the proximal tubule; TDL, thin descending limb of the loop of Henle; MAL, medullary portion of the thick ascending limb of the loop of Henle; CAL, cortical portion of the thick ascending limb of the loop of Henle; DCTb, bright-appearing portion of distal convoluted tubule; DCTg, granular-appearing portion of distal convoluted tubule; CCTl, light portion of cortical collecting tubule; MCT, medullary portion of collecting tubule; ■, control; □, salmon CT. (From Chabardès *et al.*, 1976.)

indirectly by clinical studies in intact humans (Paillard *et al.*, 1972) and directly by experiments utilizing recollection micropuncture techniques in rats (Gekle, 1972). There exist marked differences with respect to CT- and PTH-responsive adenyl cyclase. The segments sensitive to CT were found to be insensitive to PTH, and vice versa (Chabardès *et al.*, 1976), and this finding explains why most authors (Heersche *et al.*, 1974; Loreau *et al.*, 1975; Marx *et al.*, 1972), but not all (Kurokawa *et al.*, 1974; Melson *et al.*, 1970; Murad *et al.*, 1970) found that the effects of these two hormones on cAMP generation were additive when tested together. Also, marked species differences with respect to localization of CT-sensitive adenyl cyclase exist (Morel *et al.*, 1978); these sites are located more distally in the mouse nephron (bright portion of the distal convoluted tubule) than in the rabbit nephron (medullary and cortical portions of the thick ascending limb of the loop of Henle).

6. GLUCAGON

6.1. Effects of Glucagon on Serum Pi Levels

No consistent abnormality in serum Pi levels or urinary rates of Pi excretion has been observed in the rare patients with glucagon-secreting islet-cell adenomas (Case Records of the Massachusetts General Hospital, 1975). In adult patients, Butturini and Bonomini (1958) and Elrick *et al.* (1958) observed a fall in serum Pi following intravenous injection of glucagon. The hypophosphatemic effect of glucagon may paritally be due to hyperglycemia; however, if the serum glucose levels were raised, either by glucagon or by a glucose load, more marked lowering of Pi was seen after glucagon than after glucose loading, pointing to specific effects of glucagon independent of hyperglycemia (Elrick *et al.*, 1958). Presumably, the fall in serum Pi is due mainly to a shift of extracellular Pi to the intracellular space, where Pi is trapped as hexosephosphate ester subsequent to stimulation of glycogenolysis. However, indirect effects, such as increased CT secretion in response to glucagon, may also be involved. Glucagon is also known to lower serum Ca in hypercalcemic patients and was reported to inhibit bone resorption by a direct action on bone (Paloyan *et al.*, 1967; Stern and Bell, 1970).

6.2. Effects of Glucagon on Renal Handling of Pi

The information on hemodynamic effects of glucagon in the kidney is conflicting. Levy and Starr (1972) found a consistent increase in GFR and RPF associated with natriuresis after infusion of glucagon into one renal artery of dogs. In contrast, glucagon had no consistent effect on GFR and tended to increase RPF in humans or dogs in the studies of Elrick *et al.* (1958) and Staub *et al.* (1957). In the isolated perfused rat kidney, glucagon increased total renal blood flow, while the GFR remained unchanged (Franke *et al.*, 1977).

In acute experiments, after infusion of high doses (40 μg/kg) of glucagon, an increase in the urinary excretion rate of Pi was found both in humans (Butturini and Bonomini, 1958; Elrick *et al.*, 1958) and in dogs (Pullmann *et al.*, 1967; Staub *et al.*, 1957) (Fig. 5). In contrast, in the study of Saudek *et al.* (1973), no increase in urinary Pi excretion was found upon infusion of physiological doses of glucagon in healthy obese subjects.

Increased urinary excretion of Pi in the face of reduced filtered load of Pi was interpreted by Butturini and Bonomini (1958) and Elrick *et al.* (1958) as evidence of an acute effect of glucagon on net tubular transport of Pi. It was also concluded that the increased C_{Pi}/GFR was not due to concomitant hyperglycemia, since the electrolyte effect following glucagon preceded the rise in the level of blood glucose (Elrick *et al.*, 1958).

6.3. Factors Related to the Effects of Glucagon on Renal Handling of Pi

Glucagon is known to stimulate the release of CT (Paloyan *et al.*, 1967; Stern and Bell, 1970), and this effect may underlie the phosphaturia observed by some investigators. In addition, in experimental animals, serum Ca levels may fall after administration of glucagon (Stern and Bell, 1970). Since the phosphaturic response to glucagon has not been studied in PTX or TPTX individuals or animals, the role of PTH or CT in the renal phosphaturic response to glucagon cannot be definitely excluded.

It is unlikely that glucagon may alter urinary Pi excretion through an effect on the release of GH. Some investigators found no change in GH levels in normal subjects, while others reported significant increments of plasma GH in children and adults after glucagon administration (Stuart-Mason, 1972). But in none of the studies was an inhibition of GH release found which could explain a fall in tubular reabsorption of Pi.

According to Broadus *et al.* (1970), urinary cAMP excretion rises in response to glucagon exclusively due to an increase in the filtered load of cAMP. However, Gill *et al.* (1971) found evidence for an adenyl cyclase in the proximal tubule which was stimulated by glucagon and which was thought to be related to the inhibitory effect of glucagon on Na absorption. Glucagon is known to cause natriuresis (Levy and Starr, 1972; Saudek *et al.*, 1973). This effect apparently is a direct one, since the natriuresis occurred during the infusion of the hormone into the renal artery (Pullmann *et al.*, 1967); these authors suggested that this effect was mediated

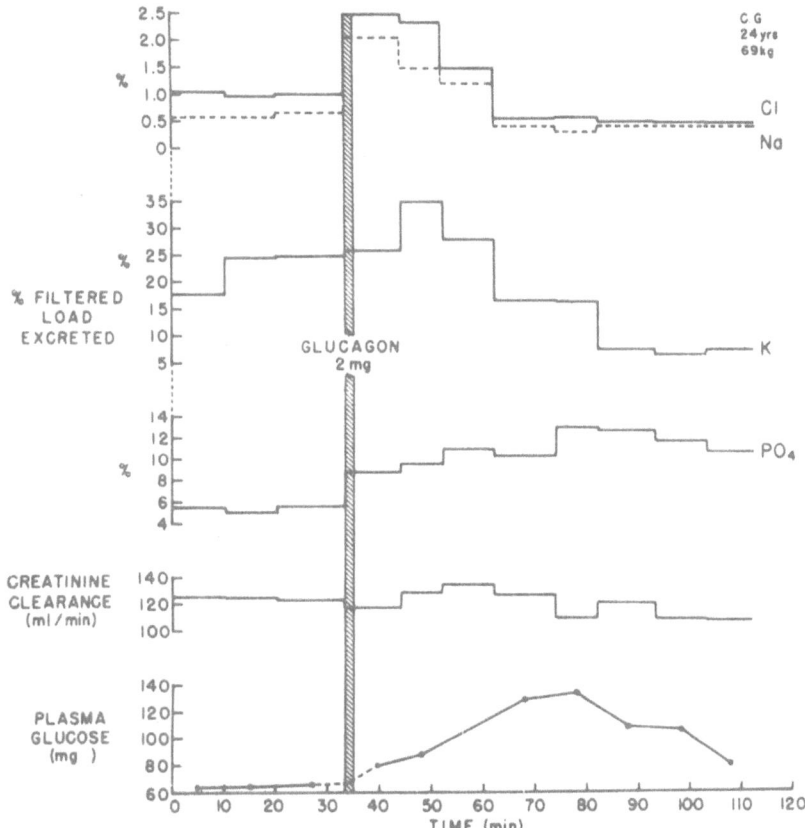

Fig. 5. Effect of glucagon on renal clearance ratios of Cl, Na, K, and PO_4; on creatinine clearance; and on plasma glucose levels. (From Elrick *et al.*, 1958.)

by decreased tubular reabsorption of Na rather than by increased GFR, but Pi was not measured in these experiments.

On the basis of available information, it is uncertain whether glucagon consistently causes a phosphaturic response and, if phosphatemia occurs, whether it is due to a direct effect of glucagon or to an indirect one.

7. INSULIN

7.1. Effects of Insulin on Serum Pi Levels

The effect of insulin on serum Pi levels was studied immediately after pure insulin preparations became available (Cori and Cori, 1931; Perlzweig *et al.*, 1923). Both in experimental animals and in humans, the administration of insulin causes a fall in serum Pi (Harrop and Benedict, 1923, 1924). Such lowering of serum Pi concentrations is related to trans-location of extracellular Pi into the intracellular space, where Pi is com-partmentalized subsequent to the synthesis of organic hexosephosphate esters. The fall in blood Pi caused by insulin is mediated, in part, by β-adrenergic receptors, since β-adrenergic blockade with propranolol sig-nificantly inhibited insulin-induced hypophosphatemia (Massara and Ca-manni, 1970) (see Fig. 7).

7.2. Effects of Insulin on Renal Handling of Pi

Excessive urinary elimination of Pi has been observed in patients with diabetes mellitus (Mandel and Lusk, 1904; Moraczewski, 1897) and in depancreatized dogs. Carbohydrate ingestion is followed by a tem-porary diminution in Pi excretion in normal individuals. In diabetic dogs, however, glucose ingestion did not lead to changes in urinary Pi excretion (Bolliger and Hartman, 1925). These data suggested an antiphosphaturic action for insulin, an effect which could be the result of a fall in blood Pi levels and its filtered load.

After acute administration of insulin, the rate of urinary excretion of Pi falls both in humans (Allen *et al.*, 1925; Butturini and Bonomini, 1958) and in experimental animals (Eggleton and Shuster, 1954). How-ever, these early investigations suggesting an antiphosphaturic action for insulin are difficult to interpret, since in these studies a number of vari-ables which are known to affect tubular transport of Pi, such as changes in the filtered load of glucose, extracellular fluid volume, serum glucagon concentration, GFR, and renal blood flow, were not controlled. In ad-dition, insulin induces hypoglycemia; the latter is known to increase sym-pathetic activity and may, by this, increase PTH secretion (Fischer *et al.*, 1973; Kukreja *et al.*, 1975). Stimulation of the secretion of PTH during hypoglycemic stress via increased epinephrine levels was clearly dem-onstrated by Shah *et al.* (1975).

In a more recent study, DeFronzo *et al.* (1975) studied the effect of insulin on the renal handling of Pi and other electrolytes while maintaining the blood glucose concentration at the fasting level by negative-feedback servocontrol of variable glucose infusion. Additional factors which might act on tubular transport of Pi, such as GFR, RPF, and plasma aldosterone and glucagon concentrations, were also monitored in the study. In water-loaded normal subjects maintained in a steady state of water diuresis, elevation in the plasma concentration of insulin to 90 and 193 μU/ml decreased urinary Pi excretion from 540 ± 43 to 230 ± 43 μg/min despite no change in blood glucose, filtered glucose, and RPF and only a slight fall in serum Pi. Since GFR remained constant, the filtered load of Pi

Table 3. Influence of Insulin on the Overall TRP by Isolated Dog Kidney[a,b]

	Control		+ Insulin		Differential values	
Plasma Pi (mg/100 ml)	19.4	(2.7)	19.4	(1.5)	0	(0.4)
GFR (ml/min/100 g)	43.9	(4.2)	41.9	(3)	−2	(2.7)
Pi filtered load (mg/min/100 g)	8.45	(0.95)	8.11	(1.79)	−0.34	(0.47)
Pi excretion (mg/min/100 g)	3.41	(0.76)	2.84	(0.69)	−0.57	(0.29)
Overall TRP (%)	63	(4)	68	(3)	+5	(2)

[a] Nizet et al. (1976).
[b] Average values of 13 comparative experiments and 56 clearance periods. Limits of confidence for $2p = 0.05$ are given in parentheses. Significance of differences is calculated from paired values.

decreased by approximately 10–15%. Thus, it remains undecided whether the change in urinary Pi excretion was secondary to changes in the filtered load of Pi or to alterations in tubular handling of Pi, although the authors felt that the magnitude of the decrement in urinary Pi was greater than that anticipated from the fall in serum Pi. Their data suggest that insulin has an antiphosphatemic action. This conclusion is further supported by the findings of Nizet et al. (1976) that perfusion of isolated dog kidney with slightly supraphysiological concentrations of porcine insulin increases TRP (Table 3). In these studies, GFR and plasma Pi did not change significantly, and extrarenal effects of insulin can obviously be excluded by the experimental protocol.

7.3. Factors Related to the Effects of Insulin on Renal Handling of Pi

Parameters of urinary acid excretion may affect Pi exretion, but they were not measured in the studies of DeFronzo et al. (1975) and Nizet et al. (1976). In the study of Butturini and Bonomini (1958), however, an acute reduction in titratable acid and ammonium associated with a slight rise in bicarbonate excretion was found subsequent to the injection of insulin. Such changes should enhance urinary Pi excretion.

McIntyre (1978) reported that insulin activates the renal 1α-hydroxylase, which should increase the circulating levels of 1,25-dihydroxycholecalciferol. The role, if any, of this observation in the effect of insulin on net tubular transport of Pi remains to be clarified.

Pharmacological doses of glucagon have been shown to be both natriuretic and phosphaturic (Butturini and Bonomini, 1958). An increase in plasma insulin concentration is known to be accompanied by reciprocal changes in circulating glucagon (Unger, 1971), and such a fall in plasma glucagon was observed in the study of DeFronzo et al. (1975). Consequently, the lowering of serum glucagon might have contributed to the observed changes in urinary Pi excretion in vivo. However, such indirect effects via glucagon can be excluded in the model of the isolated perfused kidney studied by Nizet et al. (1976).

Luft and Cerasi (1967, 1968) found that infusion of minute amounts of insulin (0–0.1 U/kg body weight) that lead to a decrease of blood glucose concentration of only about 10 mg/100 ml could induce GH release. Since GH is known to raise tubular reabsorption of Pi, such an indirect effect mediated by GH cannot be excluded in some of the early in vivo studies (Butturini and Bonomini, 1958; Eggleton and Shuster, 1954); however, serum glucose was controlled in the study of DeFronzo et al. (1975), and any such GH-mediated effect is excluded in the isolated perfused kidney preparation of Nizet et al. (1976).

In the study of DeFronzo et al. (1975), urinary Na excretion and osmolar clearance decreased, while free water clearance increased. This finding is in line with previous observations of the stimulatory effect of insulin on Na transport in amphibian epithelia (André and Crabbé, 1966; Herrera et al., 1963) and in the isolated perfused dog kidney (Nizet et al., 1971). Furthermore, there is evidence that insulin stimulates active Na transport in skeletal muscle, frog skin, bladder, and colon (Rubinstein et al., 1975). These findings suggest an action of insulin on tubular Na transport; furthermore, the effect of insulin on C_{H_2O} suggests that the action of insulin on Na excretion is due to an enhancement of Na reabsorption in the diluting segment of the distal nephron. Since it is highly controversial whether Pi reabsorption occurs at this nephron site, it remains undecided whether the effect of insulin on tubular transport of Pi is related to the effect on tubular Na handling.

In the isolated perfused rat kidney (Cohen et al., 1977), insulin increased both net utilization of glucose and decarboxylation of glucose without a concomitant increase in net lactate production. In addition, insulin increased fractional reabsorption of Na in the presence, but not in the absence, of glucose. These observations suggest that the presence of glucose and insulin-mediated metabolism of glucose are prerequisites for the action of insulin on Na transport. It is unknown whether the same pertains to the effects of insulin on Pi transport.

Such a direct effect of insulin on tubular transport processes is not surprising in view of the demonstration of insulin receptors on isolated renal tubules; however, in contrast to other polypeptide hormones, insulin does not stimulate cAMP production or gluconeogenesis in isolated proximal tubules (Guder, 1976).

The body of available evidence would suggest that insulin enhances tubular reabsorption of Pi by a direct action on renal tubules. However, the nephron site and the molecular mechanisms of this action are not known.

8. CATECHOLAMINES

8.1. Effects of Catecholamines on Serum Pi Levels

The hypophosphatemic response to epinephrine has been known since the investigations of Perlzweig *et al.* (1923) in humans and has since been documented in many species (Ellis, 1956). Such a fall in serum Pi is associated with an increase in hexosephosphate in muscle (Cori and Cori, 1931), which is presumably related to the glycogenolytic action of epinephrine. Experiments with radiophosphate showed rapid removal of Pi from plasma after administration of epinephrine (Hevesy and DalSanto, 1954), and since urinary excretion of Pi falls in response to epinephrine (Allen *et al.*, 1925; Perlzweig *et al.*, 1923), Pi is presumably shifted to the intracellular space.

In PTX animals and in those with intact parathyroid glands, Kenny (1964) observed a hypophosphatemic response after epinephrine and isoproterenol, but not after norepinephrine (Fig. 6). The hypophosphatemic response was antagonized by β-blocking agents, but not by phenoxybenzamine. Massara and Camanni (1970) were also able to completely abolish epinephrine-induced hypophosphatemia in humans by propranolol. These observations suggest that a β-adrenergic receptor mechanism is involved (Fig. 7).

8.2. Effects of Catecholamines on Renal Handling of Pi

A hypophosphaturic response to epinephrine has been consistently observed in dogs (Allen *et al.*, 1925; Nishimoto, 1929), in rabbits (Klisiechi and Pytasz, 1961), and in humans (Perlzweig *et al.*, 1923). In the study of Morey and Kenny (1964), the response of urinary Pi excretion to epinephrine was variable: Urinary Pi decreased in parathyroid-intact rats as in the studies cited above. However, urinary Pi increased in PTX rats. Since GFR and RPF were not measured, it is difficult to exclude variations in the filtered load of Pi as the cause of the observed changes in urinary Pi.

Irrespective of the PTH status, urinary Pi excretion fell after isoproterenol in the experiments of Morey and Kenny (1964) in rats. In contrast, isoproterenol had no significant effect or tended even to increase fractional excretion of Pi in dogs (Cuche *et al.*, 1976). Subsequent to the administration of phenoxybenzamine, the hypophosphaturic response to epinephrine was potentiated and quantitatively similar to that seen after isoproterenol. Consequently, the somewhat variable effects after epinephrine administration may be due to the concomitant expression of α-adrenergic and β-adrenergic activities.

After administration of norepinephrine, a consistent increase in urinary Pi excretion was found by Morey and Kenny (1964). Similarly, Cuche *et al.* (1976) found that infusion of norepinephrine in TPTX dogs decreased fractional excretion of Pi at a dose level which produced a mild increase in blood pressure without a decrease in renal hemodynamics. There was no significant change in fractional Na excretion, but since plasma Pi concentration decreased, the change in fractional Pi excretion might have been due solely to changes in the filtered load of Pi.

Dopamine elicits a phosphaturic response in dogs (Cuche *et al.*, 1976) (Table 4). After infusion of dopamine into the renal artery, an increase in fractional Pi excretion was observed both in intact and in TPTX dogs.

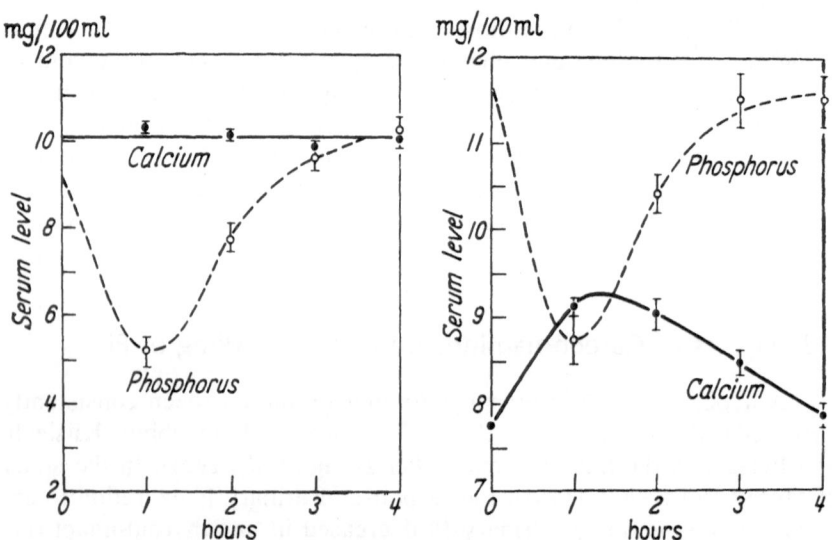

Fig. 6. Left: The effect of isoproterenol (0.5 mg/kg subcutaneously) on serum Ca and P levels in intact rats: time–response curve. The vertical bars represent the SEM. Each point represents the mean value from 9 to 13 rats. Right: The effect of isoproterenol (0.5 mg/kg subcutaneously) on serum Ca and P levels in PTX rats: time–response curve. The vertical bars represent the SEM. Each point represents the mean value from 10 to 22 rats. (From Kenny, 1964.)

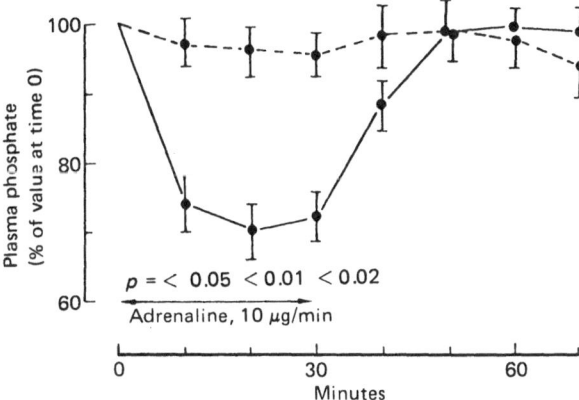

Fig. 7. Effect of propranolol on the adrenaline-induced decrease in plasma Pi. ———, adrenaline test; --------, adrenaline + propranolol test. Values of p represent the probability based on the paired t test. The vertical bars indicate the SEM of observations in six patients. (From Massara and Camanni, 1970.)

The effect of dopamine on phosphaturia could be dissociated from dopamine-induced changes in blood flow and Na excretion, since phosphaturia persisted when renal blood flow and urinary Na excretion had returned to control levels. Intrarenal infusion of the dopamine precursor dopa increased phosphaturia both in the presence and in the absence of PTH or CT.

Adrenergic nerve endings have been found in close proximity to the basolateral infoldings of the proximal tubule (Barajas, 1978). Stimulation of these nerves at frequencies which fail to affect renal hemodynamics induces antidiuresis. Denervation, on the other hand, decreases proximal tubular fluid reabsorption (DiBona, 1977). These results suggest a direct effect of catecholamines on the cells of the tubular epithelium. However, it is not known whether such effects on proximal tubular transport are related to the known phosphaturic or antiphosphaturic activities of dopamine and noradrenaline on the one hand or isoproterenol and epinephrine on the other hand.

Receptors for the various catecholamines have been demonstrated in renal tissue (Dousa and Valtin, 1976), and direct effects of catecholamines on tubular cell metabolism or tubular adenyl cyclase have been reported. Catecholamines increase gluconeogenesis from a variety of substrates in isolated tubules (Guder, 1976; Klahr et al., 1973; Kurokawa and Massry, 1973). cAMP formation and glucose production were blocked by propranolol in the study of Kurokawa and Massry (1973). However, Guder and Rupprecht (1975) concluded that catecholamine-stimulated

Table 4. Effects of Dopamine and Isoproterenol on Pi
Excretion[a,b]

FE$_{Pi}$ (%)	Plasma Pi (mM)
Dogs with intact parathyroid glands	
Group 1: Dopamine infusion (1.05 μg/kg/min) (n = 9)	
C 10.5 ± 2.2	1.95 ± 0.14
E 16.8 ± 2.7[c]	2.01 ± 0.14
PI 15.8 ± 2.1[c]	2.02 ± 0.14
Dogs with control of plasma PTH level	
Group 3: Dopamine infusion (0.88 μg/kg/min) (n = 8)	
C 17.7 ± 3.6	1.96 ± 0.08
E 24.2 ± 4.5[c]	1.93 ± 0.09
PI 23.0 ± 4.2[d]	1.92 ± 0.10
Group 4: Isoproterenol infusion (25 ng/kg/min) (n = 7)	
C 11.8 ± 4.4	1.75 ± 0.11
E 15.4 ± 4.2	1.65 ± 0.11[c]
PI 14.2 ± 5.2	1.89 ± 0.16

[a] Cuche et al. (1976).
[b] Abbreviations: FE$_{Pi}$, fractional excretion of Pi; C, E, and PI, control, experimental, and postinfusion periods, respectively.
[c] $p < 0.01$.
[d] $p < 0.05$.

gluconeogenesis was an α-adrenergic event. Catecholamines in doses that increase glucose formation lead to a decrease of PTH-stimulated cAMP formation in isolated tubules (Guder and Rupprecht, 1975). This is in contrast to previous findings of Melson et al. (1970) and Beck et al. (1972), who observed that the activation of renal cortical adenyl cyclase by PTH in vitro was not affected by propranolol, phentolamine, and epinephrine. In agreement with these latter findings, Leme et al. (1973) noted that the increment in phosphaturia with PTH was not influenced by norepinephrine, propranolol, or phentolamine. In microdissected isolated tubules, Morel et al. (1976) were unable to demonstrate activation of adenyl cyclase by isoproterenol in the proximal tubule, but found stimulation of adenyl cyclase by isoproterenol in the distal tubule and cortical collecting duct.

A dopamine-sensitive adenyl cyclase has been demonstrated in renal cortical tissue (Nakajima et al., 1974a,b). In the isolated perfused rat kidney, cAMP in the effluate increased after perfusion with dopamine, and this effect was abolished by spiroperidol, a specific antagonist to dopamine, but not by phenoxybenzamine or propranolol. In addition, dopamine increased cAMP concentrations in a rat kidney particulate preparation. It is uncertain whether such dopamine receptors and dopamine-sensitive adenyl cyclase are located in the proximal tubule.

The available evidence suggests that dopamine is phosphaturic and isoproterenol antiphosphaturic. The effects of noradrenaline on Pi excretion and tubular transport of Pi are less well defined. Catecholamines have direct effects on cAMP generation and metabolism of proximal tubules, but it remains to be shown that these effects are related to the action of these agents on tubular Pi transport.

9. GLUCOCORTICOIDS

9.1. Effects of Glucocorticoids on Serum Pi Levels

Patients with adrenocortical overfunction (Cushing's syndrome) tend to have low serum Pi levels (Gallagher *et al.*, 1973; Mills and Thomas, 1958; Nordin and Fraser, 1956; Ross *et al.*, 1966). In humans, a fall in serum Pi was noticed after acute administration of ACTH (Ingbar *et al.*, 1951) or after high doses of hydrocortisone given orally or intravenously (Anderson and Forster, 1959; Mills and Thomas, 1957; Persky *et al.*, 1955). On the other hand, Goldsmith *et al.* (1965) found that the acute infusion of supraphysiological doses of hydrocortisone had no effect on serum Pi. Also, no change in serum Pi was observed after intravenous administration of DOCA in a dose which clearly caused Na retention (Mills and Thomas, 1957).

The effect of glucocorticoids on serum Pi is observed after a latency period of more than one hour (Mills and Thomas, 1957), but the effect is then sustained for long periods of time (Wajchenberg *et al.*, 1965).

In the rat, Gemzell and Samuels (1950) observed a fall in serum Pi after administration of ACTH. Other investigators found a decrease in serum Pi after administration of cortisone (Laron *et al.*, 1957) or hydrocortisone (Williams *et al.*, 1974). The fall in serum Pi in response to cortisone was observed even in bilaterally nephrectomized rats (Thompson *et al.*, 1974), suggesting that the changes in serum Pi are mainly due to extrarenal effects of the glucocorticoids. After administration of glucocorticoids in the study of Mills and Thomas (1957), serum Pi decreased in healthy individuals without either a respiratory or metabolic alkalosis. Furthermore, Laron *et al.* (1957) observed a fall of serum Pi in PTX animals; these observations suggest that the effects of glucocorticoids on serum Pi are not mediated by changes in the acid–base state or by PTH. Cortisone does not block the hypophosphatemic response to CT. With respect to their effects on serum Pi, CT and cortisone are additive (Thompson *et al.*, 1974).

9.2. Extrarenal Effects of Glucocorticoids on Pi Metabolism

In the rat, Laron *et al.* (1957) observed increased intestinal absorption of Pi after short-term administration of cortisone, whereas Clark and Smith (1964) failed to find a change of Pi absorption in rats after short-term treatment with hydrocortisone. Caniggia and Gennari (1974) observed diminished intestinal absorption of Pi in patients on long-term steroid therapy. However, there may be differences between long- and short-term administration of glucocorticoids. Such diminution in intestinal Pi absorption parallels the well-studied decrease in intestinal absorption of Ca after glucocorticoid administration (Gallagher *et al.*, 1973; Harrison and Harrison, 1960; Kimberg *et al.*, 1971).

The fall in serum Pi after acute administration of hydrocortisone cannot be explained, at least not exclusively, by an increase in urinary Pi excretion. This is evident from the studies of Persky *et al.* (1955) and Mills and Thomas (1957) in normal subjects treated with hydrocortisone. After an acute rise, urinary Pi fell below original levels, while serum Pi levels continued to fall. Therefore, Mills and Thomas (1957) concluded that Pi was trapped intracellularly. In individuals who had been given an intravenous Pi infusion, the loss of Pi from the extracellular fluid space under the influence of cortisol could not be accounted for by the increase in urinary excretion of Pi. Such a concept finds some support in the studies of Gemzell and Samuels (1950) and Kocsis (1956); ACTH increased Pi turnover in all tissues of hypophysectomized rats, and adrenalectomy diminished significantly the uptake of radiophosphate in muscle (Gemzell and Samuels, 1950). After treatment with ACTH, increased uptake of radiophosphate into various Pi-containing fractions of the brain of normal and hypophysectomized rats was observed by Kocsis (1956). The finding of Thompson *et al.* (1974) of a fall in serum Pi in response to glucocorticoids even in nephrectomized rats also implies that loss of Pi from extracellular fluid occurs by redistribution, presumably into an intracellular compartment.

Because of such extrarenal effects, both the amount of Pi entering the extracellular fluid space (throughput) and the filtered load of Pi may change after administration of glucocorticoids.

9.3. Effects of Glucocorticoids on Renal Handling of Pi

In humans, urinary excretion of Pi increases in response to acute intravenous administration of cortisone (Anderson and Forster, 1959; Ingbar et al., 1951). Wajchenberg et al. (1965) observed a similar acute rise in urinary Pi excretion after administration of dexamethasone to normal humans. A biphasic response of urinary Pi, with an initial rise and a later fall, was found by Persky et al. (1955). In contrast, Goldsmith et al. (1965) found an acute fall in urinary Pi after intravenous infusion of hydrocortisone to normal individuals and individuals with various endocrine disorders.

In the dog (Roberts and Pitts, 1953) and in the rat (Laron et al., 1957), phosphaturia occurred after short-term administration of cortisone. Such a phosphaturic response was found both in normal and in PTX animals (Table 5). Complete starvation abolished the increment in Pi excretion, and this was attributed to high basal endogenous secretion of adrenal glucocorticoids in the fasting state (Laron et al., 1957).

In contrast to the phosphaturic response glucocorticoids, no increase in urinary Pi or fractional excretion of Pi occurred in response to DOCA. This was noted in dogs (Roberts and Pitts, 1953) as well as in humans (Mills and Thomas, 1957). In addition, Rastegar et al. (1972) failed to observe an increase in fractional Pi excretion during mineralocorticoid "escape" in humans and concluded that renal readjustment to expanding extracellular space occurred in nephron segments other than the proximal tubule, where Pi reabsorption was thought to be predominantly located.

Glucocorticoids are known to cause some increase in GFR and RPF (Gross and Möhring, 1973; Haack et al., 1977), which would cause an increase in filtered Pi and phosphaturia. However, most investigators observed a rise in urinary Pi even when serum Pi concentrations fell and concluded that glucocorticoids alter tubular handling of Pi.

A fall in C_{Pi}/C_{in} after intravenous administration of hydrocortisone was found by Goldsmith et al. (1965) and by Laidlaw et al. (1955). These investigators concluded that the decrease in C_{Pi}/GFR was due to a direct renal effect of hydrocortisone and not to inhibition of PTH or ACTH secretion, since such a decrease was demonstrable even in a patient with

Table 5. Effect of Cortisone on Serum and Urinary Pi in Starved PTX Rats[a]

	Wt. loss (%)	Serum Pi (mg/100 ml)	Urinary Pi excretion (mg/100 g wt./24 hr)	
Untreated	16.8	15.1	12	79.6
	23.8	13.0	15.6	120.0
	28.8	13.5	16.7	123.7
Treated	21.8	15.6	16.3	104.5
	20.6	13.8	13.6	98.5
	15.2	13.7	14.7	107.2

[a] Laron et al. (1957).

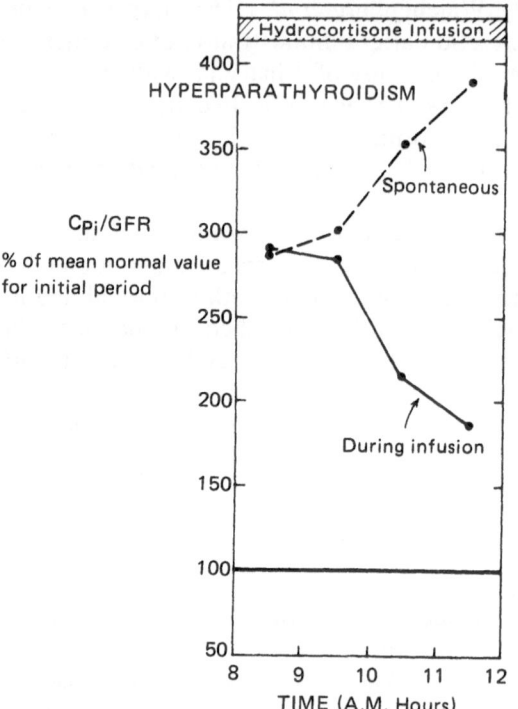

Fig. 8. Effect of hydrocortisone infusion on forenoon C_{Pi}/GFR pattern in a patient with hyperparathyroidism. (From Goldsmith *et al.*, 1965.)

hyperparathyroidism (Fig. 8) and secondary hypoadrenalism. A decrement in C_{Pi}/GFR was also observed ipsilaterally during direct infusion of hydroxycortisone into the renal artery in amounts too small to produce systemic bilateral effects (Goldsmith *et al.*, 1967). Increased C_{Pi}/C_{in} was observed by Roberts and Pitts (1953) and by Bartter (1961) after acute injection of ACTH or cortisone.

The reason for the discrepancy of results on fractional excretion of Pi is not readily apparent. Unfortunately, controlled dose–response data for glucocorticoids are not available. No information is given in some of the reports on factors that might possibly influence the phosphaturic response, for example, circadian rhythm, salt loading, dietary Pi, and parathyroid activity.

After long-term administration of glucocorticoids, Ingbar *et al.* (1951) and Thorn *et al.* (1953) found an increase in C_{Pi}/C_{in} in humans, and abnormally high urinary Pi in relation to fasting serum Pi was also found in patients on prednisolone maintenance therapy (Anderson and Forster,

1959; Gallagher *et al.*, 1973). However, in these long-term observations, secondary effects of glucocorticoids on extracellular space, PTH secretion, and vitamin D metabolism may have been present

9.4. Factors Related to the Effects of Glucocorticoids on Renal Handling of Pi

The data reported in the literature do not allow one to exclude changes in extracellular fluid space in response to glucocorticoids as being responsible for some of the observed effects on tubular Pi transport. Glucocorticoids have been shown to cause an acute increase of the extracellular fluid space; this is due to internal redistribution of Na and occurs even when a negative external Na balance is present (Haack *et al.*, 1977). Preliminary data by Relman and Schwartz (1952) showed that rigid Na restriction modified the effect of compound F acetate on excretion of Pi. In some of the clinical studies (Ingbar *et al.*, 1951), the patients were clearly volume expanded, as documented by a significant fall in hematocrit.

Glucocorticoids markedly affect net tubular hydrogen excretion and the acid–base status of the final urine (Rector, 1973). These effects have to be taken into account in the analysis of glucocorticoid effects on Pi excretion.

Long-term administration of glucocorticoids leads to a fall in serum K levels and K depletion. Renal wasting of Pi has been demonstrated in individuals with K-losing renal disease (Mahler and Stanbury, 1956), although the mechanism by which this occurs is not well defined.

Glucocorticoids have no effect on the phosphaturic response of PTH. However, a prompt and persistent stimulatory effect of glucocorticoids on PTH secretion has been demonstrated by Fucik *et al.* (1975) in humans (Fig. 9) and by Williams *et al.* (1974) in rats. Administration of cortisol causes no detectable decrease of plasma Ca in parathyroid-intact animals but causes a significant decrease of plasma Ca in PTX animals. Cortisone acetate, when given to intact rats, causes parathyroid hyperplasia and an increase in serum iPTH without a detectable change in plasma Ca. Parathyroid overactivity may be responsible, at least in part, for the hypophosphatemia observed in Cushing's syndrome (Gallagher *et al.*, 1973; Mills and Thomas, 1958; Nordin and Fraser, 1956; Ross *et al.*, 1966), and for the hypophosphatemia in renal transplant recipients maintained on glucocorticoids (David, 1977). However, the acute effects of glucocorticoids on renal handling of Pi do not depend on PTH secretion, since Laron *et al.* (1957) observed a phosphaturic response to cortisone even in PTX rats. Large doses of corticosteroids interfere with transmucosal Ca transport by mechanisms independent of the metabolism of vitamin D or of

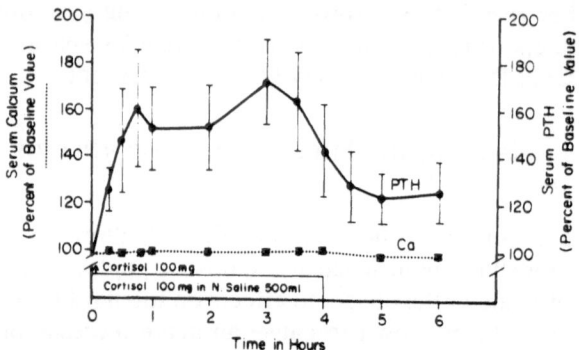

Fig. 9. Effect of cortisol infusion on serial serum Ca and PTH concentrations during the following six-hours. Values (mean ± SE) at each time period are expressed as percentages of the baseline preinfusion values (designated as 100%). Difference in PTH value from baseline: 0.5 hr, $p < 0.05$; 1, 2, 3, 3.5 hr, $p < 0.02$; other times, not significant. (From Fucik *et al.*, 1975.)

the cellular and subcellular localization of 1,25-dihydroxyvitamin D_3 on the target intestine (Kimberg *et al.*, 1971). This may contribute to the tendency to hypocalcemia and increased PTH secretion observed after administration of glucocorticoids. Such an effect of glucocorticoids on intestinal Ca transport can be clearly dissociated from stimulatory effects of glucocorticoids on renal 1α-hydroxylase (Spanos and McIntyre, 1977). These effects of glucocorticoids on PTH and vitamin D metabolism may be responsible for some of the differences between the effects of acute and chronic administration of glucocorticoids on Pi excretion.

In rat pituitary cell cultures, Kohler *et al.* (1969) found that GH synthesis was increased by physiological levels of glucocorticoids. The same was subsequently found in cultured human pituitary cells (Bridson and Kohler, 1970). However, release of GH from the pituitary may be impaired by glucocorticoids (Pecile and Müller, 1966), although other (Sakuma and Knobil, 1970) interactions between GH and glucocorticoids in various target organs have been observed (Stuart-Mason, 1972). It is not known whether such interactions also occur at the kidney and affect renal handling of Pi.

9.5. Circadian Rhythm of Pi Excretion and Glucocorticoids

There exists a marked diurnal rhythm of Pi excretion, with the troughs during the forenoon and the peaks during the afternoon and evening hours. These differences cannot be attributed to changes in GFR and can be dissociated from concomitant diurnal changes in the excretion of monovalent ions (Wesson, 1964). The changes in Pi excretion parallel those in the plasma Pi concentration. Urinary Pi excretion has been correlated with the sleep pattern (Mills and Stanbury, 1951), but a circadian rhythm persists during anesthesia (Massry *et al.*, 1973), and it is unrelated to food intake (Heaton and Hodgkinson, 1963). The role of the parathyroid glands in this phenomenon remains controversial. In hypoparathyroid patients, the circadian rhythm was found by some investigators (Lubell, 1957) to be maintained and by others (Goldsmith *et al.*, 1965) to be abolished. The rhythm persists in vitamin-D-resistant rickets (Barbour *et al.*, 1966) and in hyperparathyroidism (Goldsmith *et al.*, 1965).

Goldsmith *et al.* (1965) studied the mechanism of the forenoon phosphaturic pattern in normal subjects and in patients with various endocrine disorders. The normal pattern consisted of the excretion of a progressively increasing fraction of filtered Pi (C_{Pi}/GFR). In their study, patients with hyperparathyroidism exhibited a normal rhythm of increased amplitude, whereas patients with untreated hypoparathyroidism exhibited little or no change during the forenoon. Grossly abnormal rhythms were observed in patients with pituitary or adrenal dysfunction, whereas little variation from the normal basic rhythm was observed in patients with thyroid or testicular dysfunction. Since C_{Pi}/GFR was negatively correlated with plasma hydrocortisone concentrations, the authors concluded that the forenoon pattern of change in the fractional filtered Pi excreted was dependent upon the rhythm of plasma hydrocortisone concentration. The authors assumed that PTH, thyroid hormone, and GH set the limits within which the effect of hydrocortisone is manifested. Since other investigators failed to find a negative relation between hydrocortisone and fractional excretion of Pi (Bartter, 1961; Roberts and Pitts, 1952), the issue remains undecided.

10. ESTROGENS

10.1. Effects of Estrogens on Serum Pi Levels

Reliable data on the effect of estrogens on serum Pi or urinary handling of Pi are not available. After ovariectomy (Young and Nordin, 1967) and after natural menopause (Morgan, 1973; Young and Nordin, 1967), serum Pi levels tend to rise, but these observations could not be confirmed by other investigators (Kelley *et al.*, 1967; Szymendera and Mandajewicz, 1967). Conversely, administration of estrogens diminishes serum Pi, as observed by Albright and Reifenstein (1948), Nassim *et al.* (1956), Parfitt (1965), Young *et al.* (1968), and Recker *et al.* (1977) in studies involving mainly subjects with osteoporosis. A similar decrement in serum Pi was also observed when estrogens were given to hyperparathyroid patients (Gallagher and Wilkinson, 1973).

During pregnancy, serum Pi does not change during the first two trimesters but falls significantly during the third trimester (Tan *et al.*, 1972); this has also been attributed to the increased production of estrogens, although confirmatory evidence is lacking.

10.2. Effects of Estrogens on Extrarenal Metabolism of Pi

Estrogens have important skeletal effects, as reviewed by Rasmussen and Bordier (1974), and estrogen deficiency causes bone loss. Heany (1963) suggested a model which proposes that estrogens "set" the level of bone sensitivity to PTH. Removal of estrogens (natural or surgical menopause) should increase bone sensitivity to PTH without changing the sensitivity of its other target organs. Hence, in estrogen-deprived individuals, bone becomes a more dominant and easily accessible source of Ca to meet the needs of Ca homeostasis. The model predicts that bone remodeling will rise after menopause and that either estrogen treatment or Ca supplementation will reduce modeling. Both predictions have been confirmed in the study of Recker *et al.* (1977). The predicted decreased responsiveness of bone tissue to PTH under the influence of estrogens was directly observed in tissue culture (Orimo *et al.*, 1972). Estrogens thus cause a diminution of the net bone resorption rate. This is also suggested by the consistent decline in the urinary excretion of Ca and hydroxyproline (Riggs *et al.*, 1969). Consequently, the delivery of Ca and Pi to the extracellular fluid space is diminished. The resultant tendency for plasma Ca levels to fall causes stimulation of PTH secretion, as documented by the observation of Riggs *et al.* (1972): In osteoporotic women who had been treated with estrogens, these authors found a rise in iPTH which was inversely correlated with the fall in serum Ca.

An increase in intestinal Ca and P absorption is consistently found in pregnant women. Such maternal adjustment occurs well in advance of the time when the fetal skeleton mineralizes. This effect has been ascribed to the influence of increased estrogen secretion. However, prolonged administration of estrogens and progesterone over a seven-week period failed to increase Ca and P absorption. More recently, Heany and Skillman (1971) speculated that such maternal adjustment was due to an interaction between placental lactogen, estrogen, and PTH. It has been reported that GH and presumably also the chemically related placental lactogen stimulate renal 1α-hydroxylase and elevate circulating 1,25-dihydroxyvitamin D levels (McIntyre, 1978). This may provide a rational explanation for the changes of intestinal transport of Ca and Pi in pregnant women (Heany and Skillman, 1971).

10.3. Effects of Estrogens on Renal Handling of Pi

Estrogens have little, if any, influence on renal hemodynamics in humans, dogs, or rodents (Katz and Lindheimer, 1977).

Most studies have shown that the average urinary excretion of Pi is greater in healthy men than in healthy women at all ages. However, this is presumably not the result of a hormonal effect of estrogens, since correction for lean body mass by the use of urinary creatinine eliminates both the age and sex dependency of urinary Pi excretion rates in adults (Nordin, 1976).

Administration of estrogens decreases the urinary excretion of Pi in humans (Reifenstein et al., 1946; Young et al., 1968), probably secondary to the anabolic properties and/or to the fall in serum Pi, whereas in rats, estrogens have a phosphaturic effect (Forland, 1968), but the mechanism of this phosphaturia remains unexplained, since serum Pi, GFR, and indices of PTH secretion were not measured.

During Pi depletion, an interesting sex difference with regard to Pi balance and serum Pi levels has been reported by Dominguez et al. (1976). Female subjects had lower serum Pi levels and more markedly negative Pi balance than male individuals. It is unclear whether this is related to hormonal differences or to differences in muscle mass.

In fasting postmenopausal women, the Pi/creatinine ratio in the urine rises significantly. This was related to negative bone balance resulting from increased net bone resorption during menopause. Since there was no change in PEI, it was concluded that the rise in fasting urinary Pi was proportional to the rise in serum Pi and thus due to changes in the filtered load of Pi (Young et al., 1968). Similarly, Riggs et al. (1969) failed to observe a change in TRP after long-term administration of estrogens to osteoporotic patients. In this investigation, GFR did not change significantly, but serum Pi levels fell consistently in all individuals studied. As discussed in detail by Bijvoet (Chapter 1), PEI and TRP do not necessarily reflect the intrinsic tubular capacity to reabsorb Pi when the throughput of Pi and the filtered load of Pi change.

Several authors found normal or slightly increased urinary Pi excretion in the face of low serum Pi levels after long-term administration of estrogens and concluded that estrogens reduce net tubular reabsorption of Pi (Donaldson and Nassim, 1954; Nassim et al., 1956). Such decreased net tubular reabsorption of Pi after administration of estrogens may not necessarily be a direct effect of the hormone. The model of estrogen action on bone described above (Heany, 1963) predicts that circulating levels of PTH and 1,25-dihydroxyvitamin D_3 should be increased under the influence of estrogens. An increase in serum iPTH levels was found in the studies of Riggs et al. (1972, 1973), and decreased TRP therefore might well be secondary to changes in PTH secretion (Aitken et al., 1971; Atkins et al., 1972).

In the chicken, estrogens stimulate the renal 1α-hydroxylase (Tanaka et al., 1976). In humans, impaired production of 1,25-dihydroxyvitamin D in estrogen-deprived individuals was described by Gallagher et al. (1976), but it remains unclear how this may be related to changes in tubular handling of Pi (Chapter 7). Estrogens have potent antinatriuretic properties (Katz and Lindheimer, 1977). The magnitude of change of extracellular fluid space and its effect, if any, on tubular handling of Pi, have not been investigated.

Females usually have higher plasma GH levels during fasting, exercise, and stress than males (Frantz and Rabkin, 1965). Even a few days of estrogen therapy in men alters the GH response to stress and raises GH to the levels found in women (Merimee et al., 1966). Postmenopausal women, like men, show blunted GH responses. In view of these observations, it would appear unlikely that the effect of estrogens is mediated by GH. However, other authors found elevated GH levels in postmenopausal women (Aitken et al., 1973a) and concluded that the rise in serum Pi levels in estrogen-deprived individuals was due to the concomitant increase in circulating GH levels.

Receptors with high affinity for estrogens have been demonstrated in kidneys of various species (DeVries et al., 1972; Li et al., 1974). These estradiol–macromolecular complexes differ from those formed with aldosterone and are found both in cytosol and nuclei. These receptors may be located in the proximal tubule, where the majority of estrogen-induced ultrastructural changes have also been described (Katz and Lindheimer, 1977). DeVries et al. (1972) suggested a role for these receptors in mediating the known antinatriuretic effect of estrogens. Estrogens failed to affect Na or K excretion in acute experiments (Fimognari et al., 1967) but had Na-retaining properties when chronically administered (Johnson et al., 1972). It has not been established whether the effects of estrogens on Pi excretion are related to, or dependent upon, their antinatriuretic properties.

During pregnancy, a variety of reabsorptive functions in the proximal tubule are impaired, for example, reabsorption of glucose and amino acids (Hytten, 1976). Surprisingly, no information on tubular reabsorption of Pi during pregnancy is available, although one would anticipate that it might be decreased in parallel with reduction of net reabsorption of other substances in the proximal tubule. On the other hand, serum concentrations of human placental lactogen, which is chemically quite similar to GH, are increased in pregnancy. This hormone might increase the tubular reabsorptive capacity for Pi as does GH. This question obviously requires further clarification.

The evidence available would suggest that estrogens, at least when administered on a long-term basis, diminish net tubular reabsorption of Pi. The mechanism of this phosphaturic effect of estrogens has not been clearly analyzed, but it appears to be related to an estrogen-mediated increase in circulating PTH. The rise in circulating PTH appears to be secondary to the diminished responsiveness of bone to the action of PTH.

11. VARIOUS OTHER HORMONES

11.1. Angiotensin II

In healthy individuals, angiotensin II causes antidiuresis and antinatriuresis (Bock and Krecke, 1958). This action is independent of ADH, since it is also observed in patients with central or renal diabetes insipidus (Brodehl and Gellissen, 1966). Both changes in intrarenal hemodynamics (Gross *et al.*, 1964) and direct tubular actions of angiotensin II (Healy *et al.*, 1965) have been proposed for the effect of angiotensin II on Na and water reabsorption. Angiotensin II may have a direct action on tubular Na reabsorption which is dose dependent: At low concentrations, tubular Na reabsorption is increased, whereas at high concentrations, tubular reabsorption of Na is decreased.

The action of angiotensin II on tubular transport of Pi is controversial. Gantt and Carter (1964) described an acute antiphosphaturic action of angiotensin II in humans. This observation was confirmed by Brodehl and Gellissen (1966), who infused angiotensin II (0.02 μg/kg/min) in children and found an increase in Tm_{Pi}/GFR. Serum Pi levels and GFR did not change consistently in this study. In contrast, Gekle and von Carlowitz (1973) failed to observe consistent changes in tubular transport of Pi, measured as $(TF/P)_{Pi}/(TF/P)_{in}$, in recollection micropuncture studies of the rat. However, angiotensin II caused a consistent increase in serum Pi, and the authors concluded that the effect of angiotensin II was secondary to changes in the filtered load of Pi. In both the study of Gekle and von Carlowitz (1973) and that of Heidenreich *et al.* (1964), a rapid, transient, dose-dependent rise in serum Pi was observed. It was accompanied by a decrease of hepatic glycogen content and an increase of blood glucose. The action of angiotensin II was not due to concomitant changes in glucocorticoid secretion, since it was also observed in adrenalectomized animals, nor to changes in α-sympathetic activity or glucagon secretion, since it was also observed in animals with pharmacological α-blockade or in pancreatectomized animals. An effect on hepatic perfusion can be excluded, since it was also observed in tissue slices.

In patients with essential hypertension or renovascular hypertension, phosphaturia was observed by Heidland *et al.* (1971). This was associated with a slight decrease in plasma Pi levels and an increase in C_{Pi}/GFR. The phosphaturia was ascribed to altered tubular handling of Na in hypertensive subjects; however, it is difficult to exclude secondary hyperparathyroidism in these individuals, since RPF and GFR were slightly reduced.

11.2. "Natriuretic Hormone"

A variety of "natriuretic factors" have been described which are thought to produce natriuresis in individuals with volume expansion independent of changes in renal hemodynamics, aldosterone secretion, and ADH secretion. The physiologic role, if any, of such factors remains to be established. In a series of experiments, Bricker *et al.* (1968) isolated from the serum of uremic subjects a fraction which inhibited Na reabsorption in the proximal tubule of uremic rats, as demonstrated by recollection micropuncture studies (Weber *et al.*, 1974), and which reduced short-circuit current in the toad bladder (Favre *et al.*, 1975). The effect of this fraction on tubular Pi transport was not reported.

11.3. Prostaglandins (Bartter's Syndrome)

Bartter's syndrome is thought to be associated with excessive secretion of renal medullary prostaglandins (Verberckmoes *et al.*, 1976). No systematic studies on Pi transport in this presumed prostaglandin-excess syndrome have been reported. It is of note, however, that during indomethacin medication, Tm_{Pi}/GFR increases in Bartter's syndrome (Donker *et al.*, 1977). This finding points to an increase in proximal tubular reabsorption of Pi when excess prostaglandin secretion is inhibited. It remains undecided whether the effect is due to a direct action of prostaglandins on tubular transport of Pi or whether it is secondary to changes in proximal tubular reabsorption in response to alterations of the extracellular fluid volume.

12. TUMORAL HYPERPHOSPHATURIA

Oncogenic osteomalacia is a clinical syndrome which may be due to circulating phosphaturic factors (Aschinberg *et al.*, 1977; Drezner and Feinglos, 1977; Salassa *et al.*, 1970). Several cases of adult-onset hypophosphatemic osteomalacia made spectacular recoveries after removal of small benign sclerosing hemangiomas. In each case, the removal of the tumor was followed by an increase in the serum Pi to high normal levels and relief of clinical symptoms. Roentgenographic evidence for healing of osteomalacia was found, and iPTH levels were increased. It was speculated that such cases of adult-onset hypophosphatemic osteomalacia are related to the presence of nonendocrine tumors that elaborate a humoral substance (other than PTH) which markedly increases the renal clearance of Pi, resulting in hypophosphatemia and failure of skeletal mineralization (Salassa et al., 1970). Other than sclerosing hemangioma, such changes were found in association with giant-cell granuloma (Prader et al., 1959), osteoid tumor (McCance, 1947), cavernous hemangioma, and giant-cell tumor. Aschinberg et al. (1977) observed a similar syndrome in a boy with epidermal nevus syndrome. After excision of several fibroangiomas, all biochemical and radiological abnormalities were resolved. A homogenate of excised tissue induced excessive phosphaturia in a six-week-old puppy, again suggesting that rickets was induced by a phosphaturic substance extractable from the tumors. Drezner and Feinglos (1977) found a similar syndrome in a patient with a giant-cell neoplasm of iliac bone. Complete resolution of the biochemical abnormalities and healing of bone pathology was observed after oral administration of physiological amounts of 1,25-dihydroxyvitamin D_3. The causal role of the tumor was proved by demonstrating that resection was accompanied by roentgenographic evidence of bone healing and restoration to normal of serum Pi, Tm_{Pi}, Ca and Pi balance, aminoaciduria, and calcemic response to exogenous PTH. Severe renal Pi wasting without a measurable increase in PTH, which responded to physiological doses of 1,25-dihydroxyvitamin D_3, was interpreted as evidence of elaboration by the tumor of a factor that inhibited the synthesis of the vitamin D metabolite.

13. REFERENCES

Adams, P. H., Jowsey, J., Kelly, P. J., Riggs, B. L., Kinney, V. R., and Jones, J. D., 1967, Effects of hyperthyroidism on bone and mineral metabolism in man, *Q. J. Med.* **141**:1.

Aitken, J. M., Hart, D. M., and Smith, D. A., 1971, The effect of long-term administration on calcium and phosphorus homeostasis in oophorectomized women, *Clin. Sci.* **41**:233.

Aitken, J. M., Gallagher, M. J. D., Hart, D. M., Newton, D. A. G., and Craig, A., 1973a, Plasma growth hormone and serum phosphorus concentrations in relation to the menopause and to estrogen therapy, *J. Endocrinol.* **59**:593.

Aitken, J. M., Hart, D. M., and Lindsay, R., 1973b, Oestrogen replacement therapy for prevention of osteoporosis after oophorectomy, *Br. Med. J.* **3**:515.

Albright, F., and Reifenstein, E. C., Jr., 1948, *The Parathyroid Gland and Metabolic Bone Disease: Selected Studies* pp. 393–450, Williams and Wilkins, Baltimore.

Albright, F., Bauer, W., and Aub, J. C., 1931, Studies of calcium and phosphorus metabolism. VIII. The influence of the thyroid gland and parathyroid hormone upon the total acid–base metabolism, *J. Clin. Invest.* **10**:187.

Aldred, J. P., Stubbs, R. W., Hermann, W. R., Zeedyk, R. A., and Bastian, J. W., 1970a, Effects of porcine calcitonin on some urine electrolytes in the rat, *Acta Endocrinol. (Copenhagen)* **65**:737.

Aldred, J. P., Klezynski, R. R., and Bastian, J. W., 1970b, Effects of acute adminstration of porcine and salmon calcitonin on urine electrolyte excretion in rats, *Proc. Soc. Exp. Biol. Med.* **134**:1175.

Aldred, J. P., Klezynski, R. R., Stubbs, R. K., and Bastian, J. W., 1971, Requirement of the adrenal for certain urine electrolyte effects of salmon calcitonin in rats, *Proc. Soc. Exp. Biol. Med.* **137**:1145.

Allen, F. N., Dickson, B. R., and Markowitz, J., 1925, The relationship of phosphate and carbohydrate metabolism, *Am. J. Physiol.* **70**:333.

Altenähr, E., and Kampf, E., 1976, Parathyroid function in rats treated with growth hormone, *Virchows Arch. Pathol. Anal. Physiol.* **371**:363.

Anderson, J., and Forster, J. B., 1959, Effect of cortisone on urinary phosphate excretion in man, *Clin. Sci.* **18**:437.

Anderson, J. B., and Talmage, R. V., 1973, The effect of calcium infusion and calcitonin on plasma phosphate in sham-operated and thyroparathyroidectomized dogs, *Endocrinology* **93**:1222.

André, R., and Crabbé, J., 1966, Stimulation by insulin of active sodium transport by toadskin: Influence of aldosterone and vasopressin, *Arch. Int. Physiol. Biochem.* **74**:538.

Ardaillou, R., 1975, Kidney and calcitonin, *Nephron* **15**:250.

Ardaillou, R., Milhaud, G., Rousselet, F., Vuagnat, P., and Richet, G., 1967a, Effet de la thyrocalcitonine sur l'excrétion rénale du sodium et du chlore chez l'homme normal, *C. R. Acad. Sci.* **264**:3037.

Ardaillou, R., Vuagnet, P., Milhaud, G., and Richet, G., 1967b, Effet de la thyrocalcitonine sur l'excrétion rénale des phosphates, du calcium et des ions H^+ chez l'homme, *Nephron* **4**:298.

Ardaillou, R., Isaac, R., Nivez, M. P., Kuhn, J. M., Cazor, J. L., and Fillastre, J. P., 1976, Effect of salmon calcitonin on renal excretion of adenosine $3',5'$-monophosphate in man, *Horm. Metabl. Res.* **8**:136.

Arruda, J. A. L., Stipanuk, S., Walter, R., and Kurtzman, N. A., 1977, Effects of vasopressin administration on sodium excretion and plasma phosphate concentration, *Proc. Soc. Exp. Biol. Med.* **155**:308.

Arruda, J. A. L., Nascimento, L., and Kurtzman, N. A., 1978, Interaction of arginine vasopressin and parathyroid hormone on renal bicarbonate handling, *Miner. Electrolyte Metab.* **1**:139.

Aschinberg, L. C., Solomon, L. M., Zeis, P. M., Justice, P., and Rosenthal, I. M., 1977, Vitamin D-resistant rickets associated with epidermal nevus syndrome: Demonstration of a phosphaturic substance in the dermal lesions, *Pediatrics* **91**:56.

Atkins, D., Zanelli, J. M., Peacock, M., and Nordin, B. E. C., 1972, The effect of oestrogens on the response of bone to parathyroid hormone *in vitro*, *J. Endocrinol.* **54**:107.

Aub, J. C., Bauer, W., Heath, C., and Ropes, M., 1929, Studies of calcium and phosphorus metabolism. Effects of thyroid hormone and thyroid disease, *J. Clin. Invest.* **7**:97.

Aurbach, G. D., 1976, Hormone receptors in the kidney, in: *Membranes and Disease* (L. Bolis, J. Hoffman, and A. Leaf, eds.), pp. 241–299, Raven Press, New York.

Barajas, L., 1978, Innervation of the renal cortex, *Fed. Proc. Fed. Am. Soc. Exp. Biol.* **37**:1192.

Barbour, B. H., Kronfield, S. J., and Pawlicki, A. M., 1966, Studies on the mechanism of phosphorus excretion in vitamin D resistant rickets, *Nephron* **3**:40.

Barlet, J. P., 1972, Effect of porcine, salmon and human calcitonin on urinary excretion of some electrolytes in sheep, *J. Endocrinol.* **55**:153.

Barlet, J. P., Copp, D. H., and Robinson, C. J., 1971, Effect of porcine, salmon and human calcitonin in cows and sheep, *Horm. Metab. Res.* **3**:363.

Bartter, F. C., 1961, The effect of the parathyroid on phosphate excretion, in: *The Para-*

thyroids (R. O. Greep and R. V. Talmage, eds.), pp. 388–405, C. C. Thomas, Springfield, Ill.

Batts, A. A., Bennett, L. L., Garcia, J., and Stein, J., 1954, The effect of growth hormone on muscle potassium and on extracellular fluid, *Endocrinology* **55**:456.

Beck, J. C., McGarry, E. E., Dyrenfurth, I., and Venning, E. H., 1957, Metabolic effects of human and monkey growth hormone in man, *Science* **125**:884.

Beck, N. P., Reed, S. W., Murdaugh, H. V., and Davis, B. B., 1972, Effects of catecholamines and their interaction with other hormones on cyclic 3',5'-adenosine monophosphate of the kidney, *J. Clin. Invest.* **41**:939.

Beisel, W. R., Zerzan, C. J., Jr., Rubini, M. E., and Blythe, W. B., 1958, Phosphaturesis: A direct renal effect of triiodothyronine, *Am. J. Physiol.* **195**:357.

Belforte, L., Camanni, F., Chiodini, P. G., Liuzzi, A., Massary, F., Molinatti, G. M., Muller, E. E., and Silvestrini, F., 1977, Long-term treatment with 2-Br-alphaergocryptine in acromegaly, *Acta Endocrinol.* **85**:235.

Bijvoet, O. L. M., 1969, Relation of plasma phosphate concentration to renal tubular reabsorption of phosphate, *Clin. Sci.* **37**:23.

Bijvoet, O. L. M., 1976, The importance of the kidneys in phosphate homeostasis, in: *Phosphate Metabolism, Kidney and Bone* (L. Avioli, P. Bordier, H. Fleisch, S. Massry, and E. Slatopolsky, eds.), pp. 421–474, Nouvelle Imprimerie Fournié, Toulouse.

Bijvoet, O. L. M., and Froeling, P. C. A. M., 1973, Calcitonin, parathyroid hormone, and the kidney, in: *Clinical Aspects of Metabolic Bone Disease* (B. Frame and A. M. Parfitt, eds.), pp. 184–192, Excerpta Medica, Amsterdam.

Bijvoet, O. L. M., and Jansen, A. P., 1967, Thyrocalcitonin in Paget's disease, *Lancet* **2**:471.

Bijvoet, O. L. M., and Majoor, C. L. H., 1965, The renal tubular reabsorption of phosphate in thyrotoxicosis, *Clin. Chim. Acta* **11**:181.

Bijvoet, O. L. M., and Morgan, B., 1970, The tubular reabsorption of phosphate in man, in: *Phosphate et Métabolisme Phosphocalcique* (D. J. Hioco, ed.), pp. 153–180, Sandoz Editions, Paris.

Bijvoet, O. L. M., van der Sluys Veer, J., and Jansen, A. P., 1968, Effects of calcitonin on patients with Paget's disease, thyrotoxicosis or hypercalcemia, *Lancet* **1**:876.

Bijvoet, O. L. M., van der Sluys Veer, J., and DeVries, H. R., 1971, Natriuretic effect of calcitonin in man, *N. Engl. J. Med.* **284**:681.

Bijvoet, O. L. M., van der Sluys Veer, J., Greven, H., and Schellekens, A. M. P., 1972, Influence of calcitonin on renal excretion of sodium and calcium, in: *Parathyroid Hormone and the Calcitonin* (R. V. Talmage and P. L. Munson, eds.), pp. 284–298, Excerpta Medica, Amsterdam.

Bock, K. D., and Krecke, H.-J., 1958, Die Wirkung von synthetischem Hypertensin II auf die PAH- und Insulin-Clearance, die renale Hämodynamik und die Diurese beim Menschen, *Klin. Wochenschr.* **36**:69.

Bollinger, A., and Hartman, F. W., 1925, Curve of inorganic blood phosphates during sugar tolerance test; significance in diagnosis and prognosis, *J. Am. Med. Assoc.* **85**:653.

Bommer, J., and Ritz, E., 1974, The effect of thyroxine on renal phosphorus handling, *Eur. J. Clin. Invest.* **4**:381.

Bommer, J., Ritz, E., and Krempien, B., 1973, Bone cell metabolism in experimental hyper- and hypothyroidism, *Eur. J. Clin. Invest.* **3**:215.

Bommer, J., Ritz, E., and Schmid-Gayk, H., 1975, Serum and urinary phosphate in thyrotoxic patients. Hypoparathyroidism or hyperparathyroidism? in: *Phosphate Metabolism, Kidney and Bone* (L. Avioli, P. Bordier, H. Fleish, S. Massry, and E. Slatopolsky, eds.), pp. 413–419, Nouvelle Imprimerie Fournié, Toulouse.

Bommer, J., Ritz, E., and Gengenbach, E., 1976, Parathyroid activity in hyperthyroidism, *Calcif. Tissue Res. (Suppl)* **21**:288.

Bommer, J. Bonjour, J.-P., Ritz, E., and Fleish, H., 1979, Parathyroid-independent change in the renal handling of phosphate in hyperthyroid rats, *Kidney Int.* **15**:325.

Bonjour, J.-P., Preston, C., and Fleisch, H., 1977, Effect of 1,25-dihydroxy-vitamin D_3 on the renal handling of Pi in thyroparathyroidectomized rats, *J. Clin. Invest.* **60**:1419.

Bordier, P., Miravet, L., Matrajt, H., Hioco, D., and Ryckewaert, A., 1967, Bone changes in adult patients with abnormal thyroid function (with special reference to ^{45}Ca kinetics and quantitative histology), *Proc. R. Soc. Med.* **60**:1132.

Borle, A. B., 1969, Effects of thyrocalcitonin on calcium transport in kidney cells, *Endocrinology* **85**:194.

Borle, A. B., 1975, Regulation of cellular calcium metabolism and calcium transport by calcitonin, *J. Membr. Biol.* **21**:125.

Bortz, W., Eisenberg, E., Bowers, C. Y., and Pont, M., 1961, Differentiation between thyroid and parathyroid causes of hypercalcaemia, *Ann. Intern. Med.* **54**:610.

Boucher, B. J., 1972, The assay of human growth hormone and its clinical application, in: *Human Growth Hormone* (A. S. Mason, ed.), pp. 94–143, Heinemann, London.

Bouillon, R., and de Moor, P., 1974, Parathyroid function in patients with hyper- or hypothyroidism, *J. Clin. Endocrinol. Metab.* **38**:999.

Braumann, H., Smets, P., and Corvilain, J., 1973, Comparative study of growth hormone response to hypoglycemia in normal subjects and in patients with primary myxedema or hyperthyroidism before and after treatment, *J. Clin. Endocrinol. Metab.* **36**:1162.

Breitbarth, B., 1940, Studie über den Phosphorstoffwechsel bei der angeborenen Athyreose, *Z. Kinderheilkd.* **62**:52.

Bricker, N. S., Klahr, S., Purkerson, M., Schultze, R. G., Avioli, L. V., and Birge, S. J., 1968, *In vitro* assay for a humoral substance present during volume expansion and uremia, *Nature* **219**:1058.

Bridson, W. E., and Kohler, P. O., 1970, Cortisol stimulation of growth hormone production by human pituitary tissue in culture, *J. Clin. Endocrinol.* **30**:538.

Broadus, A. E., Kaminsky, N. I., Northcutt, R. C., Hardman, J. G., Sutherland, E. W., and Liddle, G. W., 1970, Effects of glucagon on adenosine 3',5'-monophosphate and guanosine 3',5'-monophosphate in human plasma and urine, *J. Clin. Invest.* **49**:2237.

Brodehl, J., and Gellissen, K., 1966, Der Einfluß des Angiotensins II auf die tubuläre Phosphatrückresorption beim Menschen, *Klin. Wochenschr.* **44**:1171.

Brooks, F. P., and Pickford, M., 1958, The effect of posterior pituitary hormones on the excretion of electrolytes in dogs, *J. Physiol.* **142**:486.

Buckalew, V. M., and Nelson, D. B., 1974, Natriuretic and sodium transport inhibitory activity in plasma of volume expanded dogs, *Kidney Int.* **5**:12.

Bullock, J. K., 1930, Physiologic variations in inorganic blood phosphorus content at different age periods; attempt to explain these in growing child, *Am. J. Dis. Child.* **40**:725.

Burman, K. D., Monchik, J. M., Earll, J. M., and Wartofsky, L., 1976, Ionized and total serum calcium and parathyroid hormone in hyperthyroidism, *Ann. Intern. Med.* **84**:668.

Butturini, U., and Bonomini, V., 1958, Über die Wirkung von Glukagon and Insulin auf Nierenfunktion, Harnausscheidung der Phosphat-, Bicarbonat- und Ammoniak-ionen und titrierbare Acidität beim Menschen, *Helv. Med. Acta* **5**:617.

Caniggia, A., and Gennari, C., 1974, Effect of 25-hydroxycholecalciferol (25-HCC) on intestinal absorption of ^{47}Ca in four cases of iatrogenic Cushing's syndrome, *Helv. Med. Acta* **37**:221.

Carter, D. J., and Heath, D. A., 1977, The effect of treatment of hyper- and hypothyroidism on urinary excretion of cyclic adenosine 3',5'-monophosphate, *Acta Endocrinol.* **84**:542.

Case Records of the Massachusetts General Hospital, 1975, Case 20, *N. Engl. J. Med.* **292**:1117.

Cattaneo, C., Martini, P. F., and Modica, A., 1964, The maximum tubular reabsorption of phosphate in acromegaly, *Acta Endocrinol.* **45**:203.

Chabardès, D., Imbert-Teboul, M., Montégut, M., Clique, A., and Morel, F., 1976, Distribution of calcitonin-sensitive adenylate cyclase activity along the rabbit kidney tubule, *Proc. Natl. Acad. Sci. U.S.A.* **73**:3608.

Chan, W. Y., and Sawyer, W. H., 1962, Natriuresis in conscious dogs during arginine vasopressin infusion and after oxytocin injection, *Proc. Soc. Exp. Biol. Med.* **110**:697.

Charbon, G. A., and Pieper, E. E. M., 1970, Influence of calcitonin on parathyroid hormone-induced augmentations of arterial hepatic and renal flow, in: *Proceedings of the 2nd International Symposium on Calcitonin* (S. Taylor and G. Foster, eds.), pp. 451–457, Springer, Inc., New York.

Clark, I., and Smith, M. R., 1964, Effects of parathyroidectomy and hydrocortisone on the intestinal absorption of calcium and phosphate, *Endocrinology* **74**:421.

Clark, J. D., and Kenny, A. D., 1969, Hog thyrocalcitonin in the dog. Urinary calcium, phosphorus, magnesium and sodium responses, *Endocrinology* **84**:1199.

Clerkin, E. P., Haas, H. G., Mintz, D. H., Meloni, C. R., and Canary, J. J., 1964, Osteomalacia in thyrotoxicosis, *Metabolism* **13**:161.

Cochran, M., Peacock, M., Sachs, G., and Nordin, B. E. C., 1970, Renal effects of calcitonin, *Br. Med. J.* **1**:135.

Cohen, J. J., Gregg, C. M., and Black, A. J., 1977, Glucose dependent effects of insulin on renal function and metabolism in the isolated perfused rat kidney, *Hoppe-Seyler's Z. Physiol. Chem.* **358**:1391.

Connors, M. H., Kaplan, S. L., Li, C. H., and Grumbach, M. M., 1973, Retention of biologic activity of human growth hormone in man after reduction and alkylation, *J. Clin. Endocrinol. Metab.* **37**:499.

Copp, D. H., 1973, Calcitonin physiology: Hormonal effects, in: *Peptide Hormones* (S. A. Berson and R. S. Yalow, eds.), p. 999, American Elsevier Publishing Company, New York.

Cori, C. F., and Cori, G. T., 1931, The influence of epinephrine and insulin injections on hexosephosphate content of muscle, *J. Biol. Chem.* **94**:581.

Corvilain, J., and Abramow, M., 1962, Some effects of human growth hormone on renal hemodynamics and on tubular phosphate transport in man, *J. Clin. Invest.* **41**:1230.

Corvilain, J., and Abramow, M., 1964, Effect of growth hormone on tubular transport of phosphate in normal and parathyroidectomized dogs, *J. Clin. Invest.* **43**:1608.

Corvilain, J., and Abramow, M., 1972, Growth and renal control of plasma phosphate, *J. Clin. Endocrinol.* **34**:452.

Courvoisier, B., DeBarros, Q., Jacot, C., and Zender, R., 1970, Effets aigus de la calcitonine porcine chez l'homme sans ostéopathie et dans la maladie de Paget, *Schweiz. Med. Wochenschr.* **100**:26.

Cuche, J. L., Marchand, G. R., Greger, R. F., Lang, F. C., and Knox, F. G., 1976, Phosphaturic effect of dopamine in dogs, *J. Clin. Invest.* **58**:71.

David, S. D., 1977, Mineral and bone homeostasis in renal failure: Pathophysiology and management, in: *Calcium Metabolism in Renal Failure and Nephrolithiasis* (S. D. David, ed.), pp. 1–76, John Wiley and Sons, New York.

Davis, J. O., Howell, D. S., Laqueur, G. L., and Peirce, E. C., 1954, II. Renal hemodynamic function, electrolyte metabolism and water exchange in adrenalectomized hypophysectomized dogs, *Am. J. Physiol.* **176**:411.

DeFronzo, R. A., Cooke, R. C., Andres, R., Faloona, G. R., and Davis, P. J., 1975, The effect of insulin on renal handling of sodium, potassium, calcium and phosphate in man, *J. Clin. Invest.* **55**:845.

DeVries, J. R., Ludens, J. H., and Fanestil, D. D., 1972, Estradiol renal receptor molecules and estradiol-dependent antinatriuresis, *Kidney Int.* **2**:95.

DiBona, G. F., 1977, Neurogenic regulation of renal tubular sodium reabsorption, *Am. J. Physiol.* **233**:73.

Dominguez, J. H., Gray, R. W., and Lehmann, J., 1976, Dietary phosphate deprivation in women and men: Effects on mineral and acid base balances, parathyroid hormone and the metabolism of 25-OH-vitamin D, *J. Clin. Endocrinol. Metab.* **43**:1056.

Donaldson, J. A., and Nassim, J. R., 1954, The artificial menopause with particular reference to the occurrence of spinal osteoporosis, *Br. Med. J.* **1**:1228.

Donker, A. J. M., de Jong, P. E., Statius van Eps, L. W., Brentjens, J. R. H., Bakker, H., and Doorenbos, H., 1977, Indomethacin in Bartter's syndrome, *Nephron* **19**:200.

Dousa, T. P., 1974, Effects of hormones on cyclic AMP formation in kidneys of nonmammalian vertebrates, *Am. J. Physiol.* **226**:1193.

Dousa, T. P., and Valtin, H., 1976, Cellular action of vasopressin in the mammalian kidney, *Kidney Int.* **10**:46.

Dreyfus, C. F., Gershon, M. D., Haymovits, A., and Nunez, E., 1976, Calcitonin: Antagonism at intestinal muscarinic receptors, *Br. J. Pharmacol.* **57**:155.

Drezner, M. K., and Feinglos, M. N., 1977, Osteomalacia due to 1-alpha-25-dihydroxycholecalciferol deficiency. Association with a giant cell tumor of bone, *J. Clin. Invest.* **60**:1046.

Durand, D., Prélot, M., and Raoul, Y., 1976, Effets précoces de l'hormone de croissance sur les phosphates sériques et urinaires du rat, *Experientia* **32**:120.

Eggleton, M. G., and Shuster, S., 1954, The effect of insulin on the excretion of glucose and phosphate by the kidney of the rat, *J. Physiol.* **124**:623.

Eisinger, A. J., Jones, N. F., Barraclough, M. A., and McSwiney, R. R., 1970a, Effect of vasopressin on the renal excretion of phosphate in man, *Clin. Sci.* **39**:687.

Eisinger, A. J., Jones, N. F., Barraclough, M. A., and McSwiney, R. R., 1970b, Effect of vasopressin on renal excretion of phosphate in normal man, *Nephron* **7**:92.

Ellis, S., 1956, The metabolic effects of epinephrine and related amines, *Pharmacol. Rev.* **8**:485.

Elrick, H., Huffman, E. R., Hlad, C. J., Whipple, N., and Staub, A., 1958, Effects of glucagon on renal function in man, *J. Clin. Endocrinol. Metab.* **18**:813.

Favre, H., Hwang, K. H., Schmidt, R. W., Bricker, N. S., and Bourgoignie, J. J., 1975, An inhibitor of sodium transport in the urine of dogs with normal renal function, *J. Clin. Invest.* **56**:1302.

Fimognari, G. M., Fanestil, D. D., and Edelman, I. S., 1967, Induction of RNA and protein synthesis in the action of aldosterone in the rat, *Am. J. Physiol.* **213**:954.

Fischer, J. A., Blum, J. W., and Binswanger, U., 1973, Acute parathyroid hormone response to epinephrine *in vivo*, *J. Clin. Invest.* **52**:2434.

Forland, M., 1968, Effect of estradiol on phosphorus excretion in intact and hypophysectomized rats, *Endocrinology* **83**:516.

Foster, G. V., Joplin, G. F., McIntyre, I., Melvin, K. E. M., and Slack, E., 1966, Effect of thyrocalcitonin in man, *Lancet* **1**:107.

Franke, H., Gronow, G., and Peterson, K., 1977, Glucagon induced functional changes of isolated perfused kidneys, *Hoppe-Seyler's Z. Physiol. Chem.* **358**:1391.

Frantz, A. G., and Rabkin, M. T., 1965, Effects of estrogen and sex difference on secretion of human growth hormone, *J. Clin. Endocrinol.* **25**:1470.

Fraser, R., and Harrison, M., 1960, The effect of growth hormone on urinary calcium secretion, *Ciba Found. Colloq. Endocrinol. (Proc.)* **13**:135.

Friedland, J. A., Williams, G. A., Bowser, E. N., Henderson, W. J., and Hopfeins, E.,

1965, Effect of hyperthyroidism on intestinal absorption of calcium in the rat, *Proc. Soc. Exp. Biol. Med.* **120**:20.

Friedman, J., and Raisz, L. G., 1965, Thyrocalcitonin: Inhibitor of bone resorption in tissue culture, *Science* **150**:1465.

Frick, A., 1968, Reabsorption of inorganic phosphate in the rat kidney, *Pflügers Arch. Gesamte Physiol. Menschen Tiere* **304**:351.

Frizel, D., Malleson, A., and Marks, V., 1967, Plasma levels of ionized calcium and magnesium in thyroid disease, *Lancet* **1**:1360.

Fucik, R. F., Kukreja, S. C., Hargis, G. K., Bowser, E. N., Henderson, W. J., and Williams, G. A., 1975, Effect of glucocorticoids on function of the parathyroid glands in man, *J. Clin. Endocrinol. Metab.* **40**:152.

Gallagher, J. C., and Wilkinson, R., 1973, The effect of ethinyloestradiol on calcium and phosphorus metabolism of post-menopausal women with primary hyperparathyroidism, *Clin. Sci.* **45**:785.

Gallagher, J. C., Aaron, J., Horsman, A., Wilkinson, R., and Nordin, B. E. C., 1973, Corticosteroid osteoporosis, *J. Clin. Endocrinol. Metab.* **2**:355.

Gallagher, J. C., Riggs, B. L., Eisman, J., Arnaud, S. B., and DeLuca, H. F., 1976, Impaired production of 1,25-dihydroxy-vitamin D in post-menopausal osteoporosis, *Clin. Res.* **24**:580A (Abstract).

Gantt, C. L., and Carter, W. J., 1964, Acute effects of angiotensin on calcium, phosphorus, magnesium and potassium excretion, *Can. Med. Assoc. J.* **90**:287.

Gekle, D., 1972, Der Einfluß von synthetischem Calcitonin auf die proximal-tubuläre Phosphatresorption, *Klin. Wochenschr.* **50**:527.

Gekle, D., and von Carlowitz, B., 1973, Micropuncture investigations on the effect of angiotensin on the inorganic phosphate reabsorption in the proximal tubule of the rat, *Pflügers Arch.* **342**:73.

Gellissen, K., and Brodehl, J., 1965, Clearance-Untersuchungen bei Säuglingen mit angeborene Athyreosen, *Klin. Wochenschr.* **43**:1063.

Gemzell, C. A., and Samuels, L. T., 1950, The effect of hypophysectomy, adrenalectomy and of ACTH administration on the phosphorus metabolism of rats, *Endocrinology* **47**:48.

Gershberg, H., 1960, Metabolic and renotropic effects of human growth hormone in disease, *J. Clin. Endocrinol. Metab.* **20**:1107.

Gershberg, H., and Gash, J., 1956, Effect of growth hormone on sulfate Tm, urea clearance and fasting blood glucose, *Proc. Soc. Exp. Biol. Med.* **91**:46.

Gershberg, H., and Hecht, A., 1957, Growth hormone secretion during acute hypocalcemia—a non-specific response to stress, in: *Proceedings of the 52nd Meeting of the Endocrine Society*, June, 1957, St. Louis, Mo., (Abstract).

Gill, J. R., Casper, A. G. T., Jr., and Tate, J., 1971, Renal effects of adenosine 3',5'-cyclic monophosphate and dibutyryl adenosine 3',5'-cyclic monophosphate, *J. Clin. Invest.* **50**:1231.

Goldsmith, R. S., Siemsen, A. W., Mason, A. D., Jr., and Forland, M., 1965, Primary role of plasma hydrocortisone concentration in the regulation of the normal forenoon pattern of urinary phosphate excretion, *J. Clin. Endocrinol.* **25**:1649.

Greenwood, F. C., Hunter, W. M., and Marrian, V. J., 1964, Growth-hormone levels in children and adolescents, *Br. Med. J.* **1**:25.

Grehn, S., Seybold, K., Reiners, C., Borner, W., and Moll, E., 1973, Veränderungen der Skelettmineralisation durch Schilddrüsenerkrankungen. Messungen der Knochendichte und -dicke mit einem ^{125}I-Profilscanner, *Med. Klin. (Munich)* **68**:306.

Gross, F., and Möhring, J., 1973, Renal pharmacology, with special emphasis on aldosterone and angiotensin, *Annu. Rev. Pharmacol.* **13**:57.

Gross, F., Schaechtelin, G., Brunner, H., and Peters, G., 1964, The role of renin–angiotensin system in blood pressure regulation and kidney function, *Can. Med. Assoc. J.* **90**:258.

Guder, W. G., 1976, Hormonal regulation of renal gluconeogenesis in isolated tubule fragments, in: *Current Problems in Clinical Biochemistry: 6. Renal Metabolism in Relation to Renal Function* (U. Schmidt and U. C. Dubach, eds.), pp. 202–213, Hans Huber, Bern.

Guder, W. G., and Rupprecht, A., 1975, Metabolism of isolated kidney tubules. Independent actions of catecholamines on renal cyclic adenosine $3',5'$-monophosphate levels and gluconeogenesis, *Eur. J. Biochem.* **52**:283.

Haack, D., Möhring, J., Möhring, B., Petri, M., and Hackenthal, E., 1977, Comparative study on development of corticosterone and DOCA hypertension in rats, *Am. J. Physiol.* **233**:F403.

Haas, H. G., and Dambacher, M. A., 1968, Thyrocalcitonin effects in man, *Helv. Med. Acta* **34**:327.

Haas, H. G., Dambacher, M. A., Guncaga, J., and Lauffenburger, T., 1971, Renal effects of calcitonin and parathyroid extract in man, *J. Clin. Invest.* **50**:2689.

Haddad, J. G., Jr., Birge, S. J., and Avioli, L. V., 1970, Effects of prolonged thyrocalcitonin administration on Paget's disease of bone, *N. Engl. J. Med.* **283**:549.

Hamilton, C. R., 1970, Effects of synthetic salmon calcitonin in patients with Paget's disease of bone, *Am. J. Med.* **56**:315.

Harden, R. McG., Harrison, M. T., Alexander, W. D., and Nordin, B. E. C., 1964, Phosphate excretion and parathyroid function in thyrotoxicosis, *J. Endocrinol.* **28**:281.

Harrell, A., Bindermann, I., and Rodan, G. A., 1973, The effect of calcium concentration on calcium uptake by bone cells treated with thyrocalcitonin (TCT) hormone, *Endocrinology* **92**:550.

Harrison, H. E., and Harrison, H. C., 1960, Transfer of Ca^{45} across intestinal wall *in vitro* in relation to action of vitamin D and cortisol, *Am. J. Physiol.* **199**:265.

Harrop, G. A., Jr., and Benedict, E. M., 1923, The role of phosphate and potassium in carbohydrate metabolism following insulin administration, *Proc. Soc. Exp. Biol. N.Y.* **20**:430.

Harrop, G. A., Jr., and Benedict, E. M., 1924, The participation of inorganic substances in carbohydrate metabolism, *J. Biol. Chem.* **59**:683.

Healy, J. K., Barcena, C., and Schreiner, G. E., 1965, Effect of angiotensin on maximal tubular transport of PAH and glucose in dogs, *Am. J. Physiol.* **209**:651.

Heany, R. P., 1963, Evaluation and interpretation of calcium-kinetic data in man, *Clin. Ortop.* **31**:153.

Heany, R. P., and Skillman, T. G., 1971, Calcium metabolism in normal human pregnancy, *J. Clin. Endocrinol. Metab.* **33**:661.

Heaton, F. W., and Hodgkinson, A., 1963, External factors affecting diurnal variation in electrolyte excretion with particular reference to calcium and magnesium, *Clin. Chim. Acta* **8**:246.

Heersche, J. N. M., Marcus, R., and Aurbach, D. G., 1974, Calcitonin and the formation of $3',5'$-AMP in bone and kidney, *Endocrinology* **94**:241.

Heidenreich, O., Kook, Y., Baumeister, L., and Reus, E., 1964, Stoffwechselwirkungen von synthetischem Angiotensin II, *Arch. Int. Pharmacodyn.* **148**:309.

Heidland, A., Hennemann, R., Hensler, R., Heidbreder, E., and Gekle, D., 1971, Untersuchungen zur Pathophysiologie der renalen Phosphatxkretion bei essentieller und renovasculärer Hypertonie, Pyelonephritis und Glomerulonephritis, *Klin. Wochenschr.* **49**:1121.

Henneman, P. H., Forbes, A. P., Moldawer, M., Dempsey, E. F., and Carroll, E. L., 1960, Effects of human growth hormone in man, *J. Clin. Invest.* **39**:1223.

Herrera, F. C., Whittembury, G., and Planchart, A., 1963, Effect of insulin on short-circuit current across isolated frog skin in the presence of calcium and magnesium, *Biochim. Biophys. Acta* **66**:170.

Hevesy, G., and DalSanto, G., 1954, Effect of adrenalin on the interaction between plasma and tissue constituents, *Acta Physiol. Scand.* **32**:339.

Hirsch, P. F., Sliwowski, A., Orimo, H., Darago, L. S., and Mewborn, Q. A., Jr., 1973, On the mode of the hypocalcemic action of thyrocalcitonin and its enhancement of phosphate in rats, *Endocrinology* **93**:12.

Humphreys, M. H., Freidler, R. M., and Earley, L. E., 1970, Natriuresis produced by vasopressin or hemorrhage during water diuresis in the dog, *Am. J. Physiol.* **219**:658.

Hytten, F. E., 1976, Renal physiology in normal pregnancy, in: *The Kidney in Pregnancy* (R. R. de Alvarez, ed.), pp. 23–45, John Wiley and Sons, New York.

Ichikawa, I., and Brenner, B. M., 1977, Evidence for glomerular actions of ADH and dibutyryl cyclic AMP in rat, *Am. J. Physiol.* **233**:102.

Ikkos, D., Luft, R., and Gemzell, C. A., 1959, The effect of human growth hormone in man, *Acta Endocrinol.* **32**:341.

Indech, M., and Jowsey, J., 1971, Secondary hyperparathyroidism produced in kittens repeatedly given porcine calcitonin, *Endocrinology* **88**:1489.

Ingbar, S. H., Kass, E. H., Burnett, C. H., Relman, A. S., Burrows, B. A., and Sisson, J. H., 1951, The effects of ACTH and cortisone on the renal tubular transport of uric acid, phosphorus, and electrolytes in patients with normal renal and adrenal function, *J. Lab. Clin. Med.* **38**:533.

Ismail-Beigi, F., and Edelman, J. S., 1971, The mechanism of the calorigenic action of the thyroid hormone. Stimulation of $Na^+ + K^+$ activated adenosine triphosphatase activity, *J. Gen. Physiol.* **57**:710.

Johnson, J. A., Davis, J. O., Brown, P. R., Wheeler, P. D., and Witty, R. T., 1972, Effects of estradiol on sodium and potassium balances in adrenalectomized dogs, *Am. J. Physiol.* **233**:194.

Jones, J. E., Desper, P. C., Shane, S. R., and Flink, E. B., 1966, Magnesium metabolism in hyperthyroidism and hypothyroidism, *J. Clin. Invest.* **45**:891.

Juan, D., Liptak, P., and Gray, T. K., 1976, Absorption of inorganic phosphate in the human jejunum and its inhibition by salmon calcitonin, *J. Clin. Endocrinol. Metab.* **43**:517.

Katz, A. I., and Lindheimer, M. D., 1973, Renal sodium- and potassium-activated adenosine triphosphatase and sodium reabsorption in the hypothyroid rat, *J. Clin. Invest.* **52**:796.

Katz, A. I., and Lindheimer, M. D., 1977, Actions of hormones on the kidney, *Annu. Rev. Physiol.* **39**:97.

Katz, A. I., Emmanouel, D. S., and Lindheimer, M. D., 1975, Thyroid hormone and the kidney, *Nephron* **15**:223.

Keating, F. R., Jones, J. D., Elveback, L. R., and Randall, R. V., 1969, The relation of age and sex to distribution of values in healthy adults of serum calcium, inorganic phosphorus, magnesium, alkaline phosphatase, total proteins, albumin and blood urea, *J. Lab. Clin. Med.* **73**:825.

Kelly, P., Jowsey, J., Riggs, B. L., and Elveback, L. R., 1967, Relationship between serum phosphate concentration and bone resorption in osteoporosis, *J. Lab. Clin. Med.* **69**:110.

Kenny, A. D., 1964, Effect of catecholamines on serum calcium and phosphorus levels in intact and parathyroidectomized rats, *Naunyn-Schmiedeberg's Arch. Exp. Pathol. Pharmakol.* **248**:144.

Kenny, A. D., and Heiskell, C. A., 1965, Effect of crude thyrocalcitonin on calcium and phosphorus metabolism in rats, *Proc. Soc. Exp. Biol. Med.* **120**:269.

Kikuyama, S., Nagasawa, H., Yanai, R., and Yamanouchi, K., 1974, Effect of perinatal hypothyroidism on pituitary secretion of growth hormone and prolactin in rats, *J. Endocrinol.* **62**:213.

Kimberg, D. V., Baerg, R. D., Gershon, E., and Graudusius, R. T., 1970, Effect of cortisone treatment on the active transport of calcium by the small intestine, *J. Clin. Invest.* **50**:1309.

Kivirikko, K. I., Laitinen, O., and Lamberg, B. A., 1965, Value of urine and serum hydroxyproline in the diagnosis of thyroid disease, *J. Clin. Endocrinol.* **25**:1347.

Klahr, S., Nawar, T., and Schoolwerth, A. C., 1973, Effects of catecholamines on ammoniagenesis and gluconeogenesis by renal cortex *in vitro*, *Biochim. Biophys. Acta* **304**:161.

Klisiechi, A., and Pytasz, M., 1961, Über die Rolle einiger Neurohormone auf die renale Phosphatausscheidung, *Helv. Physiol. Pharmacol. Acta* **58**:81.

Kocsis, J. J., 1956, Uptake of P^{32} into various phosphorus-containing fractions in the brain of normal, hypophysecomized and ACTH-treated hypophysectomized rats, *Endocrinology* **59**:591.

Kohler, P. C., Frohman, L. A., Bridson, W. E., Vanha-Pertula, T., and Hammond, J. M., 1969, Cortisone induction of growth hormone synthesis in a clonal line of rat pituitary tumor cells in culture, *Science* **166**:633.

Krane, S. M., 1971, in: *The Thyroid* (S. C. Werner and S. H. Ingbar, eds.), pp. 598–615, Harper and Row, New York.

Kukreja, S. C., Hargis, G. K., Bowser, N. E., Henderson, W. J., Fisherman, E. W., and Williams, G. A., 1975, Role of adrenergic stimuli in parathyroid hormone secretion in man, *J. Clin. Endocrinol. Metab.* **40**:478.

Kurokawa, K., and Massry, S. G., 1973, Evidence for stimulation of renal gluconeogenesis by catecholamines, *J. Clin. Invest.* **52**:961.

Kurokawa, K., Nagata, N., Sasaki, M., and Nakane, K., 1974, Effects of calcitonin on the concentration of cyclic adenosine 3',5'-monophosphate in rat kidney *in vivo* and *in vitro*, *Endocrinology* **94**:1514.

Kurtzman, N. A., Rogers, W. P., Boonjarern, S., and Arruda, J. A. L., 1975, The effect of infusion of pharmacologic amounts of vasopressin on renal electrolyte excretion, *Am. J. Physiol.* **228**:890.

Laidlaw, J. C., Dingman, J. F., Arons, W. L., Finkenstaedt, J. T., and Thorn, G. W., 1955, Comparison of metabolic effects of cortisone and hydrocortisone in man, *Ann. N.Y. Acad. Sci.* **61**:315.

Langer, B., Peytremann, A., Ruffener, C., and Jenny, M., 1971, Effets comparés de l'administration d'une dose unique de calcitonine synthétique (de type humaine et de type saumon) chez l'homme normal et les sujets atteints de la maladie de Paget ou d'hypercalcémie, *Schweiz. Med. Wochenschr.* **101**:69.

Laron, Z., Crawford, J. D., and Klein, R., 1957, Phosphaturic effect of cortisone in normal and parathyroidectomized rats, *Proc. Soc. Exp. Biol. Med.* **96**:649.

Laron, Z., Pertzelan, A., and Karp, M., 1968, Pituitary dwarfism with high serum levels of growth hormone, *Isr. J. Med. Sci.* **4**:883.

Le Grimellec, C., and Lechêne, C., 1970, Renal effects of thyroid calcium infusion in parathyroidectomized rats: Electron probe analysis, in: *Proceedings of the 4th Annual Meeting of the American Society of Nephrology*, p. 90 (Abstract).

Leme, C. E., Liberman, B., and Wajchenberg, B. L., 1973, Effect of norepinephrine, propranolol and phentolamine on the phosphaturic action of bovine parathyroid extract in man, *Nephron* **11**:365.

Lerner, R. L., and Kurokawa, K., 1977, Binding and degradation of insulin by isolated rat renal cortical tubules, *Clin. Res.* (Abstract).

Levy, M., and Starr, N. L., 1972, The mechanism of glucagon-induced natriuresis in dogs, *Kidney Int.* **2**:76.

Li, J. J., Talley, D. J., Li, S. A., and Villee, C. A., 1974, An estrogen binding protein in the renal cytosol of intact, castrated and estrogenized golden hamsters, *Endocrinology* **95**:1134.

Loreau, N., Lepreux, C., and Ardaillou, R., 1975, Calcitonin-sensitive adenylate cyclase in rat renal tubular membranes, *Biochem. J.* **150**:305.

Loreau, N., Cosyns, J.-P., Lepreux, C., Verroust, P., and Ardaillou, R., 1977, Renal calcitonin receptors and adenylate cyclase in rats immunized against tubular basement membrane, *Kidney Int.* **12**:184.

Lubell, D., 1957, The spontaneous diurnal variation of urinary phosphate excretion and its relation to the parathyroid hormone test, *Helv. Paediatr. Acta* **12**:179.

Luft, R., and Cerasi, E., 1967, Human growth hormone as a regulator of blood glucose concentration and as a diabetogenic substance, *Acta Endocrinol. (Copenhagen) Suppl.* **124**:9.

Luft, R., and Cerasi, E., 1968, Human growth hormone in blood glucose homeostasis, in: *Growth Hormone* (A. Pecile and E. E. Müller, eds.), p. 373, Excerpta Medica, Amsterdam.

Mahler, R. F., and Stanbury, S. W., 1956, Potassium losing renal disease. Renal and metabolic observations on a patient sustaining renal wastage of potassium, *Q. J. Med.* **25**:21.

Malamos, B., Sfikakis, P., and Pandos, P., 1969, The renal handling of phosphate in thyroid disease, *J. Endocrinol.* **45**:269.

Mandel, A. R., and Lusk, G., 1904, Stoffwechselbeobachtungen an einem Falle von Diabetes mellitus mit besonderer Berücksichtigung der Prognose, *Dtsch. Arch Klin. Med.* **8**:472.

Martin, T. J., and Melick, R. A., 1969, The acute effects of porcine calcitonin in man, *Aust. Ann. Med.* **18**:258.

Martinez-Maldonado, M., Eknoyan, G., and Suki, W. N., 1971, Natriuretic effects of vasopressin and cyclic AMP: Possible site of action in the nephron, *Am. J. Physiol.* **220**:2013.

Marx, S. J., and Aurbach, G. D., 1975, Renal receptors for calcitonin: Coordinate occurrence with calcitonin-activated adenylate cyclase, *Endocrinology* **97**:448.

Marx, S. J., Woodard, C. J., and Aurbach, G., 1972, Calcitonin receptors of kidney and bone, *Science* **178**:999.

Massara, F., and Camanni, F., 1970, Propranolol block of adrenalin-induced hypophosphataemia in man, *Clin. Sci.* **38**:245.

Massry, S. G., Coburn, J. W., and Kleeman, C. R., 1969, The influence of extracellular volume expansion on renal phosphate reabsorption in the dog, *J. Clin. Invest.* **48**:1237.

Massry, S. G., Coburn, J. W., and Kleeman, C. R., 1970, Evidence for suppression of parathyroid gland by hypermagnesemia, *J. Clin. Invest.* **49**:161.

Moraczewski, W. V., 1897, Stoffwechselversuch bei Diabetes Mellitus, *Zentralbl. Inn. Med.* **36**:921.

Mazzuoli, G. F., Coen, G., and Antonozzi, I., 1967, Longterm observation of the effect of thyroidectomy in patients with elevated thyroid thyrocalcitonin content, in: *Calcitonin. Proceedings of the Symposium on Thyrocalcitonin and the C Cells* (S. Taylor, ed.), pp. 364–372, Heinemann, London.

McCance, R. A., 1947, Osteomalacia with Looser's nodes (Milkman's syndrome) due to a raised resistance to vitamin D acquired about the age of 15 years, *Q. J. Med.* **16**:33.

McIntyre, I., 1978, Le rôle du rein dans le métabolisme de la vitamine D, in: *Actualités néphrologiques de l'hôpital Necker* (J. Hamburger, J. Crosnier, and J. L. Funck-Brentano, eds.), pp. 151–161, Flammarion Medicine–Sciences, Paris.

Meema, H. E., and Schatz, D. L., 1970, Simple radiologic demonstration of cortical bone loss in thyrotoxicosis, *Radiology* **97**:9.

Melson, G. L., Chase, L. R., and Aurbach, G. D., 1970, Parathyroid hormone-sensitive adenyl cyclase in isolated renal tubules, *Endocrinology* **86**:511.

Melvin, K. E. M., and Tashjian, A. H., Jr., 1968, The syndrome of excessive thyrocalcitonin produced by medullary carcinoma of the thyroid, *Proc. Natl. Acad. Sci. U.S.A.* **59**:1216.

Merimee, T. J., Burgess, J. A., and Rabinowitz, D., 1966, Sex determined hormone responses to amino acid stimulation, *J. Clin. Endocrinol.* **26**:79.

Meunier, P. J., Bianchi, G. G. S., Edouard, C. M., Bernard, J. C., Courpron, P., and Vignon, G. E., 1972, Bony manifestations of thyrotoxicosis, *Orthop. Clin. North Am.* **3**:745.

Meyer, R. A., Jr., and Meyer, M. H., 1975, Thyrocalcitonin injection to rats increases the liver inorganic phosphate, *Endocrinology* **96**:1048.

Milhaud, G., and Mouhktar, M. S., 1966, Antagonistic and synergistic actions of thyrocalcitonin and parathyroid hormone on the levels of calcium and phosphate in the rat, *Nature (London)* **211**:1186.

Milhaud, G., Mouhktar, M. S., Cherian, G., and Perault, A. M., 1966, Effect de l'administration de thyrocalcitonine sur les principaux paramètres du métabolisme du calcium du rat normal et du rat thyroparathyroïdectomisé, *C. R. Acad. Sci.* **262**:511.

Milhaud, G., Mouhktar, M. S., Perault-Staub, A. M., Coutres, G., Ardaillou, R., Bloch-Michel, H., Garel, J. M., Klingler, E., Tubiana, M., and Sizonenko, P. C., 1970, Studies in thyrocalcitonin, in: *Proceedings of the 2nd International Symposium on Calcitonin* (S. Taylor and G. Foster, eds.), pp. 182–184, Springer, New York.

Mills, J. N., and Stanbury, S. W., 1951, Intrinsic diurnal rhythm in urinary electrolyte output, *J. Physiol.* **115**:18.

Mills, J. N., and Thomas, S., 1957, The acute effect of adrenal hormones and carbohydrate metabolism upon plasma phosphate and potassium concentrations in man, *J. Endocrinol.* **16**:164.

Mills, J. N., and Thomas, S., 1958, Acute effects of cortisone and cortisol upon renal function in man, *J. Endocrinol.* **17**:41.

Morel, F., Imbert, M., and Chabardès, D., 1976, Measurement of hormone dependent adenylate cyclase activity in single pieces of rabbit kidney tubules, in: *Current Problems in Clinical Biochemistry: 6. Renal Metabolism in Relation to Renal Function* (U. Schmidt and U. C. Dubach, eds.), pp. 214–222, Hans Huber, Bern.

Morel, F., Chabardès, D., and Imbert-Teboul, M., 1978, Heterogeneity of hormonal control in the distal nephron, in: *Proceedings of the 8th International Congress of Nephrology*, (R. Barcelo, M. Bergeron, S. Carrière, J. H. Dirks, K. Drummond, R. D. Guttmann, G. Lemieux, J.-G. Mongeau, and J. F. Seely, eds.), pp. 209–218, Karger, Basel.

Morey, E. R., and Kenny, A. D., 1964, Effects of catecholamines on urinary calcium and phosphorus in intact and parathyroidectomized rats, *Endocrinology* **75**:18.

Morgan, D. B., 1973, *Osteomalacia, Renal Osteodystrophy and Osteoporosis*, C. C. Thomas, Springfield, Ill.

Mosekilde, L., Melson, F., Bagger, J. P., Myhre-Jensen, O., and Schartz-Sørensen, N., 1977, Bone changes in hyperthyroidism: Interrelationships between bone morphometry, thyroid function and calcium–phosphorus metabolism, *Acta Endocrinol.* **85**:515.

Murad, F., Brewer, H. B., Jr., and Vaughan, M., 1970, Effect of thyrocalcitonin on adenosine 3′,5′-cyclic phosphate formation by rat kidney and bone, *Proc. Natl. Acad. Sci. U.S.A.* **65**:446.

Nakajima, T., Naitoh, F., and Kuruma, I., 1974a, Elevation of adenosine 3′,5′-monophosphate in the perfusate of rat kidney after addition of dopamine, *Eur. J. Pharmacol.* **45**:195.

Nakajima, T., Naitoh, F., and Kuruma, I., 1974b, Dopamine-sensitive adenylate cyclase in the rat kidney particulate preparation, *Eur. J. Pharmacol.* **41**:163.

Nassim, J. R., Saville, P. D., and Mulligan, L., 1956, The effect of stilboestrol on urinary phosphate excretion, *Clin. Sci.* **15**:367.

New, M. I., Schwartz, E., Parks, G. A., Landey, S., and Wiedemann, E., 1972, Pseudohypopituitary dwarfism with normal plasma growth hormone and low serum sulfation factor, *J. Pediatr.* **20**:620.

Nishimoto, H., 1929, On relation between carbohydrate metabolism and inorganic phosphates, *Jpn. J. Exp. Med.* 7:207.

Nizet, A., Lefebvre, P., and Crabbé, J., 1971, Control by insulin of sodium, potassium and water excretion by the isolated dog kidney, *Pflügers Arch.* 323:11.

Nizet, A., Lefebvre, P., Luyckx, A., and Crabbé, J., 1976, Hormone and non-specific humoral factors in the interferences between sodium, glucose and phosphate handling by the dog kidney, in: *Current Problems in Clinical Biochemistry: 6. Renal Metabolism in Relation to Renal Function* (U. Schmidt and U. C. Dubach, eds.), pp. 262–272, Hans Huber, Bern.

Noble, H. M., and Matty, A. J., 1967, The effect of thyroxine on the movement of calcium and inorganic phosphate through the small intestine of the rat, *J. Endocrinol.* 37:111.

Nordin, B. E. C., 1973, *Metabolic Bone and Stone Disease,* pp. 40–41, Churchill Livingstone, London.

Nordin, B. E. C., 1976, *Calcium, Phosphate and Magnesium Metabolism,* Churchill Livingstone, London.

Nordin, B. E. C., and Fraser, R., 1956, The indirect assessment of parathyroid function, in: *Ciba Foundation Symposium on Bone Structure and Metabolism* (G. E. W. Wolstenholme and C. M. O'Connor, eds.), pp. 226–238, Churchill, London.

Nordin, B. E. C., and Fraser, R., 1960, Assessment of urinary phosphate excretion, *Lancet* 1:947.

Ogata, E., Kishikawa, T., and Nishiki, K., 1975, Calcitonin action and elevation of adenylate energy charge in rat kidney *in situ, J. Physiol. Soc. Jpn.* 35:391.

Orimo, H., Fujita, T., and Yoshikawa, M., 1972, Increases sensitivity of bone to parathyroid hormone in ovariectomized rats, *Endocrinology* 90:760.

Paillard, F., Ardaillou, R., Malendin, H., and Fillastre, J. P., 1972, Renal effects of salmon calcitonin in man, *J. Lab. Clin. Med.* 80:200.

Pak, C. Y. C., Ruskin, B., and Casper, A., 1970, Renal effects of porcine thyrocalcitonin in the dog, *Endocrinology* 87:262.

Paloyan, E., Paloyan, D., and Harper, P. V., 1967, Glucagon-induced hypocalcemia, *Metabolism* 16:35.

Parfitt, A. M., 1965, Changes in serum calcium and phosphorus during stilboestrol treatment of osteoporosis, *J. Bone J. Surg. Br. Vol.* 47:137.

Parsons, V., and Anderson, J., 1964, The maximum renal tubular reabsorptive rate for inorganic phosphate in thyrotoxicosis, *Clin. Sci.* 27:313.

Pechet, M. M., Bobadilla, E., Carroll, E. L., and Hesse, R. H., 1967, Regulation of bone resorption and formation. Influences of thyrocalcitonin, parathyroid hormone, neutral phosphate and vitamin D, *Am. J. Med.* 43:696.

Pecile, A., and Müller, E. E., 1966, Suppressive action of corticosteroids on the secretion of growth hormone, *J. Endocrinol.* 36:401.

Perault-Staub, A. M., and Staub, J. F., 1972, Thyroid function and plasma phosphate level in rat, *Endocrinology* 90:558.

Perlzweig, W. A., Latham, E., and Keefer, C. S., 1923, The behavior of inorganic phosphate in the blood and urine of normal and diabetic subjects during carbohydrate metabolism, *Proc. Soc. Exp. Biol. Med.* 21:33.

Persky, M., Linsk, J., Isaacs, M., Jenkins, J. P., Rosenbluth, M., and Kupperman, H. S., 1955, Acute effects of intravenous hydrocortisone on glucose and insulin tolerances, and levels of serum and urinary inorganic phosphorus, *J. Clin. Endocrinol. Metab.* 15:1247.

Pfleger, K., Rummer, W., and Jacobi, H., 1958, Phosphatdurchtritt am isolierten Darm unter Dinitrophenol und Thyroxin, *Biochem. Zr.* 330:303.

Prader, A., Illig, R., Uehlinger, E., and Stadler, G., 1959, Rachitis infolge Knochentumors, *Helv. Peadiatr. Acta* 14:554.

Pullmann, T. N., Lavender, A. R., and Aho, I., 1967, Direct effects of glucagon on renal hemodynamics and excretion of inorganic ions, *Metabolism* 16:358.

Puschett, J. B., Beck, W. S., Jr., Jelonek, A., and Fernandez, P. C., 1974, Study of the renal tubular interactions of thyrocalcitonin, cyclic adenosine 3′,5′-monophosphate, 25-hydroxycholecalciferol, and calcium ion, *J. Clin. Invest.* 53:756.

Queener, S. F., and Bell, N. H., 1975, Calcitonin: A general survey, *Metabolism* 24:555.

Rabkin, R., Epstein, S., Swann, M., 1975, Effect of growth hormone on renal sodium and water excretion, *Horm. Metab. Res.* 7:139.

Raisz, L. G., 1972, Calcium, phosphate, magnesium and trace elements, in: *Clinical Disorders of Fluid and Electrolyte Metabolism* (M. H. Maxwell and C. R. Kleeman, eds.), pp. 347–401, McGraw-Hill, New York.

Rasmussen, H., 1968, Parathyroid, in: *Textbook of Endocrinology* (R. H. Williams, ed.), p. 945, W. B. Saunders, Philadelphia.

Rasmussen, H., 1971, Ionic and hormonal control of calcium homeostasis, *Am. J. Med.* 50:567.

Rasmussen, H., and Bordier, P., 1974, *The Physiological and Cellular Basis of Metabolic Bone Disease,* Williams and Wilkins, Baltimore.

Rasmussen, H., Anast, C., and Arnaud, C., 1967, Thyrocalcitonin, EGTA, and urinary electrolyte excretion, *J. Clin. Invest.* 46:746.

Rasmussen, H., Kurokawa, K., and DeLong, A., 1971, Phosphate and bone cell function, in: *Phosphate et Métabolisme Phosphocalcique* (D. J. Hioco, ed.), pp. 7–29, Expansion Scientifique Française, Paris.

Rastegar, A., Agus, Z., Connor, T. B., and Goldberg, M., 1972, Renal handling of calcium and phosphate during mineralocorticoid "escape" in man, *Kidney Int.* 2:279.

Recker, R. R., Saville, P. D., and Heany, R. P., 1977, Effect of estrogens and calcium carbonate on bone loss in postmenopausal women, *Ann. Intern. Med.* 87:649.

Rector, J. F., 1973, Acidification of the urine, in: *Handbook of Physiology. Section 8: Renal Physiology* (J. Orloff and R. W. Berliner, eds.), pp. 431–455, Williams and Wilkins, Baltimore.

Reifenstein, E. C., Kinsell, L. W., and Albright, F., 1946, Observations on the use of the serum phosphorus level as an index of pituitary growth hormone activity; the effect of estrogen therapy in acromegaly, *Endocrinology* 39:71.

Relman, A. S., and Schwartz, W. B., 1952, The metabolic effects of compound F acetate in man, *J. Clin. Invest.* 31:656.

Riggs, B. L., Jowsey, J., Kelly, P. J., Jones, J. D., and Maker, F. T., 1969, Effect of sex hormones on bone in primary osteoporosis, *J. Clin. Invest.* 48:1065.

Riggs, B. L., Jowsey, J., Goldsmith, R. S., Kelly, P. J., Hoffman, D. L., and Arnaud, C. D., 1972, Short- and long-term effects of estrogen and synthetic anabolic hormone in postmenopausal osteoporosis, *J. Clin. Invest.* 51:1959.

Riggs, B. L., Jowsey, J., Kelly, P. J., Hoffman, D. L., and Arnaud, C. D., 1973, Studies on the pathogenesis and treatment in postmenopausal and senile osteoporosis, *Clin. Endocrinol. Metab.* 2:317.

Roberts, K. E., and Pitts, R. F., 1953, The effects of cortisone and desoxycorticosterone on the renal tubular reabsorption of phosphate and the excretion of titratable acid and potassium in dogs, *Endocrinology* 52:324.

Robertson, J. D., 1942, Calcium and phophorous excretion in thyrotoxicosis and myxedema, *Lancet* 1:672.

Robinson, C. J., Martin, T. J., and McIntyre, I., 1966, Phosphaturic effect of thyrocalcitonin, *Lancet* 1:83.

Ross, E. J., Marshall-Jones, P., and Friedman, M., 1966, Cushing's syndrome: Diagnostic criteria, *Q. J. Med.* 35:149.

Roycroft, J., and Talmage, R. V., 1973, Changes due to age in the hypocalcemic and hypophosphatemic effects of salmon calcitonin in growing rats, *Proc. Soc. Exp. Biol. Med.* **144:**17.

Rubinstein, A. H., Mako, M. E., and Horwitz, D. L., 1975, Insulin and kidney, *Nephron* **15:**306.

Russell, R. G. G., and Fleisch, W., 1968, The renal effects of thyrocalcitonin in the pig and dog, in: *Calcitonin. Proceedings of the Symposium on Thyrocalcitonin and the C Cells* (S. Taylor, ed.), pp. 297–305, Heinemann, London.

Sakuma, M., and Knobil, E., 1970, Failure of high rates of glucocorticoid infusion to inhibit growth hormone secretion in the Rhesus monkey, *Endocrinology* **86:**895.

Salako, L. A., Smith, A. J., and Smith, R. N., 1971, The effects of porcine calcitonin on renal function in the rabbit, *Endocrinology* **50:**485.

Salassa, R. M., Jowsey, J., and Arnaud, C. D., 1970, Hypophosphatemic osteomalacia associated with "nonendocrine" tumors, *N. Engl. J. Med.* **283:**65.

Saudek, C. D., Boulter, P. R., and Arky, R. A., 1973, The natriuretic effect of glucagon and its role in starvation, *J. Clin. Endocrinol. Metab.* **36:**761.

Schittenhelm, A., and Eisler, B., 1928, Untersuchungen über die Wirkung des Thyroxins auf den Eiweiß-Wasser-und Mineralstoffwechsel, *Z. Gesamte Exp. Med.* **61:**239.

Senft, G., Hoffmann, M., and Schultz, G., 1968, Effects of hydration and dehydration on cyclic adenosine 3',5'-monophosphate concentration in the rat kidney, *Arch. Gesamte Physiol.* **298:**348.

Shah, J. H., Motto, G. S., Kukreja, S. C., Hargis, G. K., and Williams, G. A., 1975, Stimulation of the secretion of parathyroid hormone during hypoglycemic stress, *J. Clin. Endocrinol. Metab.* **41:**692.

Simone, P. G., and Solomon, S., 1970, Aldosterone: Effect on incorporation of leucine into the trichloroacetic acid precipitable fraction of rabbit renal cortical tissue, *Experientia* **26:**656.

Simonnet, G., Laparra, J., and Blanquet, P., 1976, Action diurétique de la calcitonine: Mise en evidence d'un effect inhibiteur sur la réabsorption du sodium dans la branche ascendante de l'anse de Henlé, *C. R. Soc. Biol.* **170:**1194.

Singhelakis, P., Alevizaki, C. C., and Ikkos, D. E., 1974, Intestinal calcium absorption in hyperthyroidism, *Metabolism* **23:**311.

Sørensen, O. H., and Hindberg, I., 1972, The acute and prolonged effect of porcine calcitonin on urine electrolyte excretion in intact and parathyroidectomized rats, *Acta Endocrinol. (Copenhagen)* **70:**295.

Spanos, E., and McIntyre, I., 1977, Effect of glucocorticoids on vitamin-D-metabolism, in: *Vitamin D—Biochemical, Chemical and Clinical Aspects Related to Calcium Metabolism* (A. W. Norman, K. Schäfer, J. W. Coburn, H. F. DeLuca, D. Fraser, H. G. Grigoleit, D. von Herrath, eds.), pp. 191–195, Walter de Gruyter, Berlin.

Sraer, J., and Ardaillou, R., 1973, Renal receptors of calcitonin, in: *Endocrinology* (S. Taylor, ed.), pp. 170–176, Heinemann, London.

Sraer, J., Ardaillou, R., and Couette, S., 1974, Increased binding of calcitonin to renal receptors in parathyroidectomized rats, *Endocrinology* **95:**632.

Staub, A., Springs, V., Stoll, F., and Elrick, H., 1957, A renal action of glucagon, *Proc. Soc. Exp. Biol. Med.* **94:**57.

Steele, T. H., and DeLuca, H. F., 1976, Influence of dietary phosphorus on renal phosphate reabsorption in the parathyroidectomized rats, *J. Clin. Invest.* **57:**867.

Stern, P. H., and Bell, N. H., 1970, Effect of glucagon on serum calcium in the rat and on bone resorption in tissue culture, *Endocrinology* **87:**111.

Streifler, C., and Harell, A., 1975, Effect of thyrocalcitonin and parathyroid hormone on adenosine triphosphatases and phosphatases of rat kidney plasma membranes, *Isr. J. Med. Sci.* **11:**1220.

Stuart-Mason, A. (ed.), 1972, *Human Growth Hormone*, Heinemann, London.
Szymendera, J., and Mandajewicz, S., 1967, Calcium metabolism after castration, *Lancet* 2:1091.
Talmage, R. V., and Anderson, J. J. B., 1974, The effect of calcitonin on ^{32}P disappearance from plasma in parathyroidectomized and nephrectomized rats, *Proc. Soc. Exp. Biol. Med.* 141:982.
Talmage, R. V., Anderson, J. J. B., and Cooper, C. W., 1972, The influence of calcitonin on the disappearance of radiocalcium and radiophophorus from plasma, *Endocrinology* 90:1185.
Tan, C. M., Raman, A., and Sinnathyray, T. A., 1972, Serum ionic calcium levels during pregnancy, *J. Obstet. Gynaecol. Br. Commonw.* 79:694.
Tanaka, Y., Castillo, L., and DeLuca, H. F., 1976, Control of renal vitamin D hydroxylases in birds by sex hormones, *Proc. Natl. Acad. Sci. U.S.A.* 73:2701.
Thalassinos, N. C., Leese, B., Latham, S. C., and Joplin, G. F., 1970, Urinary excretion of phosphate in normal children, *Arch. Dis. Child.* 45:269.
Thompson, J. S., Genaro, M. A., Palmieri, M. A., and Eliel, L. P., 1974, Dissociation of the lowering effect of calcitonin on plasma Ca and P in cortisone-treated nephrectomized rats, *Endocrinology* 94:799.
Thorn, G. W., Jenkins, D., Laidlaw, J. C., Goetz, F. C., Dingman, J. F., Arons, W. L., Streeten, D. H. P., and McCracken, B. H., 1953, Pharmacologic aspects of adrenocortical steroids and ACTH in man, *N. Engl. J. Med.* 248:141.
Todd, W. R., Chuinard, E. G., and Wood, M. T., 1939, Blood calcium and phosphorus in newborn, *Am. J. Dis. Child.* 57:1278.
Tröhler, U., Bonjour, J.-P., and Fleisch, H., 1976, Inorganic phosphate homeostasis. Renal adaption to the dietary intake in intact and thyroparathyroidectomized rats, *J. Clin. Invest.* 57:264.
Tucci, J. R., and Kopp, L., 1976, Urinary cyclic nucleotide levels in patients with hyper- and hypothyroidism, *J. Clin. Endocrinol. Metab.* 43:1323.
Ullrich, K. J., 1977, Mechanism of cellular and subcellular transport of phosphate, in: *Proceedings of 3rd International Workshop on Phosphate and Other Minerals*, Madrid, p. 21.
Unger, R., 1971, Glucagon physiology and pathophysiology, *N. Engl. J. Med.* 285:443.
Van den Brande, J. L., 1975, Plasma somatomedin, in: *Growth Hormone and Related Peptides (Proceedings of 3rd International Symposium)* (A. Pacile and E. Muller, eds.), pp. 271–285, Excerpta Medica, Amsterdam.
Velentzas, C., Oreopoulos, D. G., From, G., Porret, B., and Rapaport, A., 1977, Vitamin-D levels in thyrotoxicosis, *Lancet* 1:370.
Verberckmoes, R., van Damme, B., Clement, J., Amery, A., and Michielsen, P., 1976, Bartter's syndrome with hyperplasia of renomedullary cells: Successful treatment with indomethacin, *Kidney Int.* 9:302.
Wajchenberg, B. L., Quintao, E. R., Liberman, B., and Cintra, A. B. U., 1965, Antagonism between adrenal steroids and parathyroid hormone, *J. Clin. Endocrinol. Metab.* 25:1677.
Walling, M. W., Brasitus, T. A., and Kimberg, D. V., 1977, Effects of calcitonin and substance P on the transport of Ca, Na and Cl across rat ileum *in vitro*, *Gastroenterology* 73:89.
Weber, H., Bourgoignie, J. J., and Bricker, N. S., 1974, Effects of the natriuretic serum fraction on proximal tubular sodium reabsorption, *Am. J. Physiol.* 226:419.
Wen, S. F., 1974, The effect of vasopressin on phosphate transport in the proximal tubule of the dog, *J. Clin. Invest.* 53:660.

Wesson, L. G., 1964, Electrolyte excretion in relation to diurnal cycles of renal function. Plasma electrolyte concentration and aldosterone secretion before and during salt and water balance changes in normotensive subjects, *Medicine* **43**:547.

Wesson, L. G., 1969, *Physiology of the Human Kidney*, Grune and Stratton, New York.

White, H. L., Heinbecker, P., and Rolf, D., 1949, Enhancing effects of growth hormone on renal function, *Am. J. Physiol.* **157**:47.

Wilkins, J. N., Mayer, S. E., and Vanderlaan, W. P., 1974, The effect of hyperthyroidism and 2,4-dinitrophenol on growth hormone synthesis, *Endocrinology* **95**:1259.

Williams, C. C., Matthews, E. W., Moseley, J. M., and McIntyre, I., 1972, The effects of synthetic human and salmon calcitonins on electrolyte excretion in the rat, *Clin. Sci.* **42**:129.

Williams, G. A., Peterson, W. C., and Bowser, E. N., 1974, Interrelationship of parathyroid and adrenocortical function in calcium homeostasis in the rat, *Endocrinology* **95**:707.

Yamaguchi, M., Takei, Y., and Yamamoto, T., 1975, Effect of thyrocalcitonin on calcium concentration in liver of intact and thyroparathyroidectomized rats, *Endocrinology* **96**:1004.

Young, M. M., and Nordin, B. E. C., 1967, Effects of natural and artificial menopause on plasma and urinary calcium and phophorus, *Lancet*, **2**:118.

Young, M. M., and Nordin, B. E. C., 1969, The effect of the natural and artificial menopause on bone density and fracture, *Proc. R. Soc. Med.* **62**:242.

Young, M. M., Jasani, C., Smith, D. A., and Nordin, B. E. C., 1968, Some effects of ethinyl oestradiol on calcium and phosphorus metabolism in osteoporosis, *Clin. Sci.* **34**:411.

Ziegler, R., Lemmer, B., and Pfeiffer, E. F., 1967, Über die Einwirkung von Thyrocalcitonin auf die Phosphaturie, *Klin. Wochenschr.* **45**:34.

Zilva, J. F., and Nicholson, J. P., 1973, Plasma phosphate and potassium levels in the hypercalcemia of malignant disease, *J. Clin. Endocrinol. Metab.* **36**:1019.

Zinsman, E., and Boccino, R., 1968, Hyperthyroidism and renal tubular acidosis, *Arch. Intern. Med.* **121**:118.

7

Effects of Vitamin D and Its Metabolites on Renal Handling of Phosphate

LOUIS V. AVIOLI

1. STUDIES IN HUMANS

Although the effects of a variety of peptide and steroid hormones on phosphate reabsorption and excretion by the human kidney have been well established, there is relatively little information regarding vitamin D control of phosphate excretion in humans. On the basis of observed responses of hypoparathyroid subjects to vitamin D therapy, Albright and Reifenstein concluded in 1948 that vitamin D was phosphaturic (Albright and Reifenstein, 1948). Conversely, the demonstrations of an increase in the tubular reabsorption of phosphate in osteomalacic patients with secondary hyperparathyroidism following vitamin D administration before changes in serum calcium could be detected suggested an opposite effect (Bordier *et al.*, 1969) (Table 1).

Data accumulated in patients with pseudohypoparathyroidism have also been used to defend the hypothesis that vitamin D is essential for the phosphaturic action of parathyroid hormone (PTH). Pseudohypoparathyroidism, like idiopathic or surgically induced hypoparathyroidism, is characterized by hypocalcemia and hyperphosphatemia (Avioli, 1977). The latter chemical findings result from lowered or absent circulating PTH in patients with idiopathic or postoperative hypoparathyroidism, whereas a defect in the renal tubular cyclic AMP (cAMP) and phosphaturic response to PTH accounts for the changes in subjects with pseudohypoparathyroidism (Chase *et al.*, 1969). Recently, another variety of this disorder, so-called "pseudohypoparathyroidism type II," has been uncovered and characterized by an intact renal cAMP response to PTH despite an

Table 1. Summary of Studies on Effects of Vitamin D on the Renal Handling of Phosphate in Humans[a,b]

Reference	PTH	Vitamin D status	Sterol protocol Type	Dose	When studied	Renal excretion of phosphate	Comments
Chu et al. (1940)	+++	DEF	D_2	12.5 µg/day	Days	↓	
Klein and Gow (1953)	+++	DEF	D_3	15 mg/day	1–3 days	↓	Rachitic children
Klein and Gow (1953)	0	NL	D_3	2.5 mg/day	15 days	0	
Brickman et al. (1974)	NL	NL	$1,25(OH)_2D_3$	0.5–2.7 µg/day	Days	0	Chronic renal failure
Brickman et al. (1974)	++	NL	$1,25(OH)_2D_3$	0.5–2.7 µg/day	Days	↓	
Rusell et al. (1974)	0	NL	$1\alpha(OH)D_3$ $1,25(OH)_2D_3$	1–4 µg/day	Days	↑	Increased phosphate absorption not excluded
Llach et al. (1977)	NL	NL	$1,25(OH)_2D_3$	2.6 µg bolus	6–12 hr	0	Urinary cAMP decreased; ~PTH suppression
Levine et al. (1978)	++	NL	$1\alpha(OH)D_3$	2 µg/day	80 days	↑Tm_{PO_4}	Chronic renal failure

[a] Modified from Levine et al. (1978).
[b] Abbreviations: ↑, increased; ↓, decreased; 0, no change; ++, +++, increased to variable degrees; DEF, deficient; NL, normal; PTH, parathyroid hormone.

absent or blunted phosphaturic response (Drezner *et al.*, 1973; Rodrigues *et al.*, 1974). However, the phosphaturic response to PTH observed in patients with pseudohypoparathyroidism during vitamin D therapy (Stogmann and Fischer, 1975; Suh *et al.*, 1970) does not necessarily imply a permissive effect of the vitamin for the phosphaturic response to PTH. Reversing hypocalcemia by calcium administration alone increases phosphate clearance in hypoparathyroid patients not taking vitamin D preparations (Eisenberg, 1965), and the phosphaturic response to PTH of vitamin-D-treated individuals with pseudohypoparathyroidism is attended by a reversal of the hypocalcemia (Stogmann and Fischer, 1975; Suh *et al.*, 1970). Moreover, the phosphaturic response to PTH has also been restored to normal in type II pseudohypoparathyroidism by calcium alone without any changes in circulating PTH levels (Rodrigues *et al.*, 1974). Calcium ion appears to inhibit PTH-stimulated phosphate transport by the kidney (Beck *et al.*, 1974). Thus, the restoration of the renal response to PTH of pseudohypoparathyroid patients on vitamin D therapy with rising serum calcium levels may simply reflect the now well-established control of phosphate excretion by calcium per se (Cuche *et al.*, 1976).

Within the past decade, it has become increasingly apparent that the skeletal and intestinal responses to vitamin D are due entirely to the biological expression of a number of hydroxylated metabolites, with 25-hydroxycholecalciferol (25OHD$_3$) and 1,25-dihydroxycholecalciferol [1,25(OH)$_2$D$_3$] most significant in this regard (Avioli, 1978; DeLuca, 1978). Assuming that a renal response to vitamin D could also be mediated through these hydroxylated metabolites, a variety of attempts have been made to establish this relationship in human subjects. Although a reduction in the fractional excretion of filtered phospahte or a rise in Tm$_{PO_4}$ has been observed in patients with renal insufficiency after prolonged administration of either 1,25(OH)$_2$D$_3$ or its structurally related synthetic analogue 1α-hydroxycholecalciferol (1αOHD$_3$) (Brickman *et al.*, 1974; Madsen *et al.*, 1976) (Table 1), these changes in phosphate excretion could also be attributed to the attendant alterations in circulating calcium and the suppression of PTH release. Worth noting in this regard is that Madsen *et al.* (1977), in studies designed to evaluate the effect of 1αOHD$_3$ on phosphate excretion in parathyroidectomized (PTX) individuals, recently concluded that phosphate excretion was unaffected by 1αOHD$_3$ in the absence of PTH. Puschett *et al.* (1974), while evaluating the effects of 25OHD$_3$ in children with hypophosphatemic rickets, noted no changes in urinary electrolyte or phosphate excretion in normal individuals subjected to the same 25OHD$_3$ dosage regimen. The evidence accumulated to date provides little if any positive evidence for a direct effect of vitamin D, its biologically active hydroxylated metabolites, or its structurally related analogues on renal tubular phosphate reabsorption and excretion in humans. Previously demonstrated antiphosphaturic effects of these agents in humans should be considered a result of concomitant suppression of the phosphaturic effect of PTH and/or the attendant changes in serum calcium.

2. STUDIES IN ANIMALS

One might conclude from the confusing results obtained in human subjects that more definitive prospective studies using appropriate animal models were essential to delineate the relationship between vitamin D, its metabolites, and phosphate excretion. Harrison and Harrison (1941) were the first to report that large doses of vitamin D decreased phosphate excretion and raised Tm_{PO_4} in intact vitamin-D-deficient dogs. Subsequent observations by these same investigators indicated that in rats, the phosphaturic response to PTH was dependent on vitamin D (Harrison and Harrison, 1974). Ney et al. concluded in 1965 that in dogs, PTH was phosphaturic in the absence of vitamin D. Subsequently, Arnaud et al. (1966) demonstrated a phosphaturic response to PTH in vitamin-D-deficient rats but noted an enhanced phosphaturia when the experiment was repeated in vitamin-D-repleted rats. These authors also observed that the blunted phosphaturia of D-deficient, PTX, hypocalcemic rats to PTH reverted to normal when the hypocalcemia was corrected. In 1971, Gekle and associates reported the results of micropuncture studies performed in the proximal convolution of normal, PTX, and rachitic rats. They observed that systemic infusions of vitamin D increased the reabsorption of phosphate in the proximal tubule for the first two hours in all three experimental groups and concluded that the reabsorption mechanism was independent of PTH. However, this response was critically time dependent, since, despite continuous infusion of vitamin D and normal renal function, the fractional reabsorption of phosphate paradoxically decreased during the third and fourth hours of the experimental study. In studies designed to analyze the role of vitamin D on phosphate excretion in the D-deficient state, Steele and DeLuca (1976) and Brautbar et al. (1979) noted no defect in the renal conservation of phosphate. Conversely, Costanzo and co-workers (1974) reported that vitamin D_3 administration to acutely PTX, vitamin-D-deficient rats resulted in a decrease in phosphate excretion in animals on low-dietary-phosphate regimens.

The isolation and subsequent synthesis of the biologically active vitamin D metabolites $25OHD_3$ and $1,25(OH)_2D_3$ ultimately led to a series of investigations designed to evaluate their effect on phosphate clearance in animals and the role of PTH in this regard. In 1972, Puschett et al. (1972a), using volume-expanded, hypocalcemic, PTX dogs, showed that systemic infusions of vitamin D_3 or $25OHD_3$ produced 39–47% depressions in the percentage of filtered phosphate excreted in the urine. Furthermore, they also showed that in this experimental dog model, PTH and $25OHD_3$ produced antagonistic effects on phosphate clearance. It was later reported by these same investigators that acute systemic infusions of $1,25(OH)_2D_3$ in hypocalcemic, volume-expanded, PTX dogs in doses of 25 U (0.625 μg) induced a 40% decrease in the fractional excretion rate of phosphate, with a peak response noted by 80–120 min (Puschett et al., 1972b). The time required for the onset of the renal action of $1,25(OH)_2D_3$ (20–30 min) was shorter than that observed for vitamin D_3 (50–60 min) or $25OHD_3$ (30–40 min), In this study, an equivalent dose of $25OHD_3$ had a greater effect on phosphate excretion than $1,25(OH)_2D_3$. Two years later, Popovtzer et al. (1974) demonstrated that systemic or renal arterial infusions of either $25OHD_3$ or $1,25(OH)_2D_3$ decreased phosphate clearance in intact but not in normocalcemic, PTX rats. In contrast to the results obtained in the dog by Puschett et al. (1972a), $25OHD_3$ was ineffective in reversing the phosphaturia induced in the thyroparathyroidectomized (TPTX) rat by volume expansion. Recently, it has been demonstrated that in rats, the mechanism underlying the $25OHD_3$-enhanced tubular reabsorption of phosphate is inhibition of the PTH-induced activation of adenyl cyclase in the kidney (Popovtzer and Robinette, 1975). The effects of graded doses (systemic infusion) of PTH and $25OHD_3$ on phosphate excretion have also been evaluated in the vitamin-D-depleted, nonexpanded, TPTX hypocalcemic rat (Puschett and Beck, 1975). Whereas small doses of either substance (1.0 U $25OHD_3$ or 1.2 U PTH/hr) failed to alter phosphate excretion when administered alone, they decreased phosphate clearance when administered simultaneously. In pharmacological doses (5 U/hr), PTH induced phosphaturia in the absence of $25OHD_3$. These studies are to be contrasted with those of Pechet and Hesse (1974), who demonstrated that in the rat, $1,25(OH)_2D_3$ and the structurally related $1\alpha OHD_3$ analogue enhanced the renal tubular reabsorption of phosphate in the absence of PTH. In their studies, PTH was able to reverse the effect.

Recently, Nseir et al. (1978), stressing the enhancement of ionic tubular transport induced by $25OHD_3$ and $1,25(OH)_2D_3$, reported that vasopressin, like PTH, was permissive for the effects of the vitamin D metabolites on the renal handling of phosphate. Garabedian et al. (1976) reported a phosphaturic effect of $1,25(OH)_2D_3$ in PTX, hyperphosphatemic rats. Bonjour et al. (1977) concluded that $1,25(OH)_2D_3$ was essential for the regulation of phosphate excretion by the rat kidney and normalized the capability of the PTX animal to excrete phosphate while adapting to large variations in dietary inorganic phosphate. The latter investigators cited similar adaptive responses in hyperphosphatemic PTX animals treated with doses of 25OHD$_3$ in the range of 26,000 pmol/day. The accumulated data led Bonjour *et al.* to conclude that in rats (and humans!!) the physiological role of 1,25(OH)$_2$D$_3$ is to facilitate the renal tubule to adapt to variations in dietary phosphate loads.

Our continued interest in the biological expression of vitamin D and its metabolites prompted a series of studies designed primarily to evaluate the direct effect of vitamin D and its metabolites on phosphate clearance in the adult intact anesthesized dog following four weeks of dietary adjustment in order to insure normal circulating PTH levels. The animals were subjected to bilateral renal arterial and ureteral catheterization. When individual renal glomerular filtration rates (GFRs) had stabilized to 18–20 ml/min, the test kidney was perfused with 5 nM concentrations of either vitamin D$_3$, 25OHD$_3$, or 1,25(OH)$_2$D$_3$. The perfusing solution consisted of 20% rachitic dog serum in isotonic saline. Using 15-min clearance periods, and comparing the response of the kidney perfused with the test substance with the contralateral one perfused with the serum–saline mixture alone at an identical rate, no significant effect of vitamin D$_3$ or its metabolites was observed on GFR, phosphate or calcium clearance, or circulating phosphate and ionized calcium during a 120-min interval (Fig. 1). These results, although preliminary, are consistent with the hypothesis that, in the normocalcemic dog with intact parathyroid glands, acute perturbations in renal arterial concentrations of vitamin D, 25OHD$_3$, or 1,25(OH)$_2$D$_3$ have little effect on those intrarenal phosphate transport parameters which regulate and ultimately condition phosphate reabsorption and excretion. As noted in Table 2, similar results have been obtained by Brautbar *et al.* (N. Brautbar, B. S. Levine, and J. W. Coburn, unpublished observations) in dogs subjected to systemic infusions of biologically active vitamin D metabolites. *In vitro* studies of ^{32}PO$_4^3$ transport in proximal renal tubules isolated from rachitic rats also demonstrate no direct affect of vitamin D$_3$ or its biologically active hydroxylated metabolites in physiological concentrations on phosphate transport (Halstead *et al.*, 1973).

3. SUMMARY

The conflicting array of experimental animal data is difficult to interpret because of species differences and the failure of some investigators to appreciate the direct effect on phosphate excretion of volume expansion, which often accompanies systemic infusion studies in animals (Gradowska *et al.*, 1973; Hebert *et al.*, 1972; Schneider *et al.*, 1975). Moreover, the physiological significance of the acute response of a hypocalcemic animal to either PTH or vitamin D metabolites is tenuous at best. When

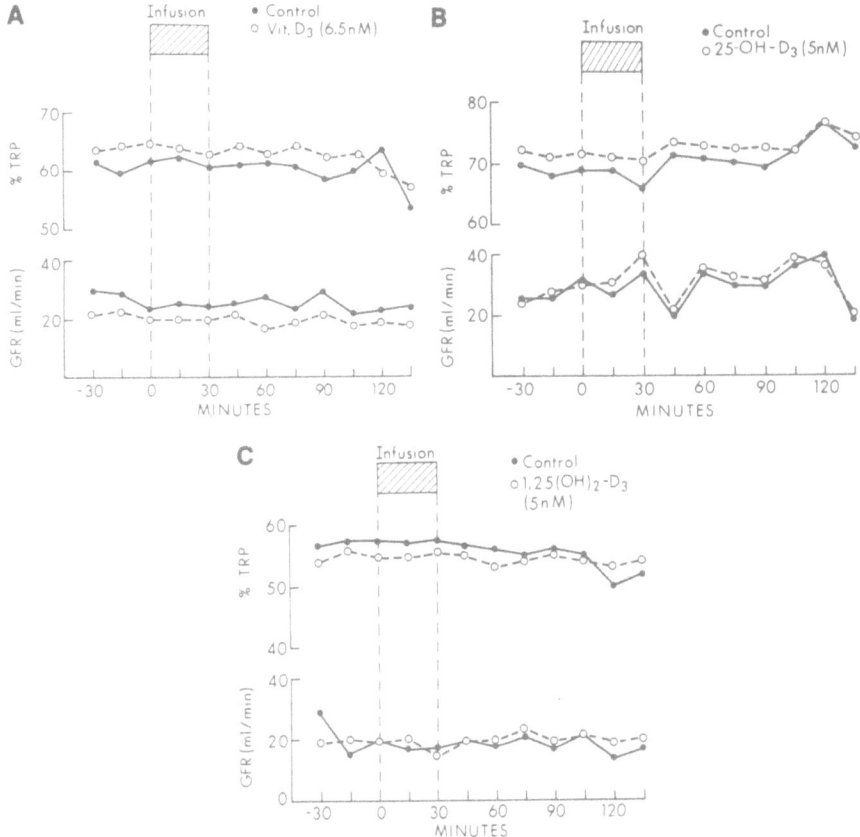

Fig. 1. Effect of vitamin D_3 (A), 25OHD$_3$ (B), and 1,25(OH)$_2$D$_3$ (C) on the tubular reabsorption of phosphate (% TRP) in the dog. The acute clearance studies were performed in adult mongrel dogs in a steady state of volume expansion. In each experiment, right and left renal arteries and ureters were catheterized. The control (20% rachitic serum in isotonic saline) and test [either vitamin D_3, 25OHD$_3$, or 1,25(OH)$_2$D$_3$] kidneys were perfused simultaneously in each experiment. Each point represents the mean of four separate experiments. Glomerular filtration rates (GFRs) were estimated using conventional endogenous creatinine clearance techniques.

hypocalcemia is acutely induced in rachitic animals with intact parathyroid glands, the stimulated release of endogenous PTH naturally blunts the response to exogenously administered PTH. In addition to these problems, phosphate clearance responses of hypocalcemic animals rendered normocalcemic by the test substance are difficult to interpret, since phosphate clearance increases in hypoparathyroid subjects (Eisenberg, 1965) and TPTX dogs (Crumb *et al.*, 1974) when the hypocalcemia is corrected by calcium infusion per se; moreover, the acute infusion of calcium into

Table 2. Effects of $1,25(OH)_2D_3$ and $24,25(OH)_2D_3$ on Fractional Excretion of Phosphate in Awake, Water-Loaded Dogs[a,b]

	Baseline C_{PO_4}/C_{cr} (ml/min)	Change in C_{PO_4}/C_{cr} from baseline value			
		1 hr	2 hr	3 hr	4 hr
Vehicle (5)[c]	7.4 ± 2.1^d	3.5 ± 4.7	16.1 ± 13.8	24.7 ± 15.6	31.8 ± 17.6
$1,25(OH)_2D_3$ 3 µg/hr (5)	16.0 ± 8.0	3.9 ± 8.0 NS	5.0 ± 17.9 NS	12.1 ± 15.6 NS	14.2 ± 16.9 NS
$1,25(OH)_2D_3$ 6 µg/hr (4)	11.1 ± 2.8	10.5 ± 3.5 NS	19.6 ± 10.6 NS	21.7 ± 7.4 NS	21.6 ± 8.5 NS
$24,25(OH)_2D_3$ 3 µg/hr (4)	8.6 ± 2.5	6.1 ± 0.8 NS	9.5 ± 1.8 NS	13.7 ± 3.2 NS	18.9 ± 2.9 NS

[a] PTE (Lilly), 3.0 U/hr, given during baseline (90 min) and continued through hr 1–4; vitamin D sterol infused during hr 1 and 2; hr 3 and 4 represent postinfusion observations.
[b] Abbreviations: C_{PO_4}/C_{cr}, ratio of phosphate clearance to creatinine clearance; NS, not significantly different from same period of vehicle infusion.
[c] Number in parentheses represents number of dogs in group.
[d] Data are mean ± SE.

the renal artery of dogs also decreased phosphate clearance (Lavender and Pullman, 1963); and, as demonstrated by Arnaud et al. (1966) in the rat, hypocalcemia may also blunt the phosphaturic response to PTH. Finally, the demonstration of phosphaturia on days following the administration of pharmalogical doses of vitamin D preparations (Crawford et al., 1955) need only reflect the well-documented effect of vitamin D metabolites on the intestinal absorption of phosphate (Avioli, 1974; Birge and Miller, 1977; Rizzoli et al., 1977). One can only conclude that at present, the experimental data derived primarily from a mixed array of animal experiments are controversial at best, offering limited insight into the permissive or direct effect (if any) of vitamin D metabolites on the renal clearance of phosphate.

ACKNOWLEDGMENT. I would like to acknowledge the capable assistance of Ms. C. Melloh in typing this manuscript.

4. REFERENCES

Albright, F., and Reifenstein, E. C. (eds.), 1948, in: *The Parathyroid Glands and Metabolic Bone Disease*, pp. 131–134, Williams and Wilkins, Baltimore.

Arnaud, C., Rasmussen, H., and Anast, C., 1966, Further studies on the interrelationship between parathyroid hormone and vitamin D, *J. Clin. Invest.* **45**:1955.

Avioli, L. V., 1977, Hyperparathyroidism, hypoparathyroidism, pseudohypoparathyroidism and pseudopseudohypoparathyroidism, in: *Scientifc Approach to Clinical Neurology*, Vol. II (E. Goldensohn and S. Appel, eds.), p. 1871, Lea anad Febiger, Philadelphia.

Avioli, L. V., 1974, A role of 1,25-dihydroxyvitamin D_3 in phosphate metabolism, *Nutr. Rev.* **32**:247

Avioli, L. V., 1978, Recent advances in vitamin D metabolism, *Arch. Intern. Med.* **138**:835.

Beck, N., Singh, H., Reed, S. W., and Davis, B. B., 1974, Direct inhibitory effect of hypercalcemia on renal actions of parathyroid hormone, *J. Clin. Invest.* **53**:717.

Birge, S. J., and Miller, R., 1977, The role of phosphate in the action of vitamin D on the intestine, *J. Clin. Invest.* **60**:980.

Bonjour, J.-P., Preston, C., and Fleisch, H., 1977, Effects of 1,25-dihydroxy-vitamin D_3 on the renal handling of Pi in thyroparathyroidectomized rats, *J. Clin. Invest.* **60**:1419.

Bordier, P., Bioco, D., Rouquier, M., Hepner, G. W., and Thompson, G. R., 1969, Effects of intravenous vitamin D on bone and phosphate metabolism in osteomalacia, *Calcif. Tissue Res.* **4**:78.

Brautbar, N., Walling, M. W., and Coburn, J. W., 1979, Interactions between vitamin D deficiency and phosphate depletion, *J. Clin. Invest.* **63**: 335.

Brickman, A. S., Coburn, J. W., and Massry, S. G., 1974, 1,25-Dihydroxyvitamin D_3 in normal man and patients with renal failure, *Ann. Intern. Med.* **80**:161.

Chase, L. R., Nelson, G. L., and Aurbach, G. D., 1969, Pseudohypoparathyroidism: Defective excretion of 3',5'-AMP in response to parathyroid hormone, *J. Clin. Invest.* **48**:1832.

Chu, H. I., Liu, S. H., Su, H. C., Yu, T. F., and Cheng, T. Y., 1940, Calcium and phosphorus in osteomalacia. Further studies on vitamin D action: Early signs of depletion and effects of minimal doses, *J. Clin. Invest.* **29**:349.

Costanzo, L. S., Sheehe, P. R., and Weiner, I. M., 1974, Renal actions of vitamin D in D-deficient rats, *Am. J. Physiol.* **226**:1490.

Crawford, J. D., Gribetz, D., and Talbot, N. B., 1955, Mechanism of renal tubular phosphate reabsorption and the influence thereon of vitamin D in completely parathyroidectomized rats, *Am. J. Physiol.* **180**:156.

Crumb, C. K., Martinez-Maldonado, M., Ecknoyan, G., and Suki, W. N, 1974, Effects of volume expansion, purified parathyroid extract and calcium on renal bicarbonate absorption in the dog, *J. Clin. Invest.* **54**:1287.

Cuche, J. L., Ott, C. E., Marchand, G. R., Diaz-Buxo, J. A., and Knox, F. G., 1976, Intrarenal calcium in phosphate handling, *Am. J. Physiol.* **230**:790.

DeLuca, H. F., 1978, Vitamin D. Metabolism and function. *Arch. Intern. Med.* **138**:836.

Drezner, N., Neelon, F. A., and Lebovitz, H. E., 1973, Pseudohypoparathyroidism type II: A possible defect in the reception of the cyclic AMP signal, *N. Engl. J. Med.* **289**:1056.

Eisenberg, E., 1965, Effects of serum calcium level and parathyroid extract on phosphate and calcium excretion in hypoparathyroid patients, *J. Clin. Invest.* **44**:942.

Garabedian, M., Pezant, E., Miravet, L., Fellot, C., and Balsan, S., 1976, 1,25-Dihydroxycholecalciferol effect on serum phosphorus homeostasis in rats, *Endocrinology* **98**:794.

Gekle, D., Stroder, J., and Rostock, D., 1971, The effect of vitamin D on renal inorganic phosphate reabsorption of normal rats, parathyroidectomized rats, and rats with rickets, *Pediatr. Res.* **5**:40.

Gradowska, L., Caglar, S., Rutherford, E., Harter, H., and Slatopolsky, E., 1973, On the mechanism of the phosphaturia of extracellular fluid volume expansion in the dog, *Kidney Int.* **3**:230.

Halstead, L., Rosenberg, E., Lee, S. W., Hahn, T., Boisseau, V., Loeb, E., and Avioli, L. V., 1973, The effect of vitamin D_3, 25-hydroxycholecalciferol, and 1,25-dihydroxycholecalciferol on the renal handling of inorganic phosphate, *Clin. Res.* **21**:885.

Harrison, H. E., and Harrison, H. C., 1941, The renal excretion of inorganic phosphate in relation to the action of vitamin D and parathyroid hormone, *J. Clin. Invest.* **20**:47.

Harrison, H. E., and Harrison, H. C., 1974, The interaction of vitamin D and parathyroid hormone on calcium, phosphorus and magnesium homeostasis in the rat, *Metabolism* **13**:952.

Hebert, C. S., Rouse, D., Eknoyan, G., Maldonado, M. M., and Suki, W. N., 1972, Decreased phosphate reabsorption by volume expansion in the dog, *Kidney Int.* **2**:247.

Klein, R., and Gow, R. C., 1953, Interaction of parathyroid hormone and vitamin D on the renal excretion of phosphate, *J. Clin. Endocrinol. Metab.* **13**:271.

Lavender, A. R., and Pullman, T. N., 1963, Changes in inorganic phosphate excretion induced by renal arterial infusion of calcium, *Am. J. Physiol.* **205**:1025.

Levine, B. S., Brautbar, N., and Coburn, J. W., 1978, Editorial: Does vitamin D affect the renal handling of calcium and phosphorus, *Miner. Electrolyte Metab.* **1**:295.

Llach, F., Coburn, J. W., Brickman, A. S., Kurokawa, K., Norman, A. W., Canterbury, J. M., and Reiss, E., 1977, Acute actions of 1,25-dihydroxyvitamin D_3 in normal man: Effect on calcium and parathyroid status, *J. Clin. Endocrinol. Metab.* **44**:1054.

Madsen, S., Olgaard, K., and Ladefoged, J., 1976, 1-Alpha-hydroxycholecalciferol-induced changes in the renal handling of phosphate and the serum parathyroid hormone level, *Acta Med. Scand.* **200**:351.

Madsen, S., Olgaard, K., and Thaysen, J. G., 1977, The effect of 1-α-hydroxycholecalciferol on the renal handling of phosphate in parathyroidectomized man, *Acta Med. Scand.* **202**:23.

Ney, R. L., Au, W. Y. W., Kelly, G., Raddi, I., and Barter, F. C., 1965, Action of parathyroid hormone in the vitamin-D deficient dog, *J. Clin. Invest.* **44**:2003.

Nseir, N. I., Szramowski, J., and Puschett, J. B., 1978, Mechanism of the renal tubular effects of 25-hydroxy and 1,25-dihydroxy vitamin D_3 in the absence of parathyroid hormone, *Miner. Electrolyte Metab.* **1**:48.

Pechet, M. M., and Hesse, R. H., 1974, Metabolic and clinical effects of pure crystalline 1α hydroxyvitamin D_3 and 1α,25 dihydroxyvitamin D_3, *Am. J. Med.* **57**:13.

Popovtzer, M. M., and Robinette, J. B., 1975, Effect of 25(OH) vitamin D_3 on urinary excretion of cyclic adenosine monophosphate, *Am. J. Physiol.* **229**:907.

Popovtzer, M. M., Robinette, J. B., DeLuca, H. F., and Holick, M. F., 1974, The acute effect of 25-hydroxycholecalciferol on renal handling of phosphorus, *J. Clin. Invest.* **53**:913.

Puschett, J. B., and Beck, W. S., 1975, Parathyroid hormone and 25-hydroxyvitamin D_3: Synergistic and antagonistic effects of renal phosphate transport, *Science* **190**:473.

Puschett, J. B., Moranz, J., and Kurnick, W. S., 1972a, Evidence for a direct action of cholecalciferol and 25-hydroxycholecalciferol on the renal transport of phosphate, sodium and calcium, *J. Clin. Invest.* **51**:373.

Puschett, J. B., Fernandez, P. C., Boyle, I. T., Gray, R. W., Omdahl, J. G., and DeLuca, H. F., 1972b, The acute renal tubular effects of 1,25-dihydroxycholecalciferol, *Proc. Soc. Exp. Biol. Med.* **141**:379.

Puschett, J. B., Genel, M., Rastegar, A., Anast, C., and DeLuca, H. F., 1974, Effects of 25-hydroxycholecalciferol on urinary electrolyte excretion in hypophosphataemic rickets, *Lancet* **2**:920.

Rizzoli, R., Fleisch, H., and Bonjour, J.-P., 1977, Role of 1,25-dihydroxyvitamin D_3 on intestinal phosphate absorption in rats with a normal vitamin D supply, *J. Clin. Invest.* **60**:639.

Rodrigues, H. J., Villarreal, H., Klahr, S., and Slatopolsky, E., 1974, Pseudohypoparathyroidism type II: Restoration of normal renal responsiveness to parathyroid hormone
   by calcium administration, *J. Clin. Endocrinol. Metab.* **39:**693.
Russell, R. G. G., Walton, F. J., Smith, R., Preston, C., Basson, R., Henderson, R. G.,
   and Norman, A. W., 1974, 1,25-Dihydroxycholecalciferol and 1α-hydroxycholecalci-
   ferol in hypoparathyroidism, *Lancet* **1:**14.
Schneider, E. G., Goldsmith, R. S., Arnaud, C. D., and Knox, F. G., 1975, Role of parathyroid of hormone in the phosphaturia of extracellular fluid volume expansion, *Kidney
   Int.* **7:**317.
Steele, T. H., and DeLuca, H. F., 1976, Influence of dietary phosphorus on renal phosphate
   reabsorption in the parathyroidectomized rat, *J. Clin. Invest.* **57:**867.
Stogmann, W., and Fischer, J. A., 1975, Pseudohypoparathyroidism: Disappearance of the
   resistance to parathyroid extract during treatment with vitamin D, *Am. J. Med.* **59:**140.
Suh, S. M., Fraser, D., and Kooh, S. W., 1970, Pseudohypoparathyroidism: Responsiveness
   to parathyroid extract induced by vitamin D_3 therapy, *J. Clin. Endocrinol. Metab.*
   30:609.

8

Effect of Urinary Alkalinization on Renal Phosphate Reabsorption

NORMAN BANK and GERHARD MALNIC

1. INTRODUCTION

A large number of physiological variables are known to influence the rate of renal tubular reabsorption of filtered phosphate and urinary excretion of phosphate. Among these is a relationship between either the pH or bicarbonate content of the tubular fluid and urine on the one hand, and phosphate reabsorption on the other. Although not all investigators agree, there is a considerable body of data which suggests that the phosphate reabsorptive rate is slowed by acute experimental maneuvers which raise the pH and/or bicarbonate concentration of tubular fluid. Much less well studied is the effect of reducing urinary pH and bicarbonate concentration on phosphate reabsorption, but such a relationship would presumably be more difficult to demonstrate, because the fraction of filtered phosphate reabsorbed under normal acid–base conditions is quite high, and urinary pH is quite low. The material discussed in this chapter will therefore focus upon the relationship between acute alkalinization of the urine and phosphate reabsorption. Observations made in clearance, micropuncture, microperfusion, and isolated-membrane studies will be discussed. The relationship between urinary pH and/or HCO_3^- and phosphate reabsorption is important mainly because it provides some insight into the basic cellular mechanisms of phosphate transport by the renal tubular epithelium.

2. CLEARANCE STUDIES

A number of clearance studies in humans, dogs, and rats have shown that urinary phosphate excretion and renal phosphate clearance rise and tubular reabsorption of phosphorus falls during experimental maneuvers which increase urinary bicarbonate excretion. Malvin and Lotspeich (1956) measured Tm for phosphate in dogs during metabolic alkalosis produced by sodium bicarbonate ($NaHCO_3$) or sodium lactate infusion, during metabolic acidosis induced by acetazolamide administration, and during acute respiratory alkalosis. In all of these experimental conditions, Tm for phosphate was significantly reduced. The effect was not related to plasma pH or HCO_3^-, since these varied widely according to the particular experimental protocol, but in all groups of animals the decrease in phosphate reabsorption was associated with an increase in urinary HCO_3^- excretion.

Mostellar and Tuttle (1964) found that acute respiratory and metabolic alkalosis in normal humans reduced plasma phosphorus concentration, and, in the case of alkalosis produced by $NaHCO_3$ infusion, urinary phosphate excretion and clearance rose. Puschett and Goldberg (1969) found that acetazolamide administration caused a rise in absolute and fractional phosphate excretion (FE_{PO_4}) in normal individuals. $NaHCO_3$ infusion sufficient to approach an "apparent tubular maximum Tm for bicarbonate" was accompanied by phosphaturia, which was somewhat smaller in magnitude than that observed with acetazolamide. Infusion of equivalent amounts of saline led to a relatively small phosphaturia as compared with $NaHCO_3$, suggesting that the effect was not due to volume expansion alone. Administration of $NaHCO_3$ and acetazolamide together resulted in a greater phosphaturia than with either alone. Fulop and Brazeau (1968) found that $NaHCO_3$ infusion in dogs increased fractional and absolute excretion of phosphorus. Similarly, acetazolamide increased FE_{PO_4} and absolute phosphate excretion consistently. Infusion of large amounts of isotonic NaCl, slightly hypertonic NaCl, or Na_2SO_4 had no significant effect on urinary phosphate, in spite of increases in sodium excretion and extracellular volume.

Jobin et al. (1977) found that the effect of acetazolamide on phosphate excretion occurred in dogs in which phosphate reabsorption had already been reduced by volume expansion and also in acidotic volume-expanded dogs. In both groups of animals, the increase in phosphate excretion with acetazolamide was associated with a rise in HCO_3^- excretion and urinary pH. It was concluded in all of these studies that alkalinization of the urine was in some way responsible for the reduction in phosphate reabsorption.

A number of other studies have shown that extracellular volume expansion per se inhibits phosphate reabsorption (Beck and Goldberg, 1974;

Frick, 1971, 1972; Gradowska *et al.*, 1973; Küntziger *et al.*, 1972; Maesaka *et al.*, 1973; Massry *et al.*, 1969; Puschett *et al.*, 1972; Schneider *et al.*, 1975), and in most of the studies cited above, volume expansion with $NaHCO_3$ could have played some role in causing the phosphaturia. Moreover, in animals with intact parathyroid glands, bicarbonate administration lowers the ionized calcium concentration in the blood (Mercado *et al.*, 1975), and the consequent stimulation of parathyroid hormone (PTH) secretion would be expected to have a potent effect on inhibiting phosphate reabsorption. In addition, hypocalcemia per se has also been shown to inhibit renal phosphate reabsorption in rats, even in the absence of PTH (Amiel *et al.*, 1976; Rasmussen *et al.*, 1967). Thus, the effect of bicarbonate infusion could be due to several physiologic changes other than alkalinization of the urine. In a recent study, Mercado *et al.* (1975) examined the effect of $NaHCO_3$ infusion on phosphate reabsorption in the dog, taking into consideration many of these variables. They found that in intact dogs, $NaHCO_3$ infusion increased FE_{PO_4} from 0.8 to 29.3%. Simultaneous administration of calcium, which prevented the fall in ionized calcium, blunted the effect of bicarbonate, so that FE_{PO_4} rose to only 4.9%. In chronically thyroparathyroidectomized (TPTX) dogs, $NaHCO_3$ infusion increased FE_{PO_4} from 0.6% to 4.5%, but in these animals, the filtered load of phosphate rose, and absolute reabsorption by the renal tubules actually increased rather than fell. Finally, in chronically TPTX dogs given a constant replacement of bovine PTH, $NaHCO_3$ and NaCl infusion produced comparable degrees of phosphaturia. The authors concluded that $NaHCO_3$ infusion does not have a significant direct effect on renal phosphate reabsorption but that the major mechanisms were mediated via PTH stimulation due to hypocalcemia and nonspecific volume expansion.

This problem was recently reinvestigated by Zilenovski *et al.* (1979) in acute and chronically parathyroidectomized (PTX) rats. Supplementary dietary phosphate was given to their animals, as it has been found that variations in dietary phosphate can change renal phosphate reabsorption, even in the absence of parathyroid glands (Steele and DeLuca, 1976; Tröhler *et al.*, 1976). In Fig. 1 are shown the effects of equivalent infusions of hypertonic NaCl or hypertonic $NaHCO_3$ on FE_{PO_4} in acutely PTX rats. During control periods before the infusion was started, FE_{PO_4} was <1%. NaCl infusion increased FE_{PO_4} to 1.4%, whereas $NaHCO_3$ infusion increased FE_{PO_4} to 12.3% (p <0.001). Glomerular filtration rate (GFR) was the same in the two groups, as was the fractional excretion of filtered sodium (FE_{Na}), suggesting that the two different salt solutions had produced a comparable degree of volume expansion. Infusion of calcium gluconate along with $NaHCO_3$ did not blunt the phosphaturia (Fig. 1), even though GFR was significantly reduced by the calcium infusion. In

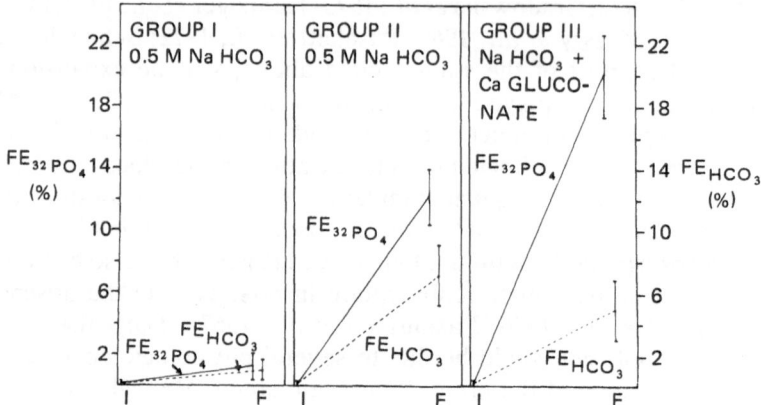

Fig. 1. Effect of hypertonic NaCl or NaHCO₃ infusion on fractional excretion (FE) of phosphate in acutely PTX rats.

Fig. 2 are shown the effects of hypertonic NaCl or NaHCO₃ on FE_{PO_4} in chronically PTX rats. These rats had developed hypocalcemia and hyperphosphatemia following PTX. FE_{PO_4} was higher than in acutely PTX rats with both NaCl and NaHCO₃ infusions, due perhaps to the low serum calcium, a high serum phosphorus, or to impairment of 1,25-dihydroxycholecalciferol synthesis in chronic PTX (Bonjour et al., 1977). Nevertheless, NaHCO₃ infusion produced a significantly greater phosphaturia than did NaCl (35.2% vs. 14.3%). In rats with intact parathyroid glands, NaHCO₃ infusion produced a considerably greater phosphaturia than in acutely PTX rats (40.1% vs. 12.3%), presumably due to stimulation of PTH secretion. Also, administration of purified bovine PTH to acutely PTX rats resulted in a FE_{PO_4} of 63.7%. These observations were interpreted to mean that PTH, either endogenous or exogenous, is a much more potent inhibitor of phosphate reabsorption than is NaHCO₃ infusion. In the rat, however, NaHCO₃ infusion does appear to inhibit phosphate reabsorption to a significant degree by a mechanism which is not dependent on PTH, extracellular volume expansion, or hypocalcemia.

The discrepancy between the observations of Mercado et al. (1975) and Zilenovski et al. (1979) may be resolved by the recent study of Steele (1977). He found that in TPTX rats, NaHCO₃ infusion did not inhibit renal phosphate reabsorption if tubular reabsorption of phosphate was initially low and the transport capacity presumably undersaturated. When tubular reabsorption was higher, due to a high-phosphorus diet or phosphorus infusion, NaHCO₃ reduced tubular reabsorption of phosphate significantly and increased FE_{PO_4}. Thus, the baseline rate of phosphate reab-

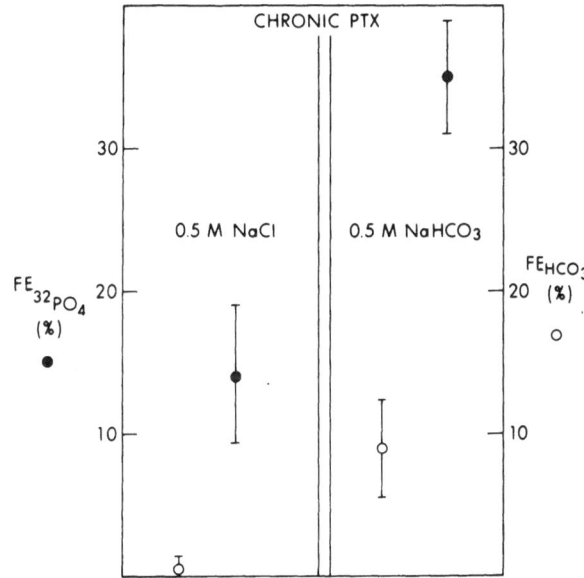

Fig. 2. Effect of hypertonic NaCl or NaHCO₃ infusion on fractional excretion (FE) of phoshate in chronically PTX rats.

sorption at the time of bicarbonate infusion seems to be important in determining whether or not alkalinization of the urine inhibits phosphate reabsorption. In the study by Zilenovski *et al.* (1979), the animals had been stabilized on a high-phosphorus intake for several days before the bicarbonate infusion.

3. MICROPUNCTURE STUDIES

The phosphaturia caused by alkalinization of the urine was studied by micropuncture techniques by a number of investigators. Beck and Goldberg (1973) measured sodium, fluid, phosphate, and calcium reabsorption in proximal tubules of the dog kidney by recollection micropuncture techniques and found a significant reduction of the reabsorption of these components of the glomerular filtrate after acetazolamide administration, both in normal and TPTX dogs. TF/UF (tubular fluid/ultrafiltrate) ratios for phosphate, measured by electron microprobe analysis, increased from a mean value of 0.56 to 0.74 in normal dogs and from 0.29 to 0.52 in TPTX dogs. These reductions in phosphate reabsorption were significantly larger than the alterations in fluid, sodium, and calcium reabsorption. Similar results were obtained by Wen (1974), who found that fractional reabsorption of phosphate measured in late proximal tubular segments of the dog was 54% of the filtered load under control conditions and 32% in acetazolamide-infused dogs.

The effect of bicarbonate infusion on proximal tubular phosphate reabsorption was studied in rats by Kuroda *et al.* (1979). Acutely and chronically PTX rats were infused with either hypertonic NaCl or $NaHCO_3$. Samples of proximal tubular fluid were analyzed for total CO_2 content, using a microcalorimetric method, and for ^{32}P and inulin. Tubular fluid HCO_3^- was calculated from the total CO_2, assuming that tubular-fluid-dissolved CO_2 was equal to that in plasma. The results in acutely PTX rats are depicted in Fig. 3. The fraction of ultrafilterable ^{32}P remaining in the tubular lumen was linearly related to the concentration of HCO_3^- in the tubular fluid ($p < 0.001$). In order to correct for differences in the site of puncture along the length of the proximal tubule, the percentage of ^{32}P remaining was plotted against the percentage of fluid reabsorbed, determined by inulin measurements (Fig. 4). The difference between NaCl infusion and $NaHCO_3$ infusion was apparent in late segments of the accessible proximal convoluted tubule. During NaCl infusion, approximately 98% of filtered phosphate was reabsorbed in the acutely PTX rats, whereas during $NaHCO_3$ infusion, approximately 83% was reabsorbed ($p < 0.001$). Absolute phosphate reabsorption in the proximal tubule was 6.8 ng/min/100 nl SNGFR (single nephron glomerular filtration rate) during NaCl infusion and 5.9 ng/min/100 nl SNGFR during $NaHCO_3$ infusion ($p < 0.02$). In chronically PTX rats, serum calcium fell to 5 mg/100 ml, and serum phosphorus rose to 13 mg/100 ml. The results obtained by

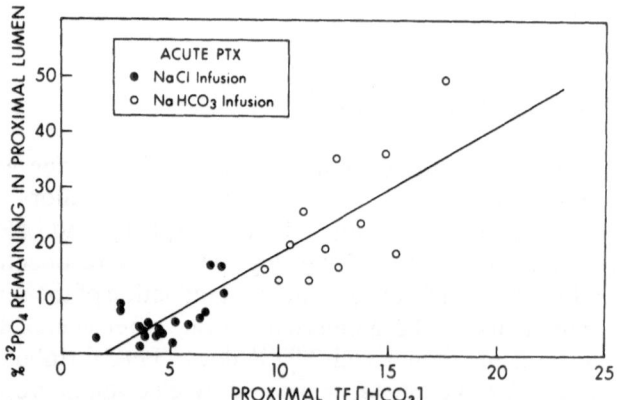

Fig. 3. Percentage of filtered phosphate remaining in proximal tubular fluid during hypertonic NaCl or $NaHCO_3$ infusion in acutely PTX rats. Data are plotted against concentration of HCO_3^- in tubular fluid.

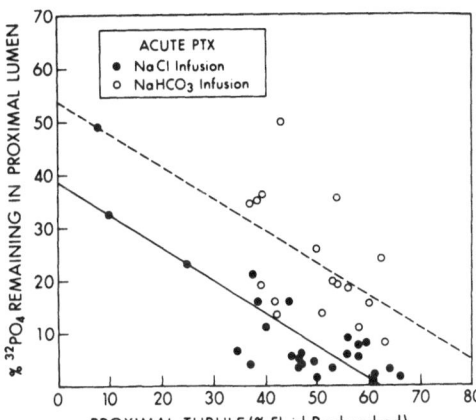

Fig. 4. Percentage of filtered phosphate remaining in proximal tubular fluid during hypertonic NaCl or NaHCO$_3$ infusion in acutely PTX rats. Data are plotted against percentage of fluid reabsorbed as an index of tubule length.

micropuncture of end-proximal tubular convolutions in these rats are depicted in Fig. 5. The fraction of filtered phosphate remaining in the tubular lumen was higher than in acutely PTX rats during both infusions. The mechanism of this reduced fractional reabsorption is not certain but could relate to hypocalcemia, hyperphosphatemia, or impaired vitamin D metabolism, all of which develop in chronically PTX rats. A clear difference was again apparent between NaCl infusion and NaHCO$_3$ infusion. The mean end-proximal ^{32}P remaining was 24% in the NaCl group and 39% in the NaHCO$_3$ group (p <0.001). Absolute phosphate reabsorption by

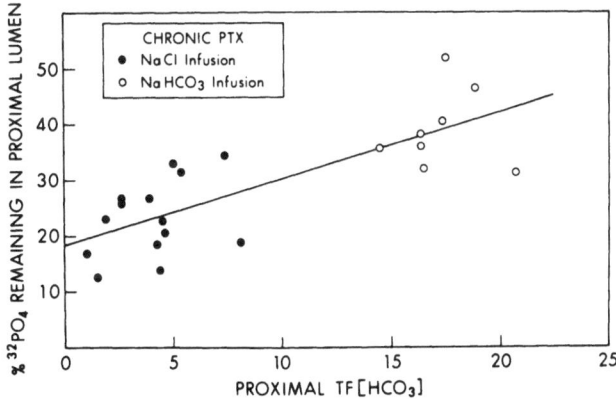

Fig. 5. Percentage of filtered phosphate remaining in proximal tubular fluid during hypertonic NaCl or NaHCO$_3$ infusion in chronically PTX rats. Data are end-proximal and are plotted against concentration of HCO$_3^-$ in tubular fluid.

the proximal tubule was 8.0 ng/min/100 nl SNGFR during NaCl infusion and 6.8 ng/min/100 nl SNGFR during $NaHCO_3$ infusion ($p < 0.05$). FE_{PO_4} in the final urine in each group was only slightly less than that remaining at the end of the accessible portions of surface proximal convoluted tubules. These observations indicate that the major site of inhibition of phosphate reabsorption during $NaHCO_3$ infusion in acutely and chronically PTX rats is the proximal convoluted tubule. It was concluded in this study that the mechanism was related in some fashion to the HCO_3^- concentration in the tubular fluid and not alterations in PTH or volume expansion. The role of hypocalcemia per se induced by $NaHCO_3$ infusion was not ruled out in the latter experiments.

4. MICROPERFUSION STUDIES

Phosphate in biologic fluids exists predominantly in two ionic forms, HPO_4^{2-} and $H_2PO_4^-$, with a ratio at pH 7.4 of approximately 4/1. Reabsorption of phosphate by the renal tubules could be indiscriminate with regard to these two forms or selective. This question was studied by Bank *et al.* (1974) by continuous microperfusion of rat proximal convoluted tubules *in vivo* with phosphate-containing solutions of widely different pH. The chemical concentration of phosphate in the perfusion fluid was 2 mmol/liter, within the physiologic range. Unidirectional efflux of trace amounts of ^{32}P from the lumen was measured, using inulin to measure water absorption. When the pH of the initial perfusion solution was in the acid range of 6.05–6.63, and 60–85% of the phosphate was in the ionic form of $H_2PO_4^-$, the ^{32}P concentration in the collected perfusate fell markedly and progressively with increasing lengths of perfused segments. This indicated a high rate of efflux and probably a fall in intraluminal chemical phosphate concentration below plasma phosphate concentration (assuming little or no influx of phosphate). When the pH of the initial perfusion solution was in the alkaline range of 7.56–7.85, and 85–92% of the phosphate was in the ionic form of HPO_4^{2-}, the ^{32}P concentration in the collected perfusate fell much less or actually rose as water was absorbed. Efflux of phosphate was much slower than with the more acid solution. The difference in efflux rates probably represented minimum differences, as the pH of the two perfusion solutions did not remain constant but tended to approach the same steady-state limiting value, probably due to the permeability of the proximal epithelium to HCO_3^- and/or H^+. When bovine PTH was administered intravenously to the rats, efflux of ^{32}P during perfusion with the acid solution was markedly reduced, whereas no clear-cut effect of PTH was seen during perfusion with the alkaline solution. It was concluded that phosphate is transported primarily in the

$H_2PO_4^-$ ionic form in the proximal tubule, probably by an active transport mechanism. The divalent anion, HPO_4^{2-} could have been reabsorbed by passive diffusion down a concentration gradient, or its reabsorption might have been dependent on conversion to $H_2PO_4^-$ by H^+ secretion. PTH appeared to specifically inhibit the transport of $H_2PO_4^-$ and to have little or no effect on HPO_4^{2-}.

When the proximal tubule is perfused with isotonic phosphate solutions (100 mM), the leak of phosphate out of the lumen is considerably slower than the rate at which tubular fluid pH changes (Cassola and Malnic, 1977). This is shown graphically in Fig. 6, where the rates of ^{32}P flux out of the tubule, as evaluated by the rate of decrease of $^{32}P/[^3H]$inulin ratios, are compared to the velocity of pH changes when alkaline or acid solutions are injected into the tubular lumen. In these experiments, proximal tubules were perfused with high concentrations of phosphate, and the overall half-times of phosphate reabsorption ranged from 32 to 66 sec, respectively, during acid (pH 5.5) and alkaline (pH 8.2) perfusions. Microperfusion experiments by Lang et al. (1977), in which much lower phosphate concentrations were used (1 mM), yielded phosphate reabsorption half-times that were considerably faster, of the order of 11 sec. This difference is due, no doubt, to the fact that at low luminal phosphate levels, the observed transport rate corresponds to that of the active reabsorptive mechanism. This process appears to be practically saturated at physiological concentrations of 2 mM, since Dennis et al. (1976) showed that increasing luminal concentrations to 3 mM in microperfusion experiments on isolated rabbit tubules does not increase the reabsorptive rate significantly. Therefore, the observed reabsorptive rate at high luminal phosphate levels is probably determined predominantly by the rate of

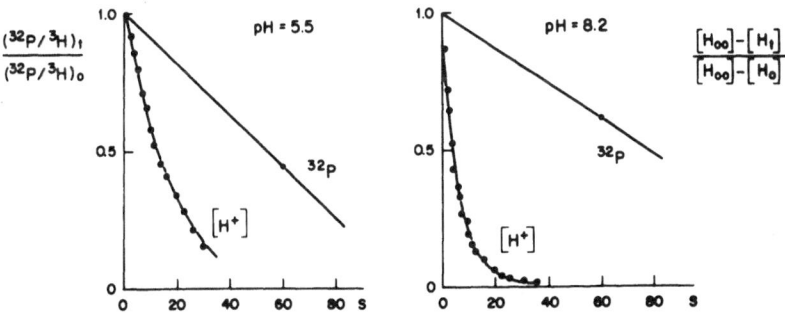

Fig. 6. Disappearance rates of ^{32}P from proximal tubular lumen (evaluated by $^{32}P/[^3H]$inulin ratios) compared to the rate of approach of H^+ concentration ($[H^+]$) to its steady-state level. Stopped-flow microperfusion with acid (pH = 5.5) and alkaline (pH = 8.2) solutions. (Data from Cassola and Malnic, 1977.)

passive reabsorption of this ion along the existing electrochemical potential gradient rather than by the active transport component.

Figure 7 shows a summary of phosphate efflux measurements obtained during stopped-flow microperfusions of proximal tubules of rat kidneys with solutions containing 100 mM phosphate at an initial pH of 5.5 and 8.0 (Cassola and Malnic, 1977). High phosphate concentrations were used in this study to produce conditions similar to those in experiments on tubular acidification and alkalinization, where a high buffering power was desirable (Giebisch et al., 1977; Malnic et al., 1972). The efflux of ^{32}P from these tubules was measured with respect to time and related to [H^3]inulin concentrations. In spite of the fact that the original pH gradients were being dissipated with time, with luminal pH changing toward its steady-state level, the half-time of phosphate efflux during perfusion with the acid solution was significantly shorter (31.9 sec) than that observed during perfusion with the alkaline solution (66 sec). The more rapid rate of disappearance of phosphate from the acid solution than from the alkaline solution can be interpreted to mean that passive diffusion of $H_2PO_4^-$ out of the lumen occurs more readily than passive diffusion of HPO_4^{2-}. After the administration of acetazolamide, the half-times of phosphate loss from the tubular lumen were not significantly different during acid and alkaline perfusions, essentially due to a prolongation of the half-times during acid perfusion. These results are in accord with those of Bank et al. (1974), who used much lower phosphate concentrations. In their study, phosphate reabsorption was inhibited by PTH during perfusion with an acid solution but was not changed significantly during perfusion with an alkaline solution. The two studies suggest that inhibition of phosphate reabsorption by acetazolamide or PTH affects primarily $H_2PO_4^-$ transport, although the mechanisms of inhibition might be different. In distal tubules studied under similar conditions, no significant phosphate loss was detected during acid or alkaline perfusions (Cassola and Malnic, 1977).

Results of other microperfusion studies on the effect of pH on phosphate reabsorption seem to conflict with the conclusions of Bank et al. (1974) and Cassola and Malnic (1977). Baumann et al. (1975b) investigated the net transport of phosphate (microchemical analysis) employing microperfusion techniques in chronically PTX rats. They studied early proximal loops, for these segments had been shown to transport phosphate at higher rates than late proximal segments (Baumann et al., 1975a). Their perfusate contained 4 mM phosphate and 51 mM raffinose in addition to the components of a mammalian Ringer's solution. This solution is an "equilibrium" solution, resulting in zero net water flux. An alkaline solution, containing 40 mM NaHCO$_3$ (pH 8.4), and an acid solution, which had its pH lowered to 6.0 by substituting 35 mM NaCl for NaHCO$_3$, were

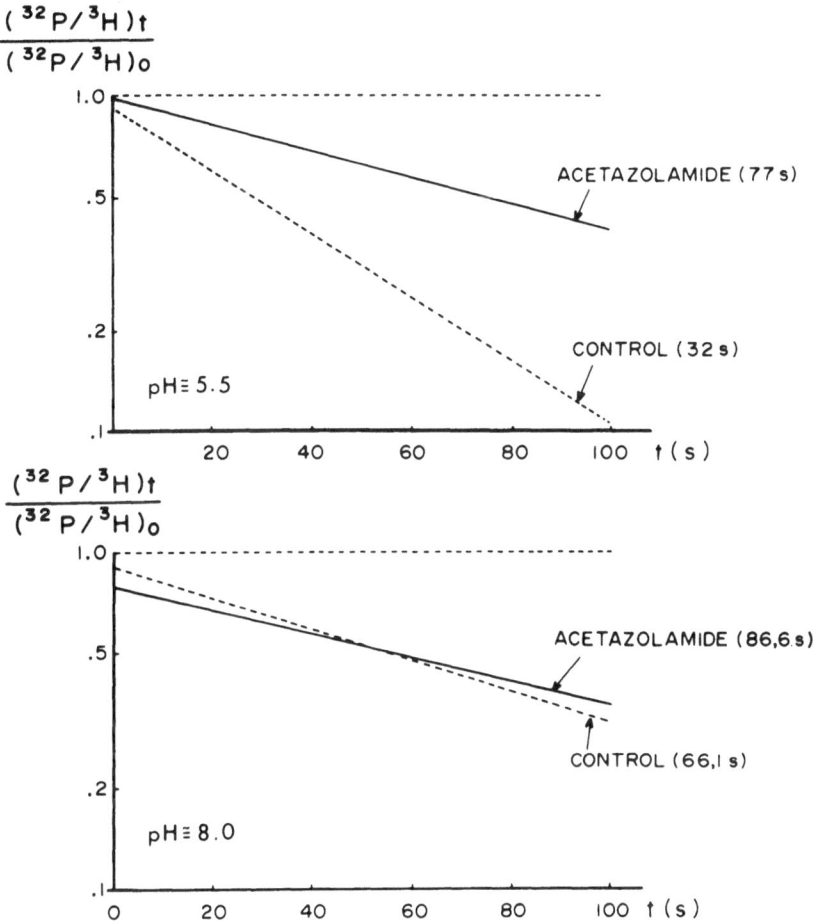

Fig. 7. Rate of ^{32}P loss from proximal tubule of the rat during stopped-flow microperfusions at pH 5.5 and 8.0 in control and acetazolamide-infused rats. Values in parentheses are half-times of phosphate disappearance. (Data from Cassola and Malnic, 1977.)

used. The pH of the collected perfusate was calculated from bicarbonate concentrations estimated from the measured anion deficit. The main findings are summarized in Table 1. Reabsorption of phosphate was significantly higher at a luminal pH between 7.4 and 7.5 than at a pH between 6.7 and 7.0. Metabolic alkalosis in PTX rats, which slowed the rate of H^+ secretion, reduced phosphate reabsorption from both perfusion solutions. On the basis of ion concentrations, the authors calculated that the potential difference (PD) was more positive (up to $+2.2$ mV) during perfusion with the acid solution than with the alkaline solution. Relative electrical negativity during perfusion with the alkaline solution could have

Table 1. Phosphate Reabsorption during Luminal Perfusion of Early Proximal Segments at Different pH Levels in Rat Kidney[c]

Rat[b]	Luminal pH[c]	HPO_4^{2-}	P_i reabsorption (pmol/cm/sec)	Number of perfused tubules
PTX	7.43–7.47	84	2.05 ± 0.18	15
PTX + cA	7.36–7.43	84	1.31 ± 0.26	12
PTX	6.74–6.90	51	0.92 ± 0.21	12
PTX + cA	6.77–7.01	57	0.60 ± 0.11	10

[a] Data from Baumann *et al.* (1975b).
[b] PTX + cA, PTX plus chronic alkalosis.
[c] Luminal pH calculated from anion deficit and rat pCO_2.

been partly responsible for the more rapid removal of HPO_4^{2-}, but the authors also suggested the possibility of a preferential tubular transport of HPO_4^{2-}. Data from the same laboratory (Ullrich *et al.*, 1977) showed that maximal transtubular phosphate gradients established in stopped-flow microperfusion experiments, during simultaneous peritubular capillary perfusion, are decreased when bicarbonate is omitted from both perfusion solutions, even when the pH is maintained at 7.4. The phosphate gradient observed after omission of bicarbonate was about half of that found under control conditions. On the other hand, when the peritubular capillaries were perfused with 10^{-3} M SITS (4-acetamido-4'-isothiocyano-2,2'-disulfonic stilbene), phosphate transport was the same as under control conditions, indicating that the reabsorption of phosphate probably does not depend specifically on peritubular bicarbonate. The mechanism of the inhibitory action of low-bicarbonate solutions is not quite clear. The authors suggested that changes in intracellular pH may mediate the observed changes in phosphate transport. Their observations may not relate specifically to the ionic species of phosphate which is reabsorbed from the tubular lumen.

Dennis and co-workers (Dennis, 1976; Dennis *et al.*, 1976, 1977) studied phosphate transport in isolated perfused segments of rabbit nephron under conditions which were somewhat similar to those of Ullrich *et al.* (1977). They perfused proximal convoluted and straight segments with low-bicarbonate rabbit serum, prepared by titration of the serum to pH 6 and subsequent adjustment of the pH to 7.4 with NaOH, a procedure yielding bicarbonate concentrations of less than 1 mM. When this solution was used as both the bathing medium and perfusion solution, they found a reduction in total-volume reabsorption (J_v) but no changes in unidirectional phosphate fluxes in either the proximal convoluted or straight segments. Lumen–bath fluxes of phosphate ($J_{PO_4}^{LB}$) were about ten times higher

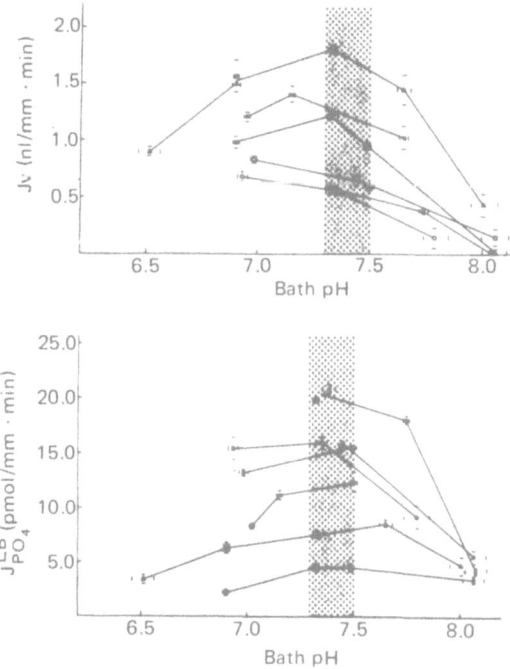

Fig. 8. Effect of variations of bath pH on rate of fluid absorption (J_V; upper graph) and on lumen-to-bath phosphate flux ($J_{PO_4}^{LB}$; lower graph) in isolated perfused rabbit proximal convoluted tubule. Shaded area represents pH range in control studies. (From Dennis *et al.*, 1976.)

than bath–lumen fluxes, showing that passive permeability of the epithelium to phosphate is low. Active transport accounted for almost all of the unidirectional efflux. Neither efflux nor influx was affected by the low-bicarbonate medium. This is apparently in disagreement with the findings of Ullrich *et al.* (1977), who found that the absence of HCO_3^- or other buffer impaired phosphate reabsorption. On the other hand, perfusion of isolated proximal convoluted tubules in baths of varying pH levels yielded the results summarized in Fig. 8 (Dennis, 1976). Both J_V and $J_{PO_4}^{LB}$ varied with bath pH and were maximal in a range of 7.3–7.5, declining both at higher and at lower pH levels. In these experiments, luminal pH was not measured, but it was assumed to vary in a manner parallel to bath pH. These results show that both fluid and phosphate reabsorption are maximal in a physiological pH range and that the active transport of phosphate from lumen to bath declines as bath pH is either raised or lowered beyond the physiological range.

Table 2. Fluid and Phosphate Transport in Proximal Convoluted and Straight Tubules of Rabbit Kidney[a,b]

	HCO_3^- serum		Low-HCO_3^- serum	
	−PTH	+PTH	−PTH	+PTH
Proximal convoluted tubule				
J_V (nl/mm/min)	1.22	0.72[c]	0.80[c]	0.77[c]
	±0.16	±0.07	±0.08	±0.09
$J_{PO_4}^{LB}$ (pmol/mm/min)	7.42	8.74	7.32	8.38
	±1.13	±1.30	±1.09	±1.36
$J_{PO_4}^{BL}$ (pmol/mm/min)	0.39	0.42	0.33	0.36
	±0.08	±0.08	±0.08	±0.08
Proximal straight tubule				
J_V (nl/mm/min)	0.63	0.45[c]	0.40[c]	0.40[c]
	±0.04	±0.04	±0.04	±0.06
$J_{PO_4}^{LB}$ (pmol/mm/min)	2.64	1.90[c]	2.50	1.85[c]
	±0.41	±0.34	±0.22	±0.23
$J_{PO_4}^{BL}$ (pmol/mm/min)	0.29	0.35	0.31	0.26
	±0.08	±0.12	±0.06	±0.05

[a] Data from Dennis et al. (1977).
[b] Abbreviations: J_V, volume reabsorption; $J_{PO_4}^{LB}$, phosphate flux, lumen to bath; $J_{PO_4}^{BL}$, phosphate flux, bath to lumen.
[c] $p < 0.01$, comparison with first column.

The experiments of Dennis et al. (1977) are summarized in Table 2. The table shows experiments in which the effect of low-HCO_3^- solutions on fluid and phosphate transport was studied in isolated rabbit tubules in the presence and absence of PTH. When proximal convoluted tubules were perfused with bicarbonate Ringer's, the addition of PTH to the bath solution inhibited fluid transport significantly. However, in low-HCO_3^- medium, J_V was reduced initially and not further affected by PTH. Phosphate transport in this segment was not affected by either low-HCO_3^- solutions or PTH. The situation with respect to J_V was similar in proximal straight segments, but $J_{PO_4}^{LB}$ was significantly reduced by PTH in this segment in HCO_3^--containing and HCO_3^--free Ringer's. Passive flux of phosphate from bath to lumen was not affected by any of these procedures. The observations are consistent with the supposition that active phosphate transport (and sodium transport) depends on the maintenance of a normal intracellular pH, mediated by the pH of the peritubular bathing solution. The data may or may not have relevance, however, with regard to the effect of intraluminal pH per se and the ionic species of phosphate transported out of the lumen, since intraluminal pH was not measured.

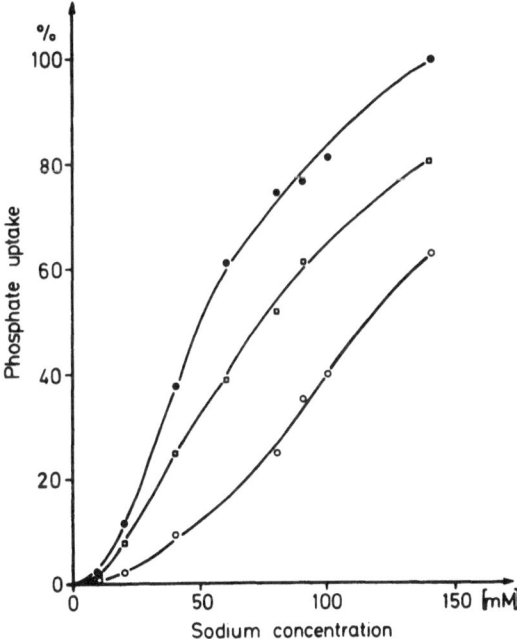

Fig. 9. Influence of sodium concentration and pH on phosphate uptake by isolated renal brush-border microvilli vesicles of rat kidney. Incubation medium at pH 8 (●), 7.4 (□), and 6 (○). Sodium was substituted by choline. Uptake is expressed as percentage of value at pH 8 and 140 mM NaCl. (From Hoffman et al., 1976.)

5. STUDIES OF LUMINAL MEMBRANE VESICLES

Hoffman et al. (1976) studied the uptake of phosphate into isolated vesicles formed from the brush border of rat kidney tubules. These authors showed a sodium dependency of phosphate uptake into these vesicles and also demonstrated a relation between the pH of the bathing medium and phosphate uptake. They studied phosphate transport (^{32}P) in solutions containing 1 mM phosphate at pH 6, 7.4, and 8 and were able to show that at increasing pH values, the initial uptake of phosphate into the vesicles also increased (Fig. 9). Figure 9 shows the stimulatory effect of sodium on phosphate uptake and also that at any given sodium concentration, the uptake was higher when the pH of the medium was higher. The authors suggested that HPO_4^{2-} was transported preferentially over $H_2PO_4^-$ by the brush-border vesicles.

The foregoing review of micropuncture, microperfusion, and isolated-vesicle data dealing with the relation between pH and phosphate transport indicates that, at present, there is no common view about the interrelationship of the two or the preferential transport of $H_2PO_4^-$ versus HPO_4^{2-}. There is no doubt that after acetazolamide administration, phosphate reabsorption along the proximal segment is decreased. Peritubular bicarbonate concentration per se, in spite of the findings of Ullrich et al. (1977), does not appear to affect phosphate fluxes in the convoluted and straight segments of the rabbit proximal tubule independently of pH, according to the studies of Dennis et al. (Dennis, 1976; Dennis et al., 1976, 1977). With respect to the influence of intraluminal pH, unidirectional ^{32}P flux from lumen to interstitium in the rat proximal tubule is increased at more acid luminal pH levels, both at physiological and elevated phosphate levels. Bath pH changes in the isolated perfused proximal tubular preparation suggest that lumen–bath flux of phosphate is maximum in the range of pH 7.3–7.5 and decreases at higher as well as lower pH, but this may relate more to intracellular pH effects than to luminal pH. The data of Baumann et al. (1975b) indicate increased phosphate transport at more alkaline intraluminal pH values, and their observations are supported by the studies in isolated brush-border vesicles (Hoffman et al., 1976). Thus, at the present time, there is evidence that intraluminal pH has an effect on the rate of phosphate reabsorption, but there is disagreement as to the mechanism of this effect and whether there is preferential transport of $H_2PO_4^-$ or HPO_4^{2-}.

6. THEORETICAL CONSIDERATIONS

6.1. Relation between H^+ and Phosphate Transport: Phosphate as a Buffer System

During the acidification of the tubular lumen, which in the mammalian kidney starts in the first segments of the proximal tubule (Gottschalk et al., 1960), the buffer systems filtered at the glomerulus will be titrated according to the isohydric principle toward the limiting luminal pH that can be generated and maintained by the tubular epithelium. This principle states that the distribution of acid and salt of the different buffer systems will be dependent on the common pH and on the respective pK:

$$pH = pK_1 + \log \frac{B_1}{A_1} = pK_2 + \log \frac{B_2}{A_2} = \ldots \qquad (1)$$

where B_1 and A_1 represent the salt and acid concentrations of the respective buffer species. Thus, the buffer species that have pK values in the range of the physiological pH along the nephron will be those responsible for the major generation of titratable acidity. Of the physio-

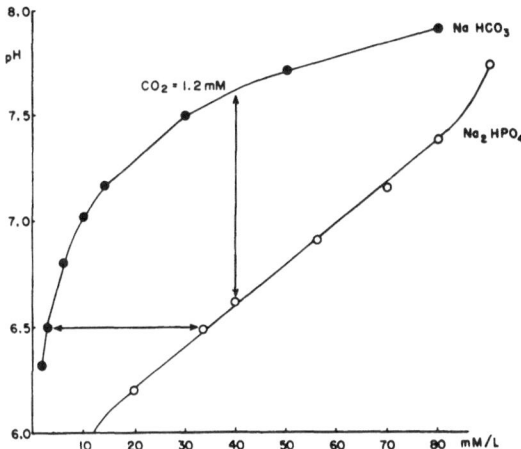

Fig. 10. Titration curves of phosphate and bicarbonate buffers, calculated by the Henderson–Hasselbalch equation. Bicarbonate is titrated at constant CO_2 concentration. Abscissa shows buffer base concentration. (From Giebisch et al., 1977.)

logical buffer systems in plasma, phosphate buffer is, after bicarbonate, the system present in significant concentrations and whose pK is nearest the physiological range. Since the tubular pH varies from a level of 7.4 at the glomerulus toward a final urinary pH of 5–6, this buffer system, with a pK of 6.8, is the most important generator of titratable acidity in the mammalian nephron. This is shown in Fig. 10 which depicts a titration curve of the phosphate buffer system. It is clearly seen that this system undergoes extensive titration within the physiological pH range. The titration curve given in this figure corresponds to the addition of acid to a vessel containing a fixed quantity of phosphate, that is, a situation in which Na_2HPO_4 is transformed into NaH_2PO_4 but where the sum of these two salts remains constant (a closed system). This would correspond to the situation in the tubular lumen only if the tubular wall were impermeable to phosphate. In the proximal tubule, filtered phosphate is reabsorbed by an active transport mechanism (Knox et al., 1973), but at more distal sites, most authors working in this field have not obtained evidence for a significant rate of reabsorption of phosphate (Cassola and Malnic, 1977; Lang et al., 1977; Staum et al., 1972; Strickler et al., 1964).

Under conditions of very high phosphate concentrations in the proximal tubule (when the active transport mechanism is presumably saturated), and in the distal nephron in general, the phosphate buffer system can be considered to be acidified in an effectively closed system, that is, in a system where the total amount of the buffer remains relatively constant. As indicated above, this is not entirely true in the proximal tubule, but the acidification rates can be corrected for the observed velocity of phosphate loss out of the lumen. The situation is entirely different for the bicarbonate buffer system. In spite of having a pK farther removed from the physiological range than phosphate, bicarbonate buffer is reabsorbed from the proximal tubule more effectively than is phosphate. This is due, in part, to the considerably higher filtered load of bicarbonate, that is, 25 mmol/liter compared with 1–2 mmol/liter of phosphate. However, even when the tubular load of these two buffers is equal (in microperfusion studies), considerably more bicarbonate will be reabsorbed until the luminal steady-state pH is established. The reason for this difference in reabsorptive rates is the high diffusibility of the acid component of the bicarbonate buffer system. The permeability of the tubular epithelium to CO_2 is much higher than to bicarbonate (Malnic and Mello Aires, 1971; Malnic and Steinmetz, 1976). Thus, bicarbonate is titrated in an effectively open system, the acid (CO_2) concentration being maintained at a constant low level in body fluids by pulmonary gas exchange. At the apparent pK of the system, 6.1, there will be equal concentrations of acid and salt. Since acid (CO_2) concentration is fixed at about 1.2 mM, at a pH of 6.1 the bicarbonate concentration will also be 1.2 mM. Figure 10 shows some of the differences between the *in vivo* titration curves of phosphate and of bicarbonate, both starting at approximately the same high concentration. At a pH of 6.5, which is approximately the pH of tubular fluid in late portions of the rat proximal tubule, and at a CO_2 concentration of 1.2 mM, a bicarbonate concentration of 3 mM is obtained by the Henderson–Hasselbalch equation:

$$pH = 6.5 = 6.1 + \log \frac{HCO_3^-}{1.2}$$

Thus, whatever the initial luminal bicarbonate concentration, it will be titrated to a level of 3 mM in the tubular fluid when a pH of 6.5 is reached. On the other hand, when 100 mM phosphate is titrated in the proximal tubule to the same pH of 6.5, a concentration of 33.3 mM $NaHPO_4$ will remain in the tubular lumen, assuming no phosphate is reabsorbed:

$$pH = 6.5 = 6.8 + \log \frac{Na_2HPO_4}{(100 - Na_2HPO_4)}$$

Thus, because of the rapid removal of CO_2, the concentration of bicarbonate falls more rapidly than that of HPO_4^{2-} when pH is reduced to the same level in the proximal tubule.

This discussion illustrates that the permeability of the tubular epithelium to the components of a buffer system is important in determining the way in which the system will be titrated in the lumen. When dealing with a buffer composed of a weak acid and its salt, the acid is poorly dissociated and therefore will tend to be more lipid soluble than the salt. In consequence, it will diffuse more easily across the tubular epithelium. This mechanism was proposed by Ullrich *et al.* (1975) to account for reabsorption of the glycodiazine buffer system. The rate of luminal disappearance of this substance was equated with the rate of H^+ secretion. The authors assumed that H^+ secretion converts the salt into the acid form, and the latter, being easily diffusible, would rapidly equilibrate with the peritubular blood concentration of this molecule. As in the case of bicarbonate, the rate of reabsorption of the salt is equivalent to that of H^+ secretion, but the moiety actually transversing the tubular epithelium is the undissociated acid, which corresponds to CO_2 for the bicarbonate buffer system.

6.2. Use of Phosphate in Renal Acidification Studies

As discussed above, phosphate buffer used in concentrations above the physiological level represents a reasonable approximation to a closed buffer system within the distal renal tubules and is a somewhat less ideal system in mammalian proximal tubules. Due to these characteristics, it has been used to determine the rate of tubular H^+ secretion in the mammalian nephron. Renal tubular acidification leads to both reabsorption of bicarbonate and to buffer titration. Both processes may be mediated by epithelial H^+ secretion, a view held by a considerable number of investigators (Rector, 1973). However, it has been proposed that bicarbonate reabsorption per se, in ionic form, may be responsible for at least a part of this process. This view is based, in part, on the finding that the administration of carbonic anhydrase inhibitors does not reduce bicarbonate transport to levels that may be attributed to uncatalyzed hydration of CO_2 in the tubular cell alone (Maren, 1967). Therefore, there has been an extensive dispute concerning the ultimate mechanisms of bicarbonate reabsorption. An essential piece of evidence regarding the mechanism of HCO_3^- reabsorption is the finding of disequilibrium pH and pCO_2 values both in the renal tubule *in vivo* (Rector *et al.*, 1965; Sohtell and Karlmark, 1976; Vieira and Malnic, 1968) and in turtle urinary bladder *in vitro* (Schilb and Brodsky, 1972; Schwartz *et al.*, 1974; Steinmetz, 1974). The importance of the measurement of these disequilibrium concentrations is based on the reactions occurring during H^+ secretion or bicarbonate reabsorption within the bicarbonate buffer system:

$$CO_2 + H_2O \underset{\text{Carbonic anhydrase}}{\overset{}{\rightleftharpoons}} H_2CO_3 \rightleftharpoons H^+ + HCO_3^- \qquad (2)$$

During H^+ secretion, this reaction is shifted to the left, and a delay in dehydration of H_2CO_3 (dependent on catalysis by the enzyme carbonic anhydrase) or of the removal of CO_2 may lead to disequilibrium concentrations of these components, that is, to an acid disequilibrium pH with higher H_2CO_3 or pCO_2 in the tubular lumen than in blood. On the other hand, primary absorption of bicarbonate ions might shift the reaction to the right, yielding an alkaline disequilibrium pH with lower H_2CO_3 or pCO_2 in the tubular lumen than in blood.

Important to the understanding of the mechanism of bicarbonate reabsorption is the comparison of this process with the rates of acidification of nonbicarbonate buffer systems. In order that titration of a buffer be equated with H^+ secretion, any reabsorption of the buffer components must be insignificant. Only then can the change in H^+ content of the buffer system, calculated by the Henderson–Hasselbalch equation, be equated with the rate of tubular secretion of H^+. Bicarbonate and phosphate acidifications are compared in Fig. 11, which gives a graphic representation of the rate at which bicarbonate approaches its steady-state level (left) and of the acidification of phosphate buffer in the proximal tubular lumen (right). The half-times of bicarbonate reabsorption are significantly shorter than those of phosphate acidification (Giebisch *et al.*, 1977); furthermore, both processes are markedly slowed by the administration of a carbonic anhydrase inhibitor.

The rate of bicarbonate reabsorption is obtained by the relation

$$J_{HCO_3} = \frac{\ln 2}{t/2} \cdot (HCO_{3_0}^- - HCO_{3_\infty}^-) \cdot r/2 \tag{3}$$

where $t/2$ is the half-time of bicarbonate reabsorption as obtained from a plot similar to that in Fig. 11; $HCO_{3_0}^-$ and $HCO_{3_\infty}^-$ are initial and steady-state bicarbonate concentrations; and r is the radius of the tubular lumen. On the other hand, the rate of H^+ secretion determined by titration of phosphate buffer is given by

$$J_H = \frac{\ln 2}{t/2} \cdot (Na_2HPO_{4_0} - Na_2HPO_{4_\infty}) \cdot r/2 \tag{4}$$

where the initial and final alkaline phosphate levels are introduced, assuming that conversion of the alkaline into the acid phosphate is due entirely to H^+ secretion (Giebisch *et al.*, 1977). This is, of course, a simplification of the real situation during tubular perfusion with phosphate. Figure 12 shows some processes other than H^+ secretion which may change luminal pH. First, absorption of the acid or alkaline salt at different velocities might change luminal pH independently of H^+ secretion. Second, since the loss of total phosphate by reabsorption will reduce the right side of equation (4), the absolute rate of H^+ secretion (J_H) at any given time will be proportional to the total amount of phosphate remaining in the tubular lumen. As discussed above, phosphate loss from the lumen

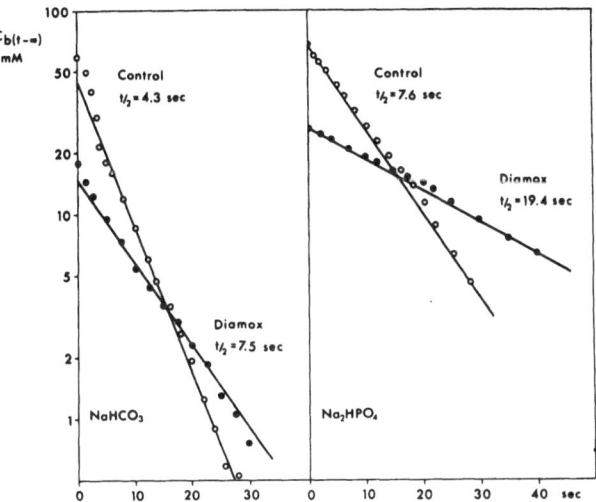

Fig. 11. Approach of luminal buffer base concentrations (C_b) to their steady-state level during proximal tubular perfusions with 100 mM bicarbonate (preequilibrated with 5% CO_2) and 100 mM phosphate solutions. $\bigcirc$, control rats; $\bullet$, acetazolamide-infused rats. (Data from Giebisch *et al.*, 1977; Malnic and Mello Aires, 1971; and Malnic *et al.*, 1972.)

is considerably slower than H^+ secretion when high luminal concentrations of the buffer are used. Therefore, H^+ secretory rates can be obtained at any time by equation (4) when total phosphate concentration at this time is known. In practice, maximal rates are obtained at time zero, as it is more convenient to use rates obtained at this time for comparison between different experimental conditions.

There are still other processes that may affect the rate of acidification of an impermeant buffer species (Fig. 12). Diffusion of CO_2 and/or HCO_3^- across the tubular epithelium might affect the luminal pH by the reaction

$$Na_2HPO_4 + H_2CO_3 \rightleftharpoons NaH_2PO_4 + NaHCO_3$$

CO_2 diffusion into the lumen will accelerate luminal acidification, while influx of bicarbonate will lead to the opposite result. Capillary perfusion with bicarbonate-free and CO_2-free Ringer's solutions, as well as perfusion experiments of isolated kidneys with such solutions, have indicated that these processes are not of major importance in the tubular acidification of intraluminal phosphate (Cassola *et al.*, 1977; Mello Aires and Malnic, 1975). Finally, diffusion of NaCl and water into isolated phosphate-containing droplets in the tubular lumen will reduce phosphate con-

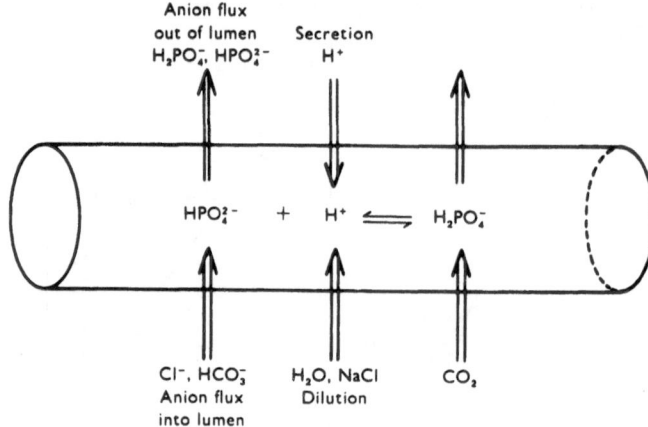

Fig. 12. Processes potentially leading to pH changes during renal tubular perfusion with phosphate buffer. (From Giebisch et al., 1977.)

centrations, leading to alterations similar to those discussed above for phosphate loss from the lumen.

Experiments such as those depicted in Fig. 11 have shown that in the proximal tubule, bicarbonate reabsorption is of the order of 9.9 nEq/cm^2/sec, while the rate of phosphate acidification is 5.2 nEq/cm^2/sec . By measuring the rates of these processes after carbonic anhydrase inhibition, it was possible to ascribe about 54% of proximal bicarbonate reabsorption to carbonic-anhydrase-dependent plus uncatalyzed H^+ generation (Cassola et al., 1977). These two components of H^+ generation could account for close to 100% of bicarbonate reabsorption in the distal tubule. During metabolic acidosis, H^+ secretion was able to account for all of bicarbonate reabsorption in both tubular segments. More recent experiments (Lucci et al., 1979; McKinney and Burg, 1977) in the isolated perfused nephron have shown practically total inhibition of bicarbonate reabsorption by carbonic anhydrase inhibitors, implying that all bicarbonate reabsorption is mediated by catalyzed H^+ secretion. In some of these experiments, however, acetazolamide concentrations of the order of 10^{-3} M were used. Such high concentrations have effects other than carbonic anhydrase inhibition; they impair cell metabolism and inhibit anion transport systems, for instance, in the red blood cell (Cousin et al., 1975; Maren, 1967; Norby et al., 1977).

The finding of complete inhibition of bicarbonate reabsorption by carbonic anhydrase inhibitors, if confirmed, would indicate that H^+ secretion alone might account for all bicarbonate reabsorption. The results obtained during stopped-flow microperfusion in vivo comparing bicarbonate with phosphate reabsorption do not necessarily imply that a specific transport system for bicarbonate ions exists. The more rapid acidification of bicarbonate buffer could be due to the highly diffusible "acid" form of the bicarbonate system, be it CO_2 or H_2CO_3, as compared with the rate of removal of $H_2PO_4^-$ (Fig. 7).

6.3. Physicochemical Properties of Anions

The idea that $H_2PO_4^-$ or HPO_4^{2-} may be reabsorbed preferentially can be considered in terms of certain general physical properties of anions. According to the lyotropic series and the Hofmeister series (Hoeber, 1947), the effectiveness of an anion to precipitate proteins from solution, to cause the gelification of colloids, to affect the ion exchange properties of macromolecules, etc., follows a sequence that is approximately common to these apparently different phenomena. In this series, divalent anions are generally more effective than monovalent anions, sulfate being in most series the more lyotropic anion (Voet, 1937). Passive ion permeability in a number of structures has also been shown to follow such series. It is well known that divalent anions are less permeant than small monovalent anions like chloride in proximal and distal nephron segments of mammalian and amphibian kidney (Boulpaep and Seely, 1971; Clapp et al., 1962; Froemter et al., 1971). This is manifested by an increase in transepithelial PD upon perfusion with solutions containing sulfate and ferrocyanide as the main anionic species. Froemter et al. (1971) have shown, furthermore, that permeability ratios in rat proximal tubule, P_{X^-}/P_{Cl^-}, are lower than free-diffusion coefficient ratios for monovalent small anions. For instance, $D_{HCO_3^-}/D_{Cl^-} = 0.59$ and $P_{HCO_3^-}/P_{Cl^-} = 0.44$; whereas $D_{SO_4^{2-}}/D_{Cl^-} = 0.42$ and $P_{SO_4^{2-}}/P_{Cl^-} = 0.25$; and $D_{Fe(CN)_6^{4-}}/D_{Cl^-} = 0.21$ and $P_{Fe(CN)_6^{4-}}/P_{Cl^-} = 0.12$. This shows that the permeability of a biological membrane to polyvalent anions is much less than its permeability to monovalent anions.

These data are compatible with the conclusion, obtained from a number of electrophysiological data, that the effective "pores" of mammalian renal tubules are lined with negative charges. This conclusion is based on the measurement of biionic potentials during perfusion with NaCl solutions. In the presence of a transepithelial NaCl gradient, the side with higher salt concentration is rendered negative, implying greater permeability of the tubular wall to cations than to anions. Streaming potentials observed during osmotically induced volume flow in rat proximal tubules also suggest the existence of such negative charges (Boulpaep and Seely, 1971; De Mello et al., 1976; Froemter et al., 1971). On the other hand, in amphibian proximal tubules, similar electrophysiological investigations have yielded evidence favoring the existence of pores lined with positive charges (Anagnostopoulos, 1973).

The behavior of phosphate ions in biological membranes depends on both their physicochemical properties in free solution and their interaction with membranes. According to Graham's law (Castellan, 1972), diffusion coefficients are related to the inverse of the square root of the molecular weight of particles:

$$D = k \cdot \frac{1}{\sqrt{Mol. wt.}}$$

where k is a proportionality coefficient. Therefore, no significant differences are expected for the diffusion coefficients of HPO_4^{2-} and $H_2PO_4^-$ in free solution. On the other hand, their limiting equivalent conductivities are markedly different, that is, 26.4–36 Ω^{-1} cm^2/Eq for $H_2PO_4^-$ against 53.4–57 Ω^{-1} cm^2/Eq for HPO_4^{2-} at 25°C (Landolt and Börnstein, 1960). Thus, while in aqueous solution, a similar diffusional mobility is expected, in an electric field, divalent phosphate movement will be affected to a much greater extent, since each particle has twice the amount of charge. The PD of the proximal tubule would thus be expected to exert a considerably greater effect on HPO_4^{2-} than on $H_2PO_4^-$. In early segments of the proximal tubule, where the lumen is electrically negative (Barratt et al., 1974), HPO_4^{2-} might move passively out of the lumen more rapidly than $H_2PO_4^-$. At more distal sites along the proximal tubule, where the lumen is electrically positive (Barratt et al., 1974), HPO_4^{2-} might be retained in the lumen and $H_2PO_4^-$ move outward more readily, presumably by active transport. Such considerations of the effect of PD might account for the different observations concerning preferential transport of $H_2PO_4^-$ versus HPO_4^{2-} in the studies by Bank et al. (1974) and by Baumann et al. (1975b). Thus, differences in the composition of the perfusion fluids, or the presence of raffinose, might have resulted in different PD values in the two studies.

Data concerning specific permeability properties of mono- and divalent phosphate salts in extrarenal tissue are scarce. In the red blood cell, whose membrane has pores with positive fixed charges, permeability to small monovalent anions is greater than that to small monovalent cations. However, this membrane shows low permeability to anions like sulfate and phosphate (Passow and Schnell, 1969). Rummel et al. (1958) have studied the effect of ambient pH on uptake and washout of ^{32}P by red blood cells. They found a maximum of both processes at a pH of 6.4–6.6; above and below this value, uptake and washout rates declined. They concluded that phosphate movement probably depended on the interaction with an enzyme-like molecule that had a pH optimum in the described range and that phosphate movement probably did not depend primarily on the form of the salt present in the medium. Similar findings are referred to by other investigators working with the red blood cell (Bielinski et al., 1969; Deuticke, 1970; Gruber and Deuticke, 1973). Studies at pH 6.6 and 8 by Schrier et al. (1970) led these authors to postulate that HPO_4^{2-} movements are predominantly passive, while $H_2PO_4^-$ transfer manifests saturation kinetics and countertransport characteristics and therefore is affected by carrier-mediated transport. This view is supported by the work of Ho and Guidotti (1975), who have identified a membrane glycoprotein responsible for phosphate transport at pH 6.42. This protein is thought to span the membrane bilayer and is the only membrane component binding to an irreversible inhibitor of phosphate transport in the red blood cell, the isothiocyanate derivative of the sulfanilate anion.

6.4. Mechanism of Action of Acetazolamide and Bicarbonate

The possibility of a common mechanism of action of acetazolamide and PTH on phosphate transport has attracted some attention. Beck and Goldberg (1973), as well as Garg (1976), did not find a carbonic anhydrase inhibitory effect of PTH in an in vitro assay system, contrary to what had been reported by Beck et al. (1975). Knox et al. (1976) studied this question further by recollection micropuncture experiments, using electron microprobe analysis of phosphate concentrations in tubular fluid. They found that in the dog, PTH increased FE_{PO_4} at the end of the cortical proximal tubule from 28 to 38% and that acetazolamide increased this excretion further to 58%. Thus, the effect of acetazolamide was additive to that of PTH, indicating that both agents act on phosphate reabsorption but apparently by independent mechanisms.

The action of PTH on the proximal tubule, causing not only phosphaturia but also bicarbonaturia has been studied (Bank and Aynedjian, 1976; Dennis, 1976; Nascimento et al., 1977). Of interest with regard to the present discussion is the proposal that the bicarbonaturia induced by PTH may be mediated by decreased plasma phosphate levels and not by a direct action of the hormone on the tubular epithelium (Gold et al., 1973). This hypothesis is based on the relationship between plasma phosphate levels and bicarbonate excretion. After phosphate depletion, urinary bicarbonate wasting was observed (Gold et al., 1973). A recent micropuncture study of this subject confirmed the relationship between plasma phosphorus and bicarbonate reabsorption both in control and TPTX dogs (Puschett and Fernandez, 1977). In these animals, absolute tubular reabsorption of bicarbonate was linearly related to serum ultrafilterable phosphorus concentration, even though serum phosphorus concentrations varied widely in the two groups. The authors suggested that the plasma level of phosphate may be one of the determining factors in bicarbonate reabsorption.

One possible explanation for the effect of acetazolamide is that intracellular pH may be increased, as suggested by the experiments of Struyvenberg et al. (1968). They found an increase of cellular pH in separated dog renal tubules from 7.32 to 7.42–7.45 when exposed to acetazolamide. Another possibility is that acetazolamide may have a specific effect on the transport mechanism of phosphate; it has been shown in other structures (red blood cell, frog cornea) that this drug may act on Cl^- transport or on Cl^-/HCO_3^- exchange (Cousin et al., 1975; Kitahara et al., 1967). Especially at high dosage levels, of the order of 10^{-3} M, acetazolamide may have a number of actions in addition to that of carbonic anhydrase inhibition, including the inhibition of cellular metabolism (Maren, 1977; Norby et al., 1977).

It has also been postulated that the effect of acetazolamide on phosphate excretion is mediated via activation of adenyl cyclase. Rodriguez et al. (1974) found that acetazolamide increased urinary excretion of cyclic AMP (cAMP) in normal and PTX rats and that the carbonic anhydrase inhibitor stimulated the activity of renal cortical adenyl cyclase in vitro. However, this hypothesis is controversial, since Sinha et al. (1977) found that acetazolamide consistently increased phosphate clearance in hypoparathyroid and pseudohypoparathyroid patients without increasing urinary cAMP excretion. Moreover, as discussed earlier, Knox et al. (1976) found that acetazolamide inhibited phosphate reabsorption predominantly in the proximal convoluted tubule, whereas PTH had a greater inhibitory effect on more distal nephron segments, and the effect of the two agents on urinary phosphate excretion was additive. These findings suggest, but do not prove, that PTH and acetazolamide inhibit phosphate reabsorption by different mechanisms. Thus, at the present time, there are data for and against the view that acetazolamide inhibits phosphate reabsorption via stimulation of renal adenyl cyclase, a mechanism which would be similar to that of PTH.

During the administration of acetazolamide, proximal tubular pH falls slightly in spite of an increase in bicarbonate concentration from about 8 to 25 mEq/liter (Rector et al., 1965; Vieira and Malnic, 1968). This change has been shown to be due to an acid disequilibrium pH caused by either an increased H_2CO_3 concentration (Rector et al., 1965; Vieira and Malnic, 1968) or the elevation of pCO_2 in tubular fluid to levels considerably higher than in plasma (Sohtell and Karlmark, 1976). The latter may result from impaired diffusion of CO_2 through the epithelium when carbonic anhydrase has been inhibited (Malnic and Mello Aires, 1971). Under these conditions, a disequilibrium state exists in which the low pH is due to accumulation of H_2CO_3 or dissolved CO_2 in the tubular fluid.

Thus, one cannot attribute the inhibition of phosphate reabsorption by acetazolamide to alkalinization of proximal tubular fluid. However, acetazolamide has another action, which is to reduce the rate of H^+ secretion by the proximal tubular cells and thereby to reduce the rate of HCO_3^- reabsorption. The result is a high concentration of HCO_3^- in the proximal tubular fluid (Rector et al., 1965; Vieira and Malnic, 1968). These high bicarbonate concentrations per se could be the cause of the reduced rate of phosphate reabsorption. However, the mechanism by which they might act is not clear. As discussed above, the work of Dennis et al. (1976) in isolated perfused rabbit nephron has shown that the lumen–bath flux of phosphate is not affected by low or normal bicarbonate concentrations as long as the fluid pH is maintained. These authors have not studied higher than normal (25 mM) bicarbonate concentrations.

A practically normal proximal pH together with high bicarbonate concentrations due to the disequilibrium situation of the bicarbonate buffer would not alter the normal proportion between HPO_4^{2-} and $H_2PO_4^-$ in the lumen, since these depend on the pH of luminal fluid, and the reactions between the components of the phosphate buffer system are practically instantaneous. Thus, the H^+ ions secreted by the acetazolamide-treated epithelium at a reduced rate would flow preferentially into phosphate buffer and would convert less HCO_3^- into CO_2 and water due to the disequilibrium situation of the bicarbonate buffer. Nevertheless, in the presence of acetazolamide, the reduced rate of H^+ secretion might make less H^+ available per unit time for titration of HPO_4^{2-} during transit of phosphate through the proximal tubule. Although a disequilibrium pH exists in the proximal tubule during administration of acetazolamide, it is not clear whether this pH remains constant along the length of the proximal tubule or falls more gradually than under control conditions. These uncertainties make it difficult to draw any conclusions about the mechanism of action of acetazolamide on phosphate reabsorption.

During bicarbonate loading, on the other hand, both HCO_3^- concentrations and pH are increased. According to the titration curves given in Fig. 10, H^+ ion secretion would be diverted predominantly into HCO_3^- reabsorption, since at a pH above 7, bicarbonate concentrations fall more rapidly than those of HPO_4^{2-}. Thus, due to the competition of the two buffers for available H^+, the increase in $H_2PO_4^-$ levels would be delayed along the proximal tubule. This effect might not occur at normal or low HCO_3^- concentrations, as indicated by the studies of Dennis et al. (1976), because the concentration of $H_2PO_4^-$ is high enough to saturate the active transport mechanism for $H_2PO_4^-$. However, the relevant alterations with both acetazolamide and bicarbonate loading might be those occurring within tubular cells. Here, both acetazolamide and bicarbonate loading increase pH (Adler et al., 1963; Struyvenberg et al., 1968).

An alternative hypothesis is that HCO_3^- competes with either $H_2PO_4^-$ or HPO_4^{2-} (or both) for sites on a common transport carrier in the luminal membrane. This seems unlikely in view of the evidence discussed above that most, if not all, HCO_3^- reabsorption is mediated by H^+ secretion rather than by transfer of the HCO_3^- ion itself.

Finally, transfer from cell to peritubular space may be affected by an anion carrier system that could be involved in both bicarbonate and phosphate transport. Recent evidence indicates that peritubular bicarbonate extrusion may be carrier mediated and depressed by acetazolamide. These conclusions are based, in part, on electrophysiological measurements of bicarbonate conductance in the basolateral membrane, which is decreased by acetazolamide (Froemter, 1975), and on microperfusion studies of peritubular capillaries which show that the equilibration of their pH with that of the cells is delayed after treatment with acetazolamide (Garcia-Filho and Malnic, 1976). It is possible that peritubular transfer of phosphate might proceed by this or a similar carrier system. In red blood cells and turtle bladder, anions (OH^-, HCO_3^-, SO_4^{2-}) are transferred across the cell membrane in exchange for chloride, a process that is inhibited by SITS and by DIDS (4,4'-diisothiocyanostilbene-2,2'-disulfonate) (Ehrenspeck and Brodsky, 1976; Knauf et al., 1977). For the proximal tubular epithelium, however, no significant effect of SITS on phosphate transport was observed (Ullrich et al., 1977).

The preceding discussion shows that the specific mechanism of the action of urinary alkalinization on phosphate reabsorption is not yet clear. The site of action of the effect might be within the tubular lumen, within the cell, or at the peritubular cell membrane. Thus, it is clear that further studies will be necessary to define the involved mechanisms more precisely.

7. CLINICAL IMPLICATIONS

Most studies on the relation between acid–base balance and phosphate excretion have been performed under acute experimental conditions. The chronic exposure of patients to elevated (0.7%) CO_2 concentrations led to decreased phosphate excretion and increased plasma phosphate levels, a finding compatible with preferential reabsorption of acid phosphate (Gray et al., 1973). The effects of alkalinization of the urine on phosphate reabsorption have been studied only under acute experimental conditions, and the observations relate more to basic mechanisms of renal phosphate transport than to long-term balance effects. The observations cannot be extrapolated to chronic situations, since a large number of other variables which influence renal phosphate excretion might dominate renal phosphate transport with long-term acid–base changes. For example, chronic acetazolamide or $NaHCO_3$ administration might have different effects on bone and other tissue phosphorus, causing release or deposition and thus altering serum phosphorus concentration. Other factors which could be influenced in long-term studies are intestinal absorption of phosphorus, PTH release, extracellular volume, renal hemodynamics, the concentration of calcium in blood, and vitamin D metabolism. All of these variables could affect phosphorus excretion in chronic studies in a manner which might either offset or augment the effect of alkalinization of the urine. Until such long-term studies have been carried out, one should not extrapolate the results of acute alkalinization experiments to clinical situations in humans.

8. REFERENCES

Adler, S., Roy, A., and Relman, A. S., 1963, Intracellular acid–base regulation. I. The response of muscle cells to changes in CO_2 tension or extracellular bicarbonate concentrations, J. Clin. Invest. 44:8.

Amiel, C., Küntziger, H., Couette, S., Coureau, C., and Bergounioux, N., 1976, Evidence for a parathyroid hormone-independent calcium modulation of phosphate transport along the nephron, J. Clin. Invest. 57:256.

Anagnostopoulos, T., 1973, Biionic potentials in the proximal tubule of Necturus kidney, J. Physiol. (London) 233:375.

Bank, N., and Aynedjian, H. S., 1976, A micropuncture study of the effect of parathyroid hormone on renal bicarbonate reabsorption, J. Clin. Invest. 58:336.

Bank, N., Aynedjian, H. S., and Weinstein, S. W., 1974, A microperfusion study of phosphate reabsorption by the rat proximal renal tubule, J. Clin. Invest. 54:1040.

Barratt, L. J., Rector, F. C., Jr., Kokko, J. P., and Seldin, D. W., 1974, Factors governing the transepithelial potential difference across the proximal tubule of the rat kidney, J. Clin. Invest. 53:454.

Baumann, K., de Rouffignac, C., Roinel, N., Rumrich, G., and Ullrich, K. J., 1975a, Renal phosphate transport: Inhomogeneity of local proximal transport rates and sodium dependence, Pflügers Arch. 356:287.

Baumann, K., Rumrich, G., Papavassiliou, F., and Kloess, S., 1975b, pH dependence of phosphate reabsorption in the proximal tubule of rat kidney, Pflügers Arch. 360:183.

Beck, L. H., and Goldberg, M., 1973, Effects of acetazolamide and parathyroidectomy on renal transport of sodium, calcium, and phosphate, Am. J. Physiol. 224:1136.

Beck, L. H., and Goldberg, M., 1974, Mechanism of the blunted phosphaturia in saline-loaded thyroparathyroidectomized dogs, Kidney Int. 6:18.

Beck, N., Kim, K. S., Wolak, M., and Davis, B. B., 1975, Inhibition of carbonic anhydrase by parathyroid hormone and cyclic AMP in rat renal cortex in vitro, J. Clin. Invest. 55:149.

Bielinski, E., Gomulkiewicz, J., and Przestalski, S., 1969, Influence of pH on the phosphate ion permeability into erythrocytes, Stud. Biophys. 13:217.

Bonjour, J.-P., Preston, C., and Fleisch, H., 1977, Effect of 1,25-dihydroxyvitamin D_3 on the renal handling of P_i in thyroparathyroidectomized rats, J. Clin. Invest. 60:1419.

Boulpaep, E. L., and Seely, J. F., 1971, Electrophysiology of proximal and distal tubules in autoperfused dog kidney, *Am. J. Physiol.* **221**:1084.

Cassola, A. C., and Malnic, G., 1977, Phosphate transfer and tubular pH during renal stopped-flow microperfusion experiments in the rat, *Pflügers Arch.* **367**:249.

Cassola, A. C., Giebisch, G., and Malnic, G., 1977, Mechanisms and components of renal tubular acidification, *J. Physiol. (London)* **267**:601.

Castellan, G. W., 1972, *Physical Chemistry*, p. 698, Addison-Wesley, Reading, Mass.

Clapp, J. R., Rector, F. C., and Seldin, D. W., 1962, Effect of unreabsorbed anions on proximal and distal transtubular potentials in rats, *Am. J. Physiol.* **202**:781.

Cousin, J. L., Motais, R., and Sola, F., 1975, Transmembrane exchange of chloride with bicarbonate ion in mammalian red blood cells: Evidence for a sulphonamide-sensitive "carrier," *J. Physiol. (London)* **253**:385.

De Mello, G. B., Lopes, A. G., and Malnic, G., 1976, Conductances, diffusion and streaming potentials in the rat proximal tubule, *J. Physiol. (London)* **260**:553.

Dennis, V. W., 1976, Influence of bicarbonate on parathyroid hormone-induced changes in fluid absorption by the proximal tubule, *Kidney Int.* **10**:373.

Dennis, V. W., Woodhall, P. B., and Robinson, R. R., 1976, Characteristics of phosphate transport in isolated proximal tubule, *Am. J. Physiol.* **231**:979.

Dennis, V. W., Bello-Reuss, E., and Robinson, R. R., 1977, Response of phosphate transport to parathyroid hormone in segments of rabbit nephron, *Am. J. Physiol.* **233**:F29.

Deuticke, B., 1970, Anion permeability of the red blood cell, *Naturwissenschaften* **57**:172.

Ehrenspeck, G., and Brodsky, W. A., 1976, Effects of 4-acetamido-4′-isothiocyano-2,2′-disulfonic stilbene on ion transport in turtle bladders, *Biochim. Biophys. Acta* **419**:555.

Frick, A., 1971, Parathormone as a mediator of inorganic phosphate diuresis during saline infusion in the rat, *Pflügers Arch. Eur. J. Physiol.* **325**:1.

Frick, A., 1972, Proximal tubular reabsorption of inorganic phosphate during saline infusion in the rat, *Am. J. Physiol.* **223**:1034.

Froemter, E., 1975, Electrophysiological studies on the mechanism of H^+/HCO_3^- transport in rat proximal tubule, in: *Proceedings of the VI International Congress of Nephrology*, Florence, Italy, p. 25 (Abstract).

Froemter, E., Mueller, C. W., and Wick, T., 1971, Permeability properties of the proximal tubular epithelium of the rat kidney studied with electrophysiological methods, in: *Electrophysiology of Epithelial Cells* (G. Giebisch, ed.), pp. 119–146, Schattauer, Stuttgart.

Fulop, M., and Brazeau, P., 1968, The phosphaturic effect of sodium bicarbonate and acetazolamide in dogs, *J. Clin. Invest.* **47**:983.

Garcia-Filho, E. M., and Malnic, G., 1976, pH in cortical peritubular capillaries of rat kidney, *Pflügers Arch.* **363**:211.

Garg, L. C., 1976, Failure of parathyroid hormone and cyclic AMP to inhibit renal carbonic anhydrase, *Pflügers Arch.* **367**:103.

Giebisch, G., Malnic, G., De Mello, G. B., and de Mello Aires, M., 1977, Kinetics of luminal acidification in cortical tubules of the rat kidney, *J. Physiol. (London)* **267**:571.

Gold, L. W., Massry, S. G., Arieff, A. I., and Coburn, J. W., 1973, Renal bicarbonate wasting during phosphate depletion. A possible cause of altered acid–base homeostasis in hyperparathyroidism, *J. Clin. Invest.* **52**:2556.

Gottschalk, L. W., Lassiter, W. E., and Mylle, M., 1960, Localization of urine acidification in the mammalian kidney, *Am. J. Physiol.* **198**:581.

Gradowska, L., Caglar, S., Rutherford, E., Harter, H., and Slatopolsky, E., 1973, On the mechanism of the phosphaturia of extracellular volume expansion in the dog, *Kidney Int.* **3**:230.

Gray, S. P., Morris, J. E. W., and Brooks, C. J., 1973, Renal handling of calcium, magneisium, inorganic phosphate and hydrogen ions during prolonged exposure to elevated carbon dioxide concentrations, *Clin. Sci. Mol. Med.* **45**:751.

Gruber, W., and Deuticke, B., 1973, Comparative aspects of phosphate transfer across mammalian erythrocyte membranes, *J. Membr. Biol.* **13**:19.

Ho, M. K., and Guidotti, G., 1975, A membrane protein from human erythrocytes involved in anion exchange, *J. Biol. Chem.* **250**:675.

Hoeber, R., 1947, *Physikalische Chemie der Zellen und Gewebe*, p. 319, Staempfli, Bern.

Hoffmann, N., Thees, M., and Kinne, R., 1976, Phosphate transport by isolated renal brush border vesicles, *Pflügers Arch.* **362**:147.

Jobin, J., Navar, T., Caron, C., and Plante, G. E., 1977, Effect of acetazolamide on renal bicarbonate reabsorption in volume-expanded dogs, *Am. J. Physiol.* **232**:F484.

Kitahara, S., Fox, K. R., and Hogben, C. A. M., 1967, Depression of chloride transport by carbonic anhydrase inhibitors in the absence of carbonic anhydrase, *Nature* **214**:836.

Knauf, P. A., Fuhrmann, G. F., Rothstein, S., and Rothstein, A., 1977, The relationship between anion exchange and net anion flow across the human red blood cell membrane, *J. Gen. Physiol.* **69**:363.

Knox, F. G., Schneider, E. G., Willis, L. R., Strandhoy, J. W., and Ott, C. E., 1973, Site and control of phosphate reabsorption by the kidney, *Kidney Int.* **3**:347.

Knox, F. G., Haas, J. A., and Lechêne, C. P., 1976, Effect of parathyroid hormone on phosphate reabsorption in the presence of acetazolamide, *Kidney Int.* **10**:216.

Küntziger, H., Amiel, C., and Gaudebout, G., 1972, Phosphate handling by the rat nephron during saline diuresis, *Kidney Int.* **2**:318.

Kuroda, S., Aynedjian, H. S., Bank, D. E., and Bank, N., 1979, Relationship between proximal tubule total CO_2 and phosphate reabsorption in acute and chronic PTX rats, *Renal Physiol.* **3**:171.

Landolt, H., and Börnstein, R., 1960, *Zahlenwerte und Funktionen*, Vol. II(7), Springer-Verlag, Berlin.

Lang, F., Greger, R., Marchand, G. R., and Knox, F. G., 1977, Stationary microperfusion study of phosphate reabsorption in proximal and distal nephron segments, *Pflügers Arch.* **368**:45.

Lucci, M. S., Warnock, D. G., and Rector, F. C., 1979, Carbonic anhydrase-dependent bicarbonate reabsorption in rat proximal tubule, *Am. J. Physiol.* **236**:58.

Maesaka, J. K., Levitt, M. F., and Abramson, R. G., 1973, Effect of saline infusion on phosphate transport in intact and thyroparathyroidectomized rats, *Am. J. Physiol.* **225**:1421.

Malnic, G., and Mello Aires, M., 1971, Kinetic study of bicarbonate reabsorption in proximal tubule of the rat, *Am. J. Physiol.* **220**:1759.

Malnic, G., and Steinmetz, P. R., 1976, Transport processes in urinary acidification, *Kidney Int.* **9**:172.

Malnic, G., Mello Aires, M., De Mello, G. B., and Giebisch, G., 1972, Acidification of phosphate buffer in cortical tubules of rat kidney, *Pflügers Arch.* **331**:275.

Malvin, R. L., and Lotspeich, W. D., 1956, Relation between tubular transport of inorganic phosphate and bicarbonate in the dog, *Am. J. Physiol.* **187**:51.

Maren, T. H., 1967, Carbonic anhydrase: Chemistry, physiology and inhibition, *Physiol. Rev.* **47**:595.

Maren, T. H., 1977, Use of inhibitors in physiological studies of carbonic anhydrase, *Am. J. Physiol.* **232**:F291.

Massry, S. G., Coburn, J. W., and Kleeman, C. R., 1969, The influence of extracellular volume expansion on renal phosphate reabsorption in the dog, *J. Clin. Invest.* **48**:1237.

McKinney, T. D., and Burg, M. B., 1977, Bicarbonate and fluid absorption by renal proximal straight tubules, *Kidney Int.* **12**:1.

Mello Aires, M., and Malnic, G., 1975, Peritubular pH and pCO_2 in renal tubular acidification, *Am. J. Physiol.* **228**:1766.

Mercado, A., Slatopolsky, E., and Klahr, S., 1975, On the mechanisms responsible for the phosphaturia of bicarbonate administration, *J. Clin. Invest.* **56**:1386.

Mostellar, M. E., and Tuttle, E. P., Jr., 1964, Effects of alkalosis on plasma concentration and urinary excretion of inorganic phosphate in man, *J. Clin. Invest.* **43**:138.

Nascimento, L., Rademacher, D. R., Arruda, J. A. L., and Kurtzman, N. A., 1977, Effect of acetazolamide and parathyroid hormone on HCO_3 and PO_4 excretion, *J. Pharmacol. Exp. Ther.* **201**:243.

Norby, L. H., Lawson, N., and Schwartz, J. H., 1977, A new mechanism for the inhibition of urinary acidification by acetazolamide, *Clin. Res.* **25**:443A.

Passow, H., and Schnell, K. F., 1969, Chemical modifiers of passive ion permeability of the erythrocyte membrane, *Experientia* **25**:460.

Puschett, J. B., and Fernandez, P. C., 1977, Relationship between serum phosphate concentration and proximal tubular bicarbonate transport, *Nephron* **19**:44.

Puschett, J. B., and Goldberg, M., 1969, The relationship between the renal handling of phosphate and bicarbonate in man, *J. Lab. Clin. Med.* **73**:956.

Puschett, J. B., Agus, Z. S., Senesky, D., and Goldberg, M., 1972, Effect of saline loading and aortic obstruction on proximal phosphate transport, *Am. J. Physiol.* **223**:851.

Rasmussen, H., Anast, C., and Arnaud, C., 1967, Thyrocalcitonin, EGTA, and urinary electrolyte excretion, *J. Clin. Invest.* **46**:746.

Rector, F. C., 1973, Acidification of the urine, in: *Handbook of Physiology, Section 8, Renal Physiology* (J. Orloff and R. W. Berliner, eds.), pp. 431–454, American Physiological Society, Washington, D.C.

Rector, F. C., Carter, N. W., and Seldin, D. W., 1965, The mechanism of bicarbonate reabsorption in the proximal and distal tubules of the kidney, *J. Clin. Invest.* **44**:278.

Rodriguez, H. J., Walls, J., Yates, J., and Klahr, S., 1974, Effects of acetazolamide on the urinary excretion of cyclic AMP and on the activity of renal adenyl cyclase, *J. Clin. Invest.* **53**:122.

Rummel, W., Pfleger, K., and Seifen, E., 1958, Die pH-Abhängigkeit der Aufnahme und Abgabe von anorganischem Phosphat am Erythrocyten, *Biochem. Z.* **330**:310.

Schilb, T. P., and Brodsky, W. A., 1972, CO_2 gradients and acidification by transport of HCO_3^- in turtle bladders, *Am. J. Physiol.* **222**:272.

Schneider, E. G., Goldsmith, R. S., Arnaud, C. D., and Knox, F. G., 1975, Role of parathyroid hormone in the phosphaturia of extracellular fluid volume expansion, *Kidney Int.* **7**:317.

Schrier, S. L., Moore, L. D., and Chiapella, A. P., 1970, Transfer of inorganic phosphate across human erythrocyte membranes, *J. Lab. Clin. Med.* **75**:422.

Schwartz, J. H., Finn, J. T., Vaughn, G., and Steinmetz, P. R., 1974, Distribution of metabolic CO_2 and the transported ion species in acidification by turtle bladder, *Am. J. Physiol.* **226**:283.

Sinha, T. K., Allen, D. O., Queener, S. F., and Bell, N. H., 1977, Effects of acetazolamide on the renal excretion of phosphate in hypoparathyroidism and pseudohypoparathyroidism, *J. Lab. Clin. Med.* **89**:1188.

Sohtell, M., and Karlmark, B., 1976, *In vivo* micropuncture pCO_2 measurements, *Pflügers Arch.* **363**:179.

Staum, B. B., Hamburger, R. J., and Goldberg, M., 1972, Tracer microinjection study of renal tubular phosphate reabsorption in the rat, *J. Clin. Invest.* **51**:2271.

Steele, T. H., 1977, Bicarbonate-induced phosphaturia, *Pflügers Arch.* **370**:291.

Steele, T. H., and DeLuca, H. F., 1976, Influence of dietary phosphorus on renal phosphate reabsorption in the parathyroidectomized rat, *J. Clin. Invest.* **57**:867.

Steinmetz, P. R., 1974, Cellular mechanism of urinary acidification, *Physiol. Rev.* **54**:890.

Strickler, J. C., Thompson, D. D., Klose, R. M., and Giebisch, G., 1964, Micropuncture study of inorganic phosphate excretion in the rat, *J. Clin. Invest.* **43**:1596.

Struyvenberg, A., Morrison, R. B., and Relman, A. S., 1968, Acid–base behavior of separated canine renal tubule cells, *Am. J. Physiol.* **214**:1155.

Tröhler, J., Bonjour, J.-P., and Fleisch, H., 1976, Inorganic phosphate homeostasis. Renal adaptation to the dietary intake in intact and thyroparathyroidectomized rats, *J. Clin. Invest.* **57**:264.

Ullrich, K. J., Rumrich, G., and Baumann, K., 1975, Renal proximal tubular buffer (glycodiazine) transport: Inhomogeneity of local transport rate, dependence on sodium effect of inhibitors and chronic adaptation, *Pflügers Arch.* **357**:149.

Ullrich, K. J., Capasso, G., Rumrich, G., Papavassiliou, F., and Kloess, S., 1977, Coupling between proximal tubular transport processes. Studies with ouabain, SITS and HCO_3^--free solutions, *Pflügers Arch.* **368**:245.

Vieira, F. L., and Malnic, G., 1968, Hydrogen secretion by rat renal cortical tubules as studied by an antimony microelectrode, *Am. J. Physiol.* **214**:710.

Voet, A., 1937, Quantitative lyotrophy, *Chem. Rev.* **20**:169.

Wen, S. F., 1974, Micropuncture studies of phosphate transport in the proximal tubule of the dog. The relationship to sodium reabsorption, *J. Clin. Invest.* **53**:143.

Zilenovski, A. M., Kuroda, S., Bhat, S., Bank, D. E., and Bank, N., 1979, Effect of sodium bicarbonate on phosphate excretion in acute and chronic PTX rats, *Am. J. Physiol.* **236**: F184.

9

Tubular Adaptation to the Supply and Requirement of Phosphate

JEAN-PHILIPPE BONJOUR and HERBERT FLEISCH

1. INTRODUCTION

Among the various fluxes of inorganic phosphate (Pi) which contribute to the setting of the plasma Pi level, the net tubular reabsorption (TR_{Pi}) is likely the largest one, at least under normal physiological conditions (Bijvoet, 1969; Bijvoet and Morgan, 1971; Nordin, 1976). Hence, a change in the net TR_{Pi} can be expected to markedly alter the plasma concentration of Pi. By altering the level of Pi in the extracellular fluid, the net TR_{Pi} probably influences the intracellular pool of Pi in the various tissues of the organism and also the amount of bone mineral. With such an impact, the tubular Pi transport could be one of the essential controlling variables in Pi homeostasis.

In order to play this controlling role, the tubular Pi transport should respond to factors which interfere with the controlled variable(s). The nature of this or these controlled variables has not been yet defined. The homeostasis of Pi is usually considered mainly in terms of the regulation of plasma Pi. The control of plasma Pi within some limits is certainly critical for maintaining an adequate [Ca] × [Pi] product in the extracellular fluids of the organism. However, the intracellular pool of Pi or at least some of its compartments may represent other variables which require a strict regulation. Indeed, Pi plays an unique intracellular role as a regulator of several metabolic pathways as well as being an essential constituent of many organic substances. Besides the ubiquitous intracellular role, Pi is a main component of bone mineral. Therefore, the amount of bone mineral might represent another variable which is tightly controlled. It is thus possible that the controlling factors of Pi homeostasis will respond to variables other than simply the plasma Pi concentration. In fact,

243

one can even envisage that the plasma Pi may be set at various levels according to the intracellular and skeletal requirements.

Whatever the exact nature of the controlled variables is, one can anticipate that fluctuations in the supply or in the demand for Pi will disturb them and provoke a response of the controlling factors. Therefore, the tubular Pi transport system should respond to variations in the supply or in the demand for Pi by changing its capacity for Pi transport according to homeostatic requirements. The purpose of this chapter is to describe the response of the renal tubule to the Pi needs of the organism and to discuss its relation to other factors known to influence the handling of Pi at the kidney level. However, before reviewing this subject, it appears appropriate to start with a note on methodology related to the assessment of the tubular capacity to transport Pi.

2. ASSESSMENT OF THE OVERALL TUBULAR CAPACITY TO TRANSPORT Pi

It is obvious that the tubular capacity to transport Pi cannot be assessed by simply measuring the clearance (C) of this ion. C_{Pi} is influenced by the glomerular filtration rate (GFR). It is thus normal to measure the amount of Pi excreted ($U_{Pi}V$) per unit of GFR or/and the fractional excretion of Pi ($FE_{Pi} = U_{Pi}V/[\text{plasma Pi}] \times GFR$). Since both C_{Pi} and FE_{Pi} can vary to a large extent in response to a small change in plasma Pi, conclusions regarding the tubular capacity to transport Pi based on the determination of FE_{Pi} at one plasma Pi concentration should be drawn with caution. For clinical purposes, an attempt has been made to correct for the influence of plasma Pi by calculating an index called the Pi excretion index (Nordin, 1976). Since TR_{Pi} is thought to be a saturable process (Pitts, 1968), the tubular maximum reabsorptive capacity relative to the GFR (Tm_{Pi}/GFR) is currently used for assessing the tubular capacity to transport Pi (Bijvoet and Morgan, 1971). At the present time, the determination of Tm_{Pi}/GFR represents probably the best way to assess abnormalities of the tubular transport capacity in clinical practice. However, it has been recently shown that, at least in the rat, there is no classical Tm_{Pi}/GFR. As will be discussed later, the net TR_{Pi} decreases with increased filtered load instead of staying constant (Boudry et al., 1975; Engle and Steele, 1975; Frick, 1968). Therefore, under those conditions in which it is impossible to demonstrate a Tm, that is, a stable maximal transport value, the tubular capacity can only be assessed by determining the urinary excretion ($U_{Pi}V/GFR$ or FE_{Pi}) at several plasma Pi concentrations. Any shift in the relationship between $U_{Pi}V/GFR$ (or FE_{Pi}) and plasma Pi should ascertain a change in the tubular capacity to transport Pi.

3. TUBULAR ADAPTATION TO THE DIETARY SUPPLY OF PHOSPHATE

It has been known for many years (Chambers *et al.*, 1956; Crawford *et al.*, 1950; Eisenberg, 1968; Goldman and Bassett, 1958; Smith and Nordin, 1964) that a restriction in the phosphate supply leads to a sharp reduction in the absolute and fractional excretion of Pi. However, the definitive proof that this phenomenon is associated with a change in the overall tubular capacity to reabsorb Pi has only recently been brought forward (Steele and DeLuca, 1976; Troehler *et al.*, 1976a). Indeed, it had been generally accepted that in the mammalian kidney, Pi was filtered at the glomerulus and reabsorbed across the proximal tubule by a system which exhibited a stable maximal transport capacity (Tm) (Pitts, 1968), with parathyroid hormone (PTH) being the predominant controller in the system. In view of this concept, the renal response to variation in the dietary supply of phosphate was usually attributed to changes in the amount of Pi filtered; and when a change in the tubular transport capacity was suspected, it was explained by an alteration in PTH secretion (Pitts, 1968). This explanation might be at least in part correct when changes in the dietary supply of phosphate are not associated with parallel variations in the supply of calcium. Under this condition, any alteration in plasma Pi tends to induce an opposite change in plasma calcium. Consequently, the release of PTH is altered. This entails a change in the tubular capacity to transport Pi, which will tend to correct the dietary-induced alteration in the plasma Pi level. However, PTH is less likely to explain the tubular Pi response when dietary calcium varies parallel to Pi. Under this condition, the tubular Pi response to PTH would be homeostatically inadequate for Pi, since the secretion of PTH is primarily modulated by calcium. Furthermore, from a teleological point of view, it is unlikely that the same hormone regulates the homeostasis of two ions which are deposited as a single salt in the skeleton when it promotes the renal retention of one but the excretion of the other. Finally, if one accepts that TR_{Pi} largely determines the setting of plasma Pi (Bijvoet, 1969; Bijvoet and Morgan, 1971; Nordin, 1976), it is logical to conceive that the action of PTH on TR_{Pi} remains under the control of some mechanism which would respond specifically to the dietary supply of phosphate.

The existence of such a tubular Pi transport mechanism which operates independently of PTH has been recently demonstrated in the growing rat. As shown in Fig. 1, the kidney responds to variations in the amount of ingested phosphate by changing its capacity to transport Pi (Steele and DeLuca, 1976; Troehler *et al.*, 1976a). The FE_{Pi} determined in rats fed a high-phosphate diet is greater than that recorded in their counterparts receiving a low-phosphate diet. This difference can be observed over a wide range of plasma Pi concentrations in both intact and thyroparathyroidectomized (TPTX) rats (Fig. 1). Thus, the capability of adaptation does not require the presence of PTH or calcitonin. Furthermore, it has been shown (Steele *et al.*, 1975) that in TPTX rats fed a diet deficient in both vitamin D and phosphate, the tubular reabsorption is virtually complete up to a very high filtered load of Pi (Fig. 2). This result strongly suggests that the tubular adaptation to a low intake of phosphate is also independent of vitamin D and its various metabolites.

An estimation of the relative potency of dietary phosphate and PTH for changing the capacity of the renal tubule to transport Pi is provided in Table 1. As indicated, the variation in dietary phosphate alters FE_{Pi} measured at similar plasma Pi concentrations 350 and 150 times in intact and TPTX rats, respectively. In contrast, removal of the parathyroid glands changes FE_{Pi} only 2–5 times (Troehler *et al.*, 1976b). Thus, it appears that the adaptation mechanism has a greater capability than PTH for changing the capacity of the tubule to transport Pi. Nevertheless, it should be kept in mind that the adaptation to a high phosphate intake is

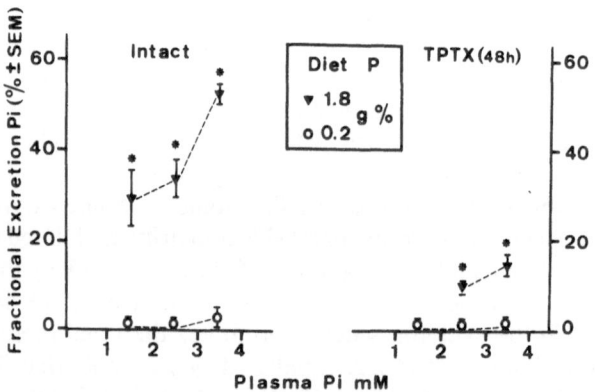

Fig. 1. Tubular adaptation to the dietary phosphate supply. FEPi was determined under acute intravenous sodium chloride and stepwise-increasing sodium phosphate infusion in intact and TPTX rats pair-fed diets containing either 0.2 or 1.8 g/100 g P for ten days. TPTX was performed 48 hours before the renal clearance study. The tubular adaptation is present in both intact and TPTX rats, although to a lesser degree in the latter conditions. *$p < 0.001$ as compared to the corresponding value measured in the group fed the low-phosphate diet. (Adapted from Troehler *et al.*, 1976a.)

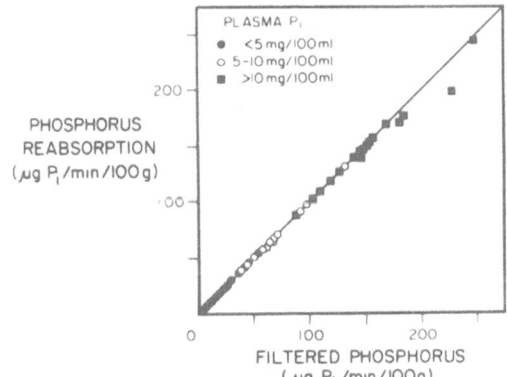

Fig. 2. Pi reabsorption, cx
pressed as a function of filtered
Pi load in vitamin-D-deficient
phosphate-depleted TPTX rats.
Irrespective of plasma Pi or filtered Pi, reabsorption was nearly
complete. (From Steele et al.,
1975.)

reduced after TPTX. The posible reason for this difference between intact
and TPTX animals will be discussed in Section 5.

Other experiments indicate that the tubular Pi adaptation to dietary
phosphate is probably independent of factors such as serum calcium, extracellular volume expansion (ECVE) tubular fluid bicarbonate concentration, and urinary pH. Indeed, the dietary-induced change in the tubular
handling of Pi can be observed in the presence of the same calcemia and
urinary pH (Troehler et al., 1976a). In intact rats, it is maintained under
marked ECVE induced by infusing either isotonic sodium chloride
(Steele, 1977a; Troehler et al., 1976a) or sodium bicarbonate solution
(Steele, 1977a). The same observation has been made in TPTX rats
(Steele, 1977a), although sodium bicarbonate loading in phosphate-deprived rats interfered with Pi reabsorption somewhat more than in intact
animals. Nevertheless, despite this interference, the dietary-induced
change in TR_{Pi} was maintained in sodium-bicarbonate-loaded TPTX rats.

No evidence has been presented so far which would indicate that the
renal adenyl cyclase system could be implicated in the phenomenon of
tubular Pi adaptation. Indeed, cyclic AMP (cAMP) excretion has been
found to be uninfluenced by the dietary restriction of phosphate intake
(Steele et al., 1976), a result that we have also observed in our laboratory
(Gloor et al., 1979).

In TPTX rats, the adaptive response to dietary phosphate is detectable three days after switching the animals from a normal to low- or high-
phosphate diets (Troehler et al., 1976a). It is quite possible that the change
could be elicited at an earlier time than 72 hours. Thus, the tubular Pi
response is an early event which does not require a severe degree of
phosphate depletion. This is in contrast to the decrease in the tubular
reabsorption of bicarbonate which appears to be only observed after prolonged and very severe phosphate deprivation. Indeed, the latter phe-

nomenon has been observed in dogs fed a diet very low (0.1 g/100 g) in phosphate for 40–160 days and receiving concomitantly an aluminum hydroxide gel (Gold et al., 1973a). A renal bicarbonate wasting has also been recently reported in intact rats fed a diet containing an extremely low amount of Pi (0.03 mg/100 g) for a period of 18–45 days (Emmet et al., 1977). With a diet fairly low in phosphate (0.07 g/100 g) given to intact or TPTX rats for 25–35 days, Steele (1977a) did not observe a change in the reabsorption of bicarbonate, whereas a marked tubular adaptation to the phosphate intake was present. The decrease in the tubular reabsorption of sodium and water (Gold et al., 1973b) appears also to require a very severe and prolonged phosphate depletion. Micropuncture studies in chronically phosphate-depleted dogs also demonstrated a decrease in proximal tubular reabsorption of sodium (Goldfarb et al., 1977). No evidence for such a change in the tubular handling of sodium and water in the whole kidney (Troehler et al., 1976a) or in the proximal tubule (Mühlbauer et al., 1977) has been found after feeding rats with a 0.2 g/100 g phosphate diet for ten days, whereas the change in TR_{Pi} was already fully expressed.

In our studies, the only tubular modification which appears to follow the same time course as Pi is the change, already described in the literature (Coburn and Massry, 1970; Massry, 1976), in the tubular reabsorption of calcium. The decrease in reabsorption of calcium after lowering the dietary intake of phosphate, and vice versa, would be consistent with a homeostatic mechanism, preventing the organism from being overloaded with calcium when its cosubstrate for mineral deposition into bone is deficient.

Table 1. Variation in the Fractional Excretion of Pi in Response to Dietary Phosphate Compared with Thyroparathyroidectomy[a,b]

Diet	$(C_{Pi}/C_{in}) \times 100$ (± SEM)		
	Sham	TPTX	Sham/TPTX
High-phosphate (1.8 g/100 g)	34.7 ± 4.4	7.1 ± 1.8	4.9
Low-phosphate (0.2 g/100 g)	0.098 ± 0.003	0.045 ± 0.009	2.2
High-low-phosphate	354	157	

[a] Adapted from Troehler et al. (1976b).

[b] FE_{Pi} (C_{Pi}/C_{in}) was measured at equal plasma Pi concentrations in rats fed high- and low-phosphate diets for ten days. Surgical TPTX or a sham operation was performed on the eighth day. On the day of the clearance measurement, animals were infused intravenously (4 ml/hr) with either isotonic sodium chloride or neutral Pi (16% NaH_2PO_4 and 84% $NaHPO_4$) at doses of 60 or 120 μmol/hr. Data were analyzed only from values of [plasma Pi] in the range between 2.25 and 2.90 mM. The mean (± SEM) values of [plasma Pi] of the four experimental groups were not significantly different: high-phosphate diet, Sham 2.54 ± 0.01 and TPTX 2.60 ± 0.07 mM; low-phosphate diet, Sham 2.46 ± 0.09 and TPTX 2.49 ± 0.11 mM.

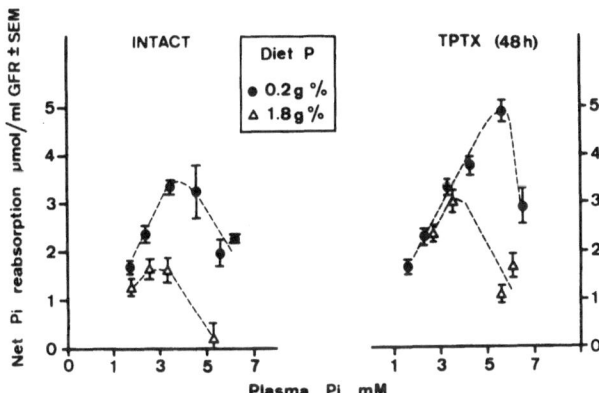

Fig. 3. Absence of stable maximal tubular Pi transport capacity in intact and TPTX rats. The net TR_{Pi} per ml of glomerular filtrate (GFR) was determined at several plasma Pi levels during acute intravenous sodium chloride and stepwise-increasing sodium phosphate infusion in intact and TPTX rats pair-fed diets containing either 0.2 or 1.8 g/100 gP. In all four conditions, a fall in the net Pi reabsorption is observed. (Adapted from Troehler *et al.*, 1976a.)

Finally, it is of importance to also note that an acute infusion of phosphate leads to a decrease in the net TR_{Pi} in intact and TPTX rats (Boudry *et al.*, 1975; Engle and Steele, 1975; Frick, 1968). When net TR_{Pi} is determined only at endogenous and elevated plasma Pi concentrations, the decrease in reabsorption seems to occur only in rats fed a normal or high-phosphate diet but not in phosphate-deprived animals (Steele, 1977a; Troehler, 1976a). However, when assessed over a wide range of plasma Pi concentrations the net TR_{Pi} falls in response to an acute phosphate loading also in intact or TPTX rats fed a low-phosphate diet (Fig. 3). Whether this PTH-independent acute response to phosphate infusion represents an early expression of the dietary phosphate adaptation or is mediated by another mechanism remains to be elucidated.

4. TUBULAR ADAPTATION TO THE PHOSPHATE DEMAND OF THE ORGANISM

As discussed above, the dietary-phosphate-induced change in the tubular capacity to transport Pi can be considered as a homeostatic response which tends to adjust the net TR_{Pi} to the needs of the organism. According to this concept, it is logical to envisage that the kidney would also adapt to variations in the demand for phosphate. In growing animals, about 80% of the phosphate ingested is taken up by the skeleton for mineralization (Irving, 1973). Thus, if a renal adaptation to the body needs is present, a decrease in the capacity of the bone to retain calcium and phosphate should elicit a change in the renal handling of Pi similar to that promoted by an increment in the dietary supply of phosphate. To test this hypothesis, we (Bonjour *et al.*, 1978a) used as a tool the diphosphonate disodium ethane-1-hydroxy-1,1-diphosphonate (EHDP). *In vitro*, EHDP is a potent inhibitor of calcium and phosphate precipitation (Fleisch *et al.*, 1970; Francis *et al.*, 1969). *In vivo*, in the growing rat, EHDP brings about a marked inhibition of bone mineral retention when given at the dose of 10 mg/kg/day (Gasser *et al.*, 1972; Schenk *et al.*, 1973). Given at the same dose for seven days, EHDP induced a marked change in the renal handling of Pi in TPTX rats. Indeed, as shown in Fig. 4, FE_{Pi} assessed at various phosphate loads is markedly higher in EHDP-treated TPTX rats than in their control counterparts. Note that administration of dichloromethane diphosphonate (Cl_2MDP), a diphosphonate which decreases bone turnover without affecting the mineral retention of the skeleton (Gasser *et al.*, 1972), does not appear to influence significantly the renal handling of Pi in TPTX rats (Fig. 4).

It seems that reducing the phosphate demand by blocking bone mineral retention with EHDP has the same influence on the renal handling

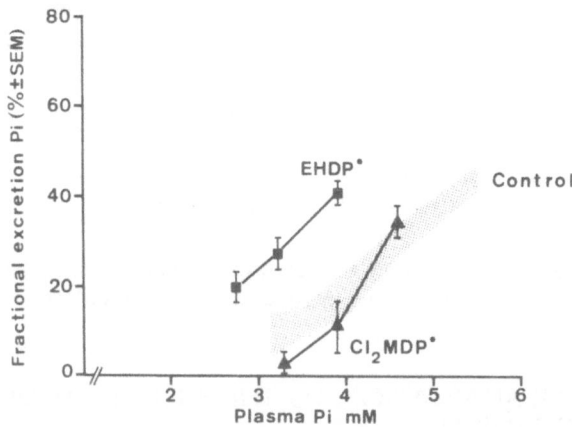

Fig. 4. Renal handling of Pi in diphosphonate-treated rats. During the seven days preceding the renal study, animals were fed a high-P (1.2 g/100 g) diet and were treated with either Cl_2MDP or EHDP (*10mg/kg/day subcutaneously for seven days). At this dosage, either diphosphonate slows down the bone turnover. However, only EHDP reduces the bone mineral retention. Assessment of the tubular capacity to transport Pi 48 hours after TPTX indicates that EHDP-but not Cl_2MDP-treated rats display a higher FE_{Pi} at various plasma Pi concentrations than that recorded in nontreated control animals (stippled area). (Adapted from Bonjour *et al.*, 1978a.)

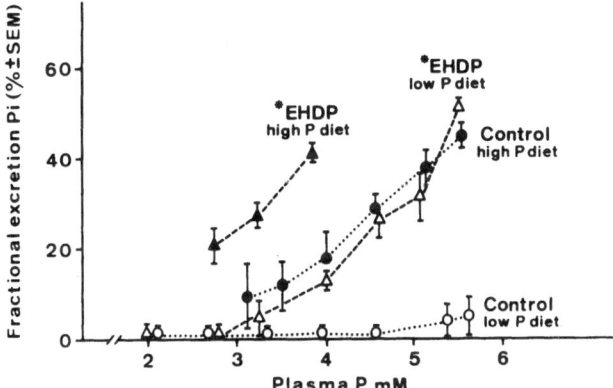

Fig. 5. Influence of EHDP and dietary phosphate on the renal handling of Pi in TPTX rats. Administration of EHDP (*10 mg/kg/day subcutaneously for seven days) to rats fed a low (0.2 g/100 g)-P diet increases FE_{Pi} to the level observed in rats fed a high (1.2 g/100 g)-P diet. The highest FE_{Pi} is observed when EHDP treatment is combined with a high-phosphate diet. (Adapted from Bonjour et al., 1978a.)

of Pi as increasing the dietary supply of phospate (Fig. 5). Like dietary phosphate, the onset of the effect of EHDP on the renal handling of Pi requires a lapse of two to three days. It appears to be specific for the tubular Pi transport system and independent of a stimulation of the adenyl cyclase system (Bonjour et al., 1978a). Furthermore, the EHDP-induced inhibition (Baxter et al., 1974; Bonjour et al., 1973; Hill et al., 1973) of the production of 1,25-dihydroxyvitamin D_3 [1,25$(OH)_2D_3$] is not responsible for the decrease in the net TR_{Pi} (Bonjour et al., 1978a) observed under the diphosphonate treatment. Therefore, although one cannot exclude that EHDP could affect the renal Pi transport through another mechanism, the data are consistent with the hypothesis that the renal response to the diphosphonate is secondary to the action of the diphosphonate on bone mineral retention. Thus, it is possible that both dietary phosphate and EHDP act through a common mechanism which responds to the phosphate needs of the organism. The fact that the kidney still displays an adaptive response to the dietary phosphate intake under EHDP treatment (Fig. 5) does not contradict this concept.

The most important physiological stimulus which affects the demand of the organism for phosphate is certainly the growth of the animal. In humans, the Tm_{Pi} is higher in children than in adults (Corvilain and Abramow, 1972). This difference may be due to growth hormone (Corvilain and Abramow, 1962, 1972). However, the increased tubular capacity to reabsorb Pi during growth could just as well be due to the same mechanism as that which responds to the supply and demand of phosphate. Accordingly, one could predict that other physiological situations in which the demand for phosphate is increased, such as pregnancy or lactation, should be associated with an increased capacity to reabsorb Pi for a given phosphate supply in the diet.

5. ROLE OF 1,25(OH)$_2$D$_3$ IN THE TUBULAR ADAPTATION IN Pi TRANSPORT

As mentioned above and depicted in Fig. 1, the adaptive response to the dietary intake of phosphate can be observed in both intact and chronically TPTX rats (Steele and DeLuca, 1976; Troehler et al., 1976a). However, the capability of the renal tubule to adapt to a high-phosphate diet is diminished in TPTX rats (Troehler et al., 1976a,b).

It is well known that TPTX or parathyroidectomy (PTX) causes a rapid and marked decrease in FE$_{Pi}$ (Bartter, 1971; Massry et al., 1973). This effect can be observed within the first 3 hours following the surgical procedure (Amiel et al., 1970). However, after the acute phase, FE$_{Pi}$ increases up to a steady-state value within 24–48 hours after PTX (Amiel and Küntziger, 1976; Amiel et al., 1970). This rise in FE$_{Pi}$ could well be interpreted as an adaptive response tending to normalize the renal handling of Pi. In chronically PTX or TPTX animals, FE$_{Pi}$ remains, nevertheless, lower than normal (Amiel et al., 1970; Bartter, 1971; Massry et al., 1973) in spite of the preservation of an operating adaptation mechanism (Troehler et al., 1976a; Steele and DeLuca, 1976). This incomplete readjustment of the tubular capacity could be attributed to the disappearance of the direct and rapid effect of PTH on the tubular Pi transport, which is probably mediated through the adenyl cyclase system (Chase and Aurbach, 1967).

Another possibility is that the lack of 1,25(OH)$_2$D$_3$, a metabolite which markedly influences phosphate homeostasis (DeLuca and Schnoes, 1976), plays a role. Indeed, removal of the parathyroid glands leads within 24 hours to a reduced production (Garabedian et al., 1972) and plasma level of 1,25(OH)$_2$D$_3$ (Hughes et al., 1975). Recently, we have obtained evidence for the latter possibility (Bonjour et al., 1977a). As shown in Figs. 6A and B, chronic administration of physiological doses of 1,25(OH)$_2$D$_3$ can normalize the renal handling of Pi in TPTX rats, restoring the ability of the tubular Pi transport system to adjust to large variations in the phosphate intake. Thus, PTH is not essential for a complete tubular Pi adaptation. It is important to underline that 1,25(OH)$_2$D$_3$ given at the same doses to intact rats does not affect the renal handling of Pi (Bonjour et al., 1977a).

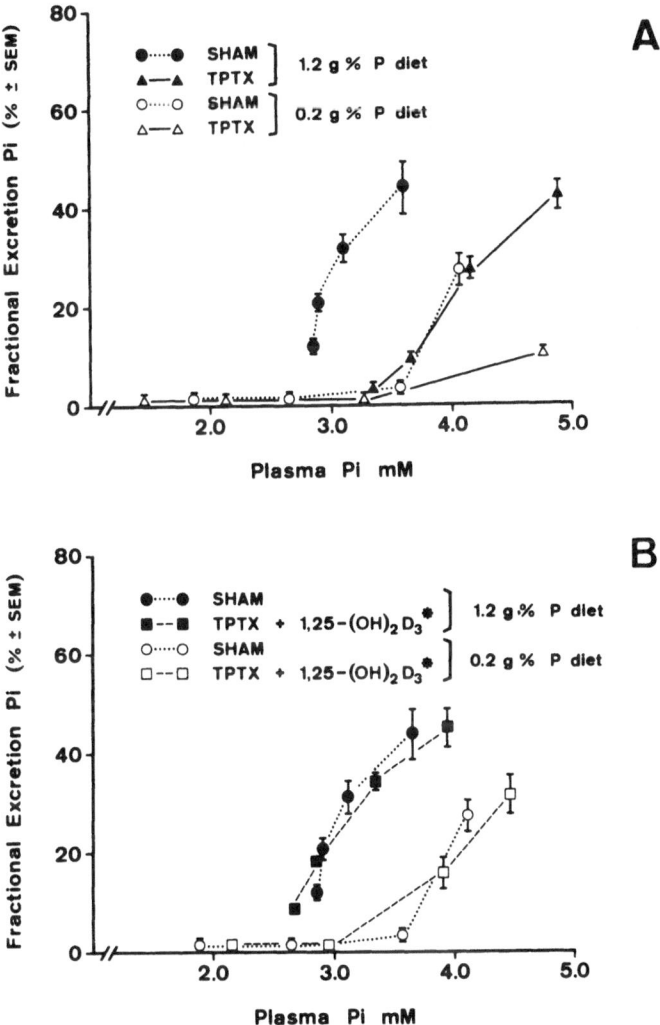

Fig. 6. Influence of 1,25(OH)$_2$D$_3$ on the renal handling of Pi. FE$_{Pi}$ was determined under acute intravenous sodium chloride and stepwise-increasing sodium phosphate infusion in (A) sham-operated and TPTX rats and (B) sham-operated and TPTX rats treated with 1,25(OH)$_2$D$_3$ (*2 × 13 pmol/day intraperitoneally for seven days). All animals were pair-fed a low- or high-phosphate diet. The renal handling of Pi in TPTX rats treated with 1,25(OH)$_2$D$_3$ is very similar to that recorded in sham-operated counterparts. (Adapted from Bonjour et al., 1977a.)

The mechanism by which $1,25(OH)_2D_3$ enhances the tubular capacity to excrete Pi does not seem to include the adenyl cyclase system. Indeed, in TPTX rats fed a high-phosphate diet, the normalization of the renal handling of Pi induced by $1,25(OH)_2D_3$ was not associated with a correction of urinary cAMP excretion (Bonjour et al., 1977a). The effect of $1,25(OH)_2D_3$ on the renal handling of Pi in TPTX rats was not accompanied by a change in the overall tubular capacity to transport calcium (Hugi et al., 1977). The effect of $1,25(OH)_2D_3$ was also maintained under marked ECVE and a conspicuous increase in the fractional excretion of sodium and was not associated with a change in urinary pH (Bonjour et al., 1977a). Thus, the chronic administration of $1,25(OH)_2D_3$ appears to affect quite selectively the tubular Pi transport system.

Among several other vitamin D metabolites tested, including $25OHD_3$, $24R,25(OH)_2D_3$, $1,24R,25(OH)_3D_3$ and $1,24S,25(OH)_3D_3$, the $1,25(OH)_2D_3$ derivative was most potent in decreasing the tubular capacity to reabsorb Pi by TPTX rats (Bonjour et al., 1978b). This selective and potent influence of $1,25(OH)_2D_3$ on the tubular Pi transport strongly suggests that this effect is of physiological significance.

Whether the renal effect is secondary to the action of the metabolite on phosphate and/or calcium metabolism and whether it could be a permissive factor for the adaptation mechanism, which, in these experimental conditions, appears to be the most important regulator of the overall tubular handling of Pi, remain to be elucidated.

6. LOCALIZATION OF THE TUBULAR ADAPTATION IN Pi TRANSPORT

6.1. Influence of Phosphate Supply

An attempt to localize the site of Pi adaptation along the nephron has been made in intact rats by free-flow micropunctures (Mühlbauer et al., 1977). This study indicates that for the same amount of Pi filtered, the amount of Pi recovered along the accessible superficial nephrons is always greater in intact rats fed a high (1.8 g/100 g)- as compared to low (0.2 g/100 g)-phosphate diet for ten days (Fig. 7). A segmental analysis (Table 2) indicates that along the superficial nephrons the effect appears to take place mainly in the first convolutions of the proximal tubule. It is interesting that in the high-phosphate diet group, the mean fractional delivery of Pi was 1.10 at the early accessible proximal convoluted tubule, although 20% of the glomerular filtrate had already been reabsorbed. This further suggested (Boudry et al., 1975) the existence of a secretory flux of Pi along the first portion of nephron. Whether the mechanism of adaptation

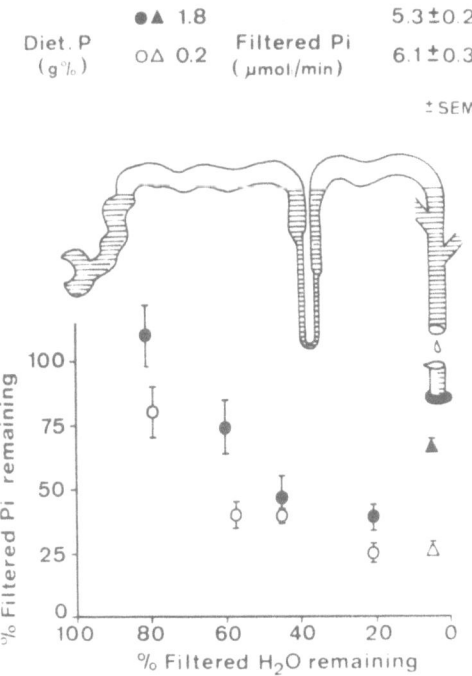

Fig. 7. Tubular localization of the adaptation to dietary phosphate in intact rats. Rats were fed a high (1.8 g/100 g)- or low (0.2 g/100 g)-P diet for ten days. Free-flow micropunctures of superficial proximal and distal convolutions were made at similar filtered loads of Pi by infusing intravenous sodium phosphate solutions. The percentage of filtered Pi remaining at puncture sties (●, ○) or in the final urine (▲, △) is plotted against that of water (plasma to tubular fluid or urine concentration ratio for inulin × 100). An approximate localization of the puncture site is provided by the schematic nephron. Along the superficial tubule, the Pi adaptation appears to take place mainly in the early proximal tubule. The results also suggest adaptation in the terminal nephron with a secretory component in rats fed a high-phosphate diet. (Adapted from Mühlbauer et al., 1977.)

in the first portion of the proximal tubule exerts its influence through this mechanism, through the rate of Pi reabsorption, or through both cannot be said at the present time.

In a recent study wherein the technique of stationary microperfusion was used, Ullrich et al. (1977) have reported that intact rats receiving a low (<0.15 g/100 g)-phosphate diet for 7–11 weeks display a higher rate of net Pi reabsorption along the entire length of the accessible proximal tubule than their counterparts with high phosphate intake (2 g/100 g diet). However, in our free-flow micropuncture study in intact rats fed experimental phosphate diets for ten days (Mühlbauer et al., 1977), the segmental analysis of the data shows that the greatest part of the accessible

Table 2. Influence of Dietary Phosphate on Segmental Tubular Transport of $Pi^{a,b}$

	Segmental delivery (μmol/min)		Net reabsorption (μmol/min)		Fractional reabsorption ($\times$ 100)	
Tubular segment	A^c	B^d	A	B	A	B
Glomerulus to "early proximal"[e]	6.07	5.34	1.21	-0.53	20	-10
"Early proximal"[e] to "late proximal"[f]	4.86	5.87	2.43	3.36	50	57
"Late proximal"[f] to "distal"[g]	2.43	2.51	1.16	0.42	48	17
"Distal"[g] to final urine[h]	1.27	2.09	0.00	-1.33	0	-64

[a] From Mühlbauer et al. (1977).
[b] The absolute and fractional contributions of each segment were calculated from the mean filtered or segmental load and the mean fractional delivery.
[c] A, 0.2 g/100 g dietary phosphate.
[d] B, 1.8 g/100 g dietary phosphate.
[e] "Early proximal": Punctures with a tubular fluid to plasma concentration ratio for inulin [$(TF/P)_{in}$] up to 1.49 were considered. The mean $(TF/P)_{in}$ was 1.26 ± 0.04 ($n = 14$) and 1.23 ± 0.03 ($n = 21$) for the rats fed 0.2 and 1.8 g/100 g dietary phosphate, respectively.
[f] "Late proximal": Punctures with a $(TF/P)_{in}$ ranging from 2.0 to 2.49 were considered. The mean $(TF/P)_{in}$ was 2.21 ± 0.04 ($n = 13$) and 2.20 ± 0.05 ($n = 12$) for the rats fed 0.2 and 1.8 g/100 g dietary phosphate, respectively.
[g] "Distal": Punctures with a $(TF/P)_{in}$ ranging from 3.5 to the highest value were considered. The mean $(TF/P)_{in}$ was 5.58 ± 0.51 ($n = 17$) and 5.42 ± 0.62 ($n = 14$) for the rats fed 0.2 and 1.8 g/100 g dietary phosphate, respectively.
[h] Only final urine of rats whose distal tubules were sampled was considered.

proximal convoluted tubule does not appear to respond to the dietary phosphate stimulus. Indeed, the net and fractional reabsorption of Pi along this segment seem even to be enhanced in the rats fed the high-phosphate diet (Table 2). It ensues that the dietary-phosphate-induced effect observed at the early proximal tubule is almost abolished further downstream the accessible proximal and distal tubule (Fig. 7). Despite a compensatory phenomenon, a marked difference in FE_{Pi} is found in the final urine. This can be due to two mechanisms. First the adaptive response is taking place along the terminal nephron. If so, it would have to be mediated to a large extent by the modulation of a secretory flux of Pi (Fig. 7, Table 2). The second possibility is that the apparent net entry of Pi along the terminal nephron is due to a functional heterogeneity between superficial and deep nephrons. This eventuality has been evoked in previous publications (Boudry et al., 1975; Knox et al., 1977; Mühlbauer et al., 1977) and is discussed in Chapter 2. These authors have demonstrated an apparent net secretion of Pi along the terminal nephron during phosphate loading in rats fed normal- to high-phosphate diets.

However, since free-flow micropunctures from distal tubules of superficial nephrons showed less Pi delivery than those from deep nephrons from the ascending limb of Henle's loop, the authors concluded this to be evidence of a functional heterogeneity between superficial and deep nephrons which could explain, at least in part, the discrepancy in Pi delivery between distal tubules and final urine. It is, however, our view that a definitive conclusion about the existence and, especially, the importance of functional heterogeneity with regard to Pi transport between the various types of nephrons cannot be drawn at the present time. Indeed, such a conclusion requires the comparison of Pi delivery at the same localization of the distal tubule of both superficial and deep nephrons and the precise quantitative evaluation of the contribution of each category of nephrons to the composition of the final urine. Since such information does not exist, the relative importance of Pi secretion along the terminal nephron to the final urinary output of Pi cannot be appreciated at the present time.

6.2. Influence of Phosphate Demand through EHDP Treatment

It is perhaps more than fortuitous that in rats treated with EHDP at doses which reduce the mineral retention of bone, one observes a change in the renal handling of Pi which can also be localized mainly in the early proximal tubule and in the terminal nephron (Bonjour *et al.*, 1977b). This result further strengthens the hypothesis that EHDP treatment influences the renal handling of Pi through the same mechanism as dietary phosphate.

7. TUBULAR ADAPTATION AND ACUTE PHOSPHATURIC RESPONSE TO PTH

7.1. Influence of Dietary Phosphate

As shown in Fig. 6B, the mechanism of the renal adaptation to dietary phosphate can fully operate in the absence of PTH when animals are supplemented with $1,25(OH)_2D_3$. Other experimental evidence indicates that the adaptation mechanism is also capable of controlling the tubular phosphaturic response to PTH. It was previously reported (Harter *et al.*, 1974) that the prior dietary intake of phosphate can markedly alter the tubular phosphaturic response to PTH without affecting the increase in cAMP excretion. This observation has been recently confirmed in two laboratories (Bonjour *et al.*, 1977b; Steele *et al.*, 1976). The blunted phosphaturic response noted in phosphate-depleted animals was initially attributed to variations in the filtered load of Pi (Harter *et al.*, 1974). However, this is not the only explanation. We have recently studied (Bonjour et al., 1978a) the phosphaturic response to PTH at various plasma Pi concentrations obtained by infusing acutely sodium phosphate solutions into rats fed low- and high-phosphate diets. At similar plasma concentration and filtered load of Pi, a blunted response was observed in the rats fed the low-phosphate diet (Fig. 8). Thus, the magnitude of the PTH-induced increase in FE_{Pi} is largely independent of the filtered load of Pi, indicating that the tubular mechanism of adaptation controls, in some way, the final expression of the PTH action on the renal transport of Pi.

7.2. Influence of EHDP

We have also observed (Bonjour et al., 1978a) that in TPTX rats fed a low-phosphate diet and treated with EHDP in doses which inhibit bone mineral retention and thus reduce the phosphate demand, the phosphaturic response is similar to that observed in the animals receiving a high-phosphate diet (Fig. 8). This result suggests that not only the supply but also the demand for phosphate by the organism can alter the acute phosphaturic response to PTH. Like dietary phosphate, EHDP treatment affects the phosphate but not the cAMP excretion in response to PTH (Bonjour et al., 1978a).

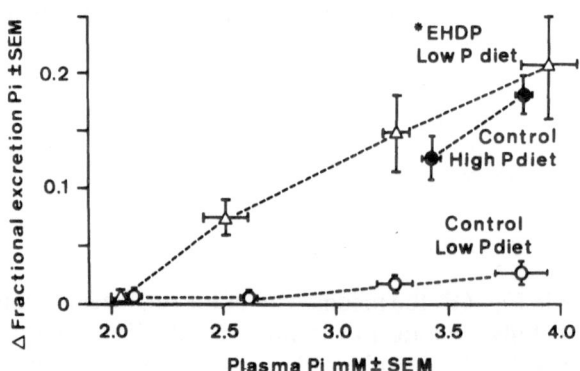

Fig. 8. Phosphaturic response to PTH in TPTX rats. Influence of dietary phosphate and EHDP. The response to PTH (2.5 IU/rat/hr) was studied at various plasma Pi concentrations obtained by infusing in TPTX rats isotonic solutions containing either 0, 5, 10, 15, or 20 mM Pi. The ordinate corresponds to the increase (Δ) in FE_{Pi} during PTH infusion. The figure illustrates the two components of the renal resistance to PTH in phosphate-depleted animals: (1) the refractoriness resulting from the low filtered load of Pi and (2) the actual tubular resistance, that is, a reduced phosphaturic response in the presence of a similar plasma concentration and filtered load of Pi. In phosphate-depleted animals, treatment with EHDP (*10 mg/kg/day subcutaneously for seven days) prevents the occurrence of the tubular resistance to PTH. (Adapted from Bonjour et al., 1978a.)

7.3. Influence of 1,25(OH)$_2$D$_3$

As discussed above, 1,25(OH)$_2$D$_3$ administered chronically to TPTX rats decreases the tubular capacity to reabsorb Pi (Figs. 6A and B). Recently, we have also observed (Gloor *et al.*, 1979) that chronic administration of small doses of 1,25(OH)$_2$D$_3$ increases the phosphaturic response to PTH in TPTX phosphate-deprived animals, but it does not alter either the increase in cAMP excretion or the hypocalciuria induced by the peptide hormone. The effect of 1,25(OH)$_2$D$_3$ on the phosphaturic response to PTH was not shared by its precursor 25(OH)D$_3$, even when given in 100-fold larger doses. These results speak again for the hypothesis that 1,25(OH)$_2$D$_3$ acts on the renal handling of Pi through the adaptation mechanism.

In the experiments described above, it appears clear that there is a relationship between the influence of factors such as dietary phosphate, EHDP, and 1,25(OH)$_2$D$_3$ treatment on the baseline tubular capacity to reabsorb Pi and their influence on the phosphaturic response to PTH. As discussed above, these three factors could exert their action through a common mechanism. This mechanism could act within the tubular segment where PTH exerts its action on Pi transport, acting at a step beyond the cAMP generation. Alternatively, the mechanism could have a different site of action from that of PTH. By acting proximally or/and distally to the site of PTH, it could alter the expression of the hormonal action in the final urine. These questions may be solved, at least in part, by localizing the site of action of these various factors along the nephron.

8. MECHANISM OF TUBULAR ADAPTATION

The nature of the mechanism underlying the renal adaptive response to the phosphate supply and probably demand is still unknown. As mentioned in the Introduction, the nature of the controlled variable(s) remains uncertain. Likewise, the transmission factor which would carry the information from the controlled to the controlling variable, that is, the tubular Pi transport, has to be defined. A humoral factor is, of course, a possibility which cannot be excluded at the present time. Recently, it has been reported (Steele, 1977b) that isolated perfused kidneys harvested from phosphate-deprived rats still display an accelerated Pi reabsorption, indicating that if a humoral agent is involved, its action is of prolonged duration. However, no definite conclusion can be drawn as to the possible existence of an extrarenally generated humoral factor as opposed to a purely intrarenal mechanism. Also unknown is the exact localization of the adaptive response in the epithelial cells of the renal tubule. Whether the response is confined to the luminal and/or basolateral plasma membranes is a question for which an answer should be found, at least for the proximal tubule. Kinne (1978), utilizing the isolated vesicles of the proximal tubule, found that the adaptation to dietary phosphate restriction is probably due to changes in the sodium–phosphate cotransport system of the brush-border membrane. These kinds of studies may eventually lead to some understanding of the molecular mechanism which controls the translocation of Pi across the renal tubule.

9. TUBULAR ADAPTATION AND DISORDERS OF THE RENAL Pi TRANSPORT

The discovery of a prevailing PTH-independent Pi transport system poses the question of whether some of the genetically transmitted or acquired defects in the tubular Pi transport may result from a dysfunction or a lack of this adaptive mechanism. One possible disease is familial X-linked hypophosphatemic rickets in humans (Scriver et al., 1976; Williams et al., 1972) and its mouse model (Eicher et al., 1976). A decrease in the tubular capacity for net TR_{Pi} is one of the salient features of this affliction. In the mouse, this decrease has been localized by free-flow micropuncture in the proximal tubule (Cowgill et al., 1977; Giasson et al., 1977), a finding which does not exclude a defective Pi reabsorption also in more distal portions of the nephron.

Another disturbance in which a defect of adaptation could possibly play a role is the "phosphate leak" which can be observed in patients with idiopathic hypercalciuria and calcium nephrolithiasis (Lemann et al., 1977; Rasmussen and Bordier, 1977; Shen et al., 1977). As in familial X-linked hypophosphatemia, the reduced TR_{Pi} cannot be explained by alteration in parathyroid function or in other factors known to influence the renal handling of Pi.

Finally, the mechanism of adaptation to the phosphate supply and requirements could also play a role in the change of FE_{Pi} which occurs in the course of chronic renal failure (Slatopolsky and Rutherford, 1976). It is generally accepted that the tubular Pi response to a progressive reduction in the nephron population results from the secondary hyperparathyroidism which develops in this condition (Slatopolsky and Rutherford, 1976). However, an increase in FE_{Pi} was also observed in TPTX dogs undergoing chronic renal failure (Swenson et al., 1975). Therefore, it appears that the kidney is able to vary its Pi transport capacity in the absence of PTH following a reduction in the number of functional renal units, as it does in response to variation in the phosphate supply or demand.

10. CONCLUSIONS

The renal tubule can adapt its Pi transport capacity to the dietary phosphate supply and to the phosphate requirement of the organism. This adaptive mechanism is more potent than PTH, is independent of the adenyl cyclase system, and also has the ability to control the tubular phosphaturic effect of the peptide hormone. Although $1,25(OH)_2D_3$ is not the factor responsible, it restores in TPTX animals the full capability for adaptation. The adaptive mechanism described appears to play a key role in phosphate homeostasis. Its nature and its relation to certain clinical disorders of tubular Pi reabsorption remain to be elucidated.

ACKNOWLEDGMENTS. Most of the experimental work presented in this review has been supported by the Swiss National Science Foundation (3.725.76), by the Procter and Gamble Company, U.S.A., and by Hoffmann–La Roche, Inc., Basel, Switzerland.

We acknowledge the invaluable secretarial help of Mrs. Brigitte Gyger and thank Mrs. Cécile Stieger for her graphical work.

11. REFERENCES

Amiel, C., and Küntziger, H., 1976, Tubular handling of phosphate, in: *Urolithiasis Research* (H. Fleisch, W. G. Robertson, L. H. Smith, and W. Vahlensieck, eds.), pp. 89–100, Plenum Press, New York.

Amiel, C., Küntziger, H., and Richet, G., 1970, Micropuncture study of handling of phosphate by proximal and distal nephron in normal and parathyroidectomized rat. Evidence for distal reabsorption, *Pflügers Arch.* **317**:93.

Bartter, F. C., 1971, Vitamin D, parathyroid hormone and the kidney, in: *The Kidney*, Vol. IV (C. Rouiller and A. Müller, eds.), pp. 249–270, Academic Press, New York.

Baxter, L. A., DeLuca, H. F., Bonjour, J.-P., and Fleisch, H., 1974, Inhibition of vitamin D metabolism by ethane-1-hydroxy-1,1-diphosphonate, *Arch. Biochem. Biophys.* **164**:655.

Bijvoet, O. L. M., 1969, Relation of plasma phosphate concentration to renal tubular reabsorption of phosphate, *Clin. Sci.* **37**:23.

Bijvoet, O. L. M., and Morgan, B., 1971, The tubular reabsorption of phosphate in man, in: *Phosphate et Métabolisme Phosphocalcique* (D. J. Hioco, ed.), pp. 153–180, Laboratoires Sandoz, Paris.

Bonjour, J.-P., DeLuca, H. F., Fleisch, H., Trechsel, U., Matejowec, L. A., and Omdahl, J. L., 1973, Reversal of the EHDP inhibition of calcium absorption by 1,25-dihydroxycholecalciferol, *Eur. J. Clin. Invest.* **3**:44.

Bonjour, J.-P., Preston, C., and Fleisch, H., 1977a, Effect of 1,25-dihydroxyvitamin D_3 on the renal handling of Pi in thyroparathyroidectomized rats, *J. Clin. Invest.* **60**:1419.

Bonjour, J.-P., Troehler, U., Mühlbauer, R., Preston, C., and Fleisch, H., 1977b, Is there a bone–kidney link in the homeostasis of inorganic phosphate (Pi)? in: *Phosphate Metabolism* (S. G. Massry and E. Ritz, eds.), pp. 319–322, Plenum Press, New York.

Bonjour, J.-P., Troehler, U., Preston, C., and Fleisch, H., 1978a, Parathyroid hormone and renal handling of Pi: Effect of dietary Pi and diphosphonates, *Am. J. Physiol.,* **234:**F497.

Bonjour, J.-P., Preston, C., Rizzoli, R., and Fleisch, H., 1978b, Vitamin D metabolites and phosphate transport, in: *Endocrinology of Calcium Metabolism* (D. H. Copp and R. V. Talmage, eds.), pp. 172–177, Excerpta Medica, Amsterdam and Oxford.

Boudry, J.-F., Troehler, U., Touabi, M., Fleisch, H., and Bonjour, J.-P., 1975, Secretion of inorganic phosphate in the rat nephron, *Clin. Sci. Mol. Med.* **48:**475.

Chambers, E. L., Jr., Gordan, G. S., Goldman, L., and Reifenstein, E. C., Jr., 1956, Tests for hyperparathyroidism: Tubular reabsorption of phosphate, phosphate deprivation and calcium infusion, *J. Clin. Endocrinol. Metab.* **16:**1507.

Chase, L. R., and Aurbach, G. D., 1967, Parathyroid function and the renal excretion of 3′,5′-adenylic acid, *Proc. Natl. Acad. Sci. U.S.A.* **58:**518.

Coburn, J. W., and Massry, S., 1970, Change in serum and urinary calcium during phosphate depletion: Studies on mechanisms, *J. Clin. Invest.* **49:**1073.

Corvilain, J., and Abramow, M., 1962, Some effect of human growth hormone on renal hemodynamics of tubular phosphate transport in man, *J. Clin. Invest.* **41:**1230.

Corvilain, J., and Abramow, M., 1972, Growth and renal control of plasma phosphate, *J. Clin. Endocrinol.* **34:**452.

Cowgill, L., Goldfarb, S., Goldberg, M., Slatopolsky, E., and Agus, Z., 1977, Nature of the renal defect in familial hypophosphatemic rickets (FHR), in: *Proceedings of the Third International Workshop on Phosphate and Other Minerals,* Madrid, p. 101 (Abstract).

Crawford, J. D., Osborne, M. M., Jr., Talbot, N. B., Terry, L. M., and Morrill, M. F., 1950, The parathyroid glands and phosphorus homeostasis, *J. Clin. Invest.* **29:**1448.

DeLuca, H. F., and Schnoes, H. K., 1976, Metabolism and mechanism of action of vitamin D, *Annu. Rev. Biochem.* **45:**631.

Eicher, E. M., Southard, J. L., Scriver, C. R., and Glorieux, F. H., 1976, Hypophosphatemia: Mouse model for human familial hypophosphatemic (vitamin D-resistant) rickets, *Proc. Natl. Acad. Sci. U.S.A.* **73:**4667.

Eisenberg, E., 1968, Effects of varying phosphate intake in primary hyperparathyroidism, *J. Clin. Endocrinol. Metab.* **28:**651.

Emmet, M., Goldfarb, S., Agus, Z., and Narins, R. G., 1977, The pathophysiology of acid–base changes in chronically phosphate-depleted rats, *J. Clin. Invest.* **59:**291.

Engle, J. E., and Steele, T. H., 1975, Renal phosphate reabsorption in the rat: Effect of inhibitors, *Kidney Int.* **8:**98.

Fleisch, H., Russell, R. G. G., Bisaz, S., Mühlbauer, R. C., and Williams, D. A., 1970, The inhibitory effect of phosphonates on the formation of calcium phosphate crystals *in vitro* and on aortic and kidney calcification *in vivo, Eur. J. Clin. Invest.* **1:**12.

Francis, M. D., Russell, R. G. G., and Fleisch, H., 1969, Diphosphonates inhibit formation of calcium phosphate crystals *in vitro* and pathological calcification *in vivo, Science* **165:**1264.

Frick, A., 1968, Reabsorption of inorganic phosphate in the rat kidney: I. Saturation of transport mechanism; II. suppression of fractional phosphate reabsorption due to expansion of extracellular fluid volume, *Pflügers Arch.* **304:**351.

Garabedian, M., Holick, M. F., DeLuca, H. F., and Boyle, I. T., 1972, Control of 25-hydroxycholecalciferol metabolism by parathyroid gland, *Proc. Natl. Acad. Sci. U.S.A.* **69:**1673.

Gasser, A. B., Morgan, D. B., Fleisch, H. A., and Richelle, L. J., 1972, The influence of two diphosphonates on calcium metabolism in the rat, *Clin. Sci.* **43:**31.

Giasson, S. D., Brunette, M. G., Danan, G., Vigneault, N., and Carriere, S., 1977, Micropuncture study of renal phosphorus transport in hypophosphatemic vitamin D resistant rickets mice, *Pflügers Arch.* **371:**33.

Gloor, H. J., Bonjour, J.-P., Caverzasio, J., and Fleisch, H., 1979, Resistance to the phosphaturic and calcemic actions of parathyroid hormone during phosphate depletion: Prevention by 1,25-dihydroxyvitamin D₃, *J. Clin. Invest.* **63**:371.

Gold, L. W., Massry, S. G., Arieff, A. I., and Coburn, J. W., 1973a, Renal bicarbonate wasting during phosphate depletion. A possible cause of altered acid–base homeostasis in hyperthyroidism, *J. Clin. Invest.* **52**:2556.

Gold, L. W., Massry, S. G., Rothman, C. M., and Coburn, J. W., 1973b, Effect of phosphate depletion on renal handling of calcium and sodium, *Clin. Res.* **21**:282.

Goldfarb, S., Westby, G. R., Goldberg, M., and Agus, Z. S., 1977, Renal tubular effects of chronic phosphate depletion, *J. Clin. Invest.* **59**:770.

Goldman, R., and Bassett, S. H., 1958, Renal regulation of phosphorus excretion, *J. Clin. Endocrinol. Metab.* **18**:981.

Harter, H. R., Mercado, A., Rutherford, W. E., Rodriguez, H., Slatopolsky, E., and Klahr, S., 1974, Effects of phosphate depletion and parathyroid hormone on renal glucose reabsorption, *Am. J. Physiol.* **227**:1422.

Hill, L. F., Lumb, G. A., Mawer, G. A., and Stanbury, S. W., 1973, Indirect inhibition of the biosynthesis of 1,25-dihydroxycholecalciferol in rats treated with a diphosphonate, *Clin. Sci.* **44**:335.

Hughes, M. R., Brumbaugh, P. F., and Haussler, M. R., 1975, Regulation of serum 1α,25-dihydroxyvitamin D₃ by calcium and phosphate in the rat, *Science* **190**:578.

Hugi, K., Preston, C., Fleisch, H., and Bonjour, J.-P., 1977, Renal handling of calcium in rats: Influence of parathyroid hormone and 1,25-dihydroxyvitamin D₃, in: *Vitamin D, Biochemical, Chemical and Clinical Aspects Related to Calcium Metabolism* (A. W. Norman, K. Schaefer, J. W. Coburn, H. F. DeLuca, D. Fraser, H. G. Grigoleit, and D. von Herrath, eds.), pp. 433–435, de Gruyter, Berlin.

Irving, J. T., 1973, *Calcium and Phosphorus Metabolism*, pp. 21–37, Academic Press, New York.

Kinne, R., 1978, Current concepts of renal proximal tubular function, *Contrib. Nephrol.* **14**:14.

Knox, F. G., Haas, J. A., Berndt, T., Marchand, G. R., and Youngberg, S. P., 1977, Phosphate transport in superficial and deep nephrons in phosphate-loaded rats, *Am. J. Physiol.* **233**:F150.

Kreusser, W. J., Kurokawa, K., Aznar, E., and Massry, S. G., 1978, Phosphate depletion: Effect on renal inorganic phosphorus and adenine nucleotides, urinary phosphate and calcium, and calcium balance, *Miner. Electrolyte Metab.* **1**:30.

Leman, J., Jr., Gray, R. W., and Wilz, D. R., 1977, Evidence for a renal PO₄ leak in patients with calcium nephrolithiasis, in: *Proceedings of the Third International Workshop on Phosphate and Other Minerals*, Madrid, p. 34 (Abstract).

Massry, S. G., 1976, Effect of phosphate depletion on renal tubular transport, in: *Phosphate Metabolism, Kidney and Bone* (L. Avioli, P. Bordier, H. Fleisch, S. Massry, and E. Slatopolsky, eds.), pp. 25–32, Armour Montagu, Paris.

Massry, S. G., Friedler, R. M., and Coburn, J. W., 1973, Excretion of phosphate and calcium. Physiology of their renal handling and relation to clinical medicine, *Arch. Intern. Med.* **131**:828.

Mühlbauer, R. C., Bonjour, J.-P., and Fleisch, H., 1977, Tubular localization of the adaptation to dietary phosphate in rats, *Am. J. Physiol.* **233**:F342.

Nordin, B. E. C., 1976, *Calcium, Phosphate and Magnesium Metabolism*, pp. 217–229, Churchill Livingstone, Edinburg.

Pitts, R. F., 1968, *Physiology of the Kidney and Body Fluids*, 2nd ed., pp. 77–78, Year Book Medical Publishers, Chicago.

Rasmussen, H., and Bordier, P., 1977, Endocrine factors in the pathogenesis of idiopathic hypercalciuria, in: *Idiopathic Urinary Bladder Stone Disease* (R. Van Reen, ed.), pp. 267–286, Fogarty International Center Proceedings, Washington.

Schenk, R., Merz, W. A., Mühlbauer, R. C., Russell, R. G. G., and Fleisch, H., 1973, Effect of ethane-1-hydroxy-1,1-diphosphonate (EHDP) and dichloromethylene diphosphonate (Cl₂MDP) on the calcification and resorption of cartilage and bone in the tibial epiphysis and metaphysis of rats, *Calcif. Tissue Res.* 11:196.

Scriver, C. R., Chesney, R. W., and McInnes, R. R., 1976, Genetic aspects of renal tubular transport: Diversity and topology of carriers, *Kidney Int.* 9:149.

Shen, F. H., Baylink, D. J., Sherrard, D. J., and Haussler, M. R., 1977, Idiopathic hypercalciuria: The "phosphate leak" hypothesis and effects of oral phosphate supplement, in: *Proceedings of the Third International Workshop on Phosphate and Other Minerals,* Madrid, p. 33 (Abstract).

Slatopolsky, E., and Rutherford, W. E., 1976, The metabolism of phosphate in chronic renal disease, in: *Phosphate Metabolism, Kidney and Bone* (L. Avioli, P. Bordier, H. Fleisch, S. Massry, and E. Slatopolsky, eds.), pp. 35–44, Armour Montagu, Paris.

Smith, D. A., and Nordin, B. E. C., 1964, The effect of a high phosphorus intake on total and ultrafiltrable plasma calcium and on phosphate clearance, *Clin. Sci.* 26:479.

Steele, T. H., 1977a, Renal response to phosphorus deprivation: Effect of the parathyroids and bicarbonate, *Kidney Int.* 11:327.

Steele, T. H., 1977b, Effect of phosphate depletion on renal transport of phosphate, in: *Proceedings of the Third International Workshop on Phosphate and Other Minerals,* Madrid, p. 45 (Abstract).

Steele, T. H., and DeLuca, H. F., 1976, Influence of dietary phosphorus on renal phosphate reabsorption in the parathyroidectomized rats, *J. Clin. Invest.* 57:867.

Steele, T. H., Engle, J. E., Tanaka, Y., Lorenc, R. S., Dudgeon, K. L., and DeLuca, H. F., 1975, Phosphatemic action of 1,25-dihydroxyvitamin D₃, *Am. J. Physiol.* 229:489.

Steele, T. H., Underwood, J. L., Stromberg, B. A., and Larmore, C. A., 1976, Renal resistance to parathyroid hormone during phosphorus deprivation, *J. Clin. Invest.* 58:1461.

Swenson, R. S., Weisinger, J. R., Ruggeri, J. L., and Reaven, G. M., 1975, Evidence that parathyroid hormone is not required for phosphate homeostasis in renal failure, *Metabolism* 24:199.

Troehler, U., Bonjour, J.-P., and Fleisch, H., 1976a, Inorganic phosphate homeostasis: Renal adaptation to the dietary intake in intact and thyroparathyroidectomized rats, *J. Clin. Invest.* 57:264.

Troehler, U., Bonjour, J.-P., and Fleisch, H., 1976b, Renal tubular adaptation to dietary phosphorus, *Nature* 261:145.

Ullrich, K. J., Rumrich, G., and Klöss, S., 1977, Phosphate transport in the proximal convolution of the rat kidney. I. Tubular heterogeneity, effect of parathyroid hormone in acute and chronic parathyroidectomized animals and effect of phosphate diet, *Pflügers Arch.* 372:269.

Williams, T. F., Winters, R. W., and Burnett, C. H., 1972, Familial (hereditary) vitamin D-resistant rickets with hypophosphatemia, in: *The Metabolic Basis of Inherited Disease* (J. B. Stanbury, J. B. Wyngaarden, and D. S. Fredrickson, eds.), pp. 1465–1485, McGraw-Hill, New York.

10

Role of Extracellular Fluid Volume Expansion and Diuretics in Renal Handling of Phosphate

MANUEL MARTINEZ-MALDONADO and
GARABED EKNOYAN

1. INTRODUCTION

One of the more remarkable functions of the kidney is maintenance of the constancy of the composition and volume (ECV) of the extracellular fluid. The understanding of the mechanisms involved in ECV homeostasis has improved colossally over the past two decades. A number of important studies during this period of time have revealed that a major site of salt and water regulation in the nephron is the proximal convoluted tubule (Jacobson and Seldin, 1977). During ECV expansion (ECVE), sodium reabsorption in the proximal convoluted tubule is depressed, whereas reabsorption is enhanced when ECV is contracted. The major determinants of proximal tubular reabsorption, in addition to a component of active sodium transport, are intrarenal hemodynamics and peritubular Starling forces. Although specific transport systems may exist for each of the constituents of glomerular filtrate, under conditions of changing ECV, bulk movement of fluid from lumen to blood or backleak from blood to lumen may take place. Considerable evidence has been presented (Boulpaep and Sackin, 1977) indicating that during ECVE, fluid backleaks through the tight junction or zona occludens of proximal tubules (or through intracytoplasmic channels). This results in retardation of sodium and water reabsorption and is measurable during micropuncture studies as a failure of the tubular fluid to plasma ratio for inulin to rise appropriately as the fluid courses from Bowman's capsule toward more distant portions of the proximal convolution (Dirks *et al.*, 1965; Rector *et al.*,

1967). The discovery that ECVE may inhibit net reabsorption of proximal tubular fluid suggested the possibility that other substances may appear in the urine as a consequence thereof. It was subsequently shown that the excretion of calcium, magnesium, phosphate, glucose, bicarbonate, uric acid, and *para*-aminohippurate could be enhanced as a result of ECVE. It is one purpose of this chapter to analyze the presently available knowledge of the effects of changes in volume on renal phosphate reabsorption. Because of the variety of factors which influence phosphate transport, it is inevitable that we will touch upon subjects which are more extensively discussed elsewhere in this volume.

2. VOLUME EXPANSION AND PHOSPHATE EXCRETION IN THE RAT AND THE DOG

The first demonstration that ECVE inhibits proximal tubular phosphate reabsorption was obtained by Frick. While examining the effect of ECVE on bicarbonate reabsorption in the rat proximal tubule, he described a concomitant inhibition of calcium and phosphate reabsorption (Frick *et al.*, 1967). Shortly thereafter, he corroborated and extended his findings in the rat (Frick, 1968), demonstrating that ECVE by Ringer's lactate in Sprague–Dawley rats resulted in marked inhibition of maximal tubular reabsorption of phosphate. In this pioneering work, it was clearly shown that a Tm for phosphate, contrary to the case for bicarbonate, did exist, since the inhibition in reabsorptive capacity produced by phosphate infusion was a result of the anion per se rather than the total volume of fluid administered. That ECVE inhibits renal phosphate reabsorption in the dog was described almost simultaneously by Massry *et al.* (1969) and by Suki *et al.* (1969). In experiments of almost identical design, these two groups of investigators showed that ECVE decreased renal phosphate reabsorption and Tm. The use of thyroparathyroidectomized (TPTX) dogs and of aortic or inferior vena cava constriction eliminated the possibility that the phosphaturia was the result of changes in the filtered load of phosphate, in plasma composition, or in parathyroid hormone (PTH) secretion. In both of these studies, TPTX was performed between 48 and 72 hr prior to the study, and all dogs were studied under pentobarbital anesthesia. In one of the studies (Massry *et al.*, 1969), TPTX dogs responded in a different fashion from intact dogs. At any level of sodium excretion, there was less phosphate excretion in TPTX than in intact dogs. From these results, one can conclude that the absence of PTH blunts or attentuates the phosphaturia of ECVE.

In another study by Beck and Goldberg (1974), in which isotonic saline expansion was used, the mean value of the relationship between sodium and phosphate in intact dogs was also similar to that of Massry's and many of Suki's TPTX dogs. In contrast, acutely and chronically TPTX dogs did not respond to saline infusion with phosphaturia. Thus, the absence of PTH under some circumstances may blunt, while elevated PTH may enhance, the phosphaturia of ECVE. Further studies in which TPTX or chemical parathyroidectomy (PTX) (Ca^{2+} infusion) was performed acutely (immediately prior to the study) showed that the phosphaturia which follows ECVE was abolished (Gradowska *et al.*, 1973; Schneider *et al.*, 1975). Acute surgical or chemical PTX may result in alterations in the kinetics of the saturable process normally responsible for phosphate transport in the nephron (Pitts and Alexander, 1944). To examine this, Hebert *et al.* (1972) measured the changes in absolute or fractional (corrected for glomerular filtration rate, GFR) tubular reabsorption of phosphate (TRP) in acutely TPTX dogs receiving phosphate infusions during ECVE. In all cases, (TRP $\times$ 100)/GFR was dminished irrespective of PTH or serum Ca^{2+} levels. These results indicate that acute PTX may contribute to blunting of the phosphaturia of ECVE by increasing the Tm, decreasing splay, or raising the renal threshold for phosphate (Hebert *et al.*, 1972). Despite natriuresis, phosphaturia was modest or trivial, suggesting that the absence of PTH enhances phosphate reabsorption somewhere in the nephron.

The most likely nephron site at which a lack of PTH may enhance phosphate reabsorption during ECVE is distal to the proximal tubule. Micropuncture and clearance studies in dogs have indicated that PTH and its presumed physiologic messenger, cyclic AMP (cAMP), exert an inhibitory effect on proximal tubular fluid (sodium) as well as phosphate reabsorption (Agus *et al.*, 1971; Wen, 1974b). Similarly, ECVE also depresses proximal sodium and phosphate reabsorption (Beck and Goldberg, 1974). Furthermore, in intact animals, the bulk of the phosphate delivered out of the proximal tubule escapes into the urine during both PTH administration and ECVE (Agus *et al.*, 1973; Beck and Goldberg, 1974; Knox and Lechêne, 1975; Puschett *et al.*, 1972; Schneider *et al.*, 1973; Wen, 1974a). Moreover, the degree of inhibition of proximal fractional sodium and fractional phosphate reabsorption was found to be similar in intact, acutely TPTX, or chronically TPTX animals (Beck and Goldberg, 1974; Knox and Lechêne, 1975). Fractional clearance of phosphate, however, was slightly increased or essentially unchanged in acutely and chronically TPTX dogs during saline loading, despite considerable increments in fractional clearance or sodium. In contrast, intact dogs developed natriuresis as well as phosphaturia in association with inhibition of proximal tubular function. It is clear that acute hypoparathyroidism must blunt the phosphaturia of ECVE distal to the last point of the proximal tubule which can be impaled for micropuncture. It is unfortunate that some authors have described the "distal nephron" as "any point between the last proximal convolution accessible to micropuncture and the urine." As recently demonstrated by Knox and his collaborators (1973, 1977), the last accessible proximal loop for micropuncture is only 60% of the total length of the proximal tubule in the dog. Although phosphate reabsorption has been shown to demonstrate different kinetic characteristics in early versus late proximal tubule in the rats (Baumann et al., 1975a,b), little is known about this specific issue in the dog. Similarly, while the pars recta of the rabbit (Dennis et al., 1977) can transport phosphate, the reabsorptive characteristics of this nephron segment in the dog are essentially unknown. In addition to intranephronal heterogeneity, superficial and deep nephrons may also be vastly different in their phosphate reabsorptive capacities. The excretion of phosphate during ECVE in acutely TPTX animals may be modified by heterogeneity of nephron function.

The rat appears to be more susceptible to the blunting effect of TPTX on the phosphaturia of ECVE. Frick (1969) was the first to demonstrate that acute PTX abolished the phosphaturia provoked by ECVE in the rat. He studied anesthetized female Sprague–Dawley rats kept on a normal diet. The rat strain, the sex of the animal, and the diet may be important in an analysis of the phosphaturia of ECVE. Female rats may show less avid proximal phosphate reabsorption, at least in Wistar rats (Harris et al., 1974), while fasting has a blunting effect on the phosphaturia of ECVE (Küntziger et al., 1972). Frick's study, however, did not examine proximal reabsorption directly. Amiel et al. (1970), on the other hand, studied by micropuncture male Sprague–Dawley rats which had undergone acute (2–3 hr prior to experiment) or chronic (6–12 days prior to study) PTX and had fasted between 15 and 18 hr prior to the experiment. The reabsorption of phosphate was determined by micropuncture with the use of ^{32}P under conditions of equilibrium of specific radioactivity between plasma and urine. It was found that considerable phosphate reabsorption occurred between the late proximal and early distal tubules but only in acutely PTX rats. The possibility that ECVE may accelerate phosphate reabsorption at distal sites must, therefore, be considered. In intact, non-volume-expanded rats, microinjection, microinfusion, and stationary microperfusion studies have not confirmed the findings of enhanced distal phosphate reabsorption (Brunette et al., 1973; Knox et al., 1973, 1977; Staum et al., 1972).

Proximal phosphate reabsorption was inhibited in the rat, as in the dog, during ECVE in studies utilizing free-flow micropuncture (Frick,

1972; Maesaka *et al.*, 1973) as well as the microinjection method (Brunette *et al.*, 1973). In the rat, as in the dog, despite some influence of increased PTH secretion (due to decreased serum Ca^{++}) on the phosphaturia, it was documented that ECVE per se can inhibit proximal tubular phosphate reabsorption (Maesaka *et al.*, 1973). In this study, it was suggested that ECVE enhances "distal" phosphate reabsorption in intact rats, but, once more, only late proximal tubular fluid and urine were compared. In an attempt to clarify this point, the same group of investigators (Maesaka *et al.*, 1976) examined the effect of ECVE on phosphate excretion in intact and acutely TPTX rats. Phosphate excretion was enhanced by ECVE in intact rats, while PTH potentiated the phosphaturia in TPTX rats. It appears that in intact rats, ECVE depresses phosphate reabsorption at a "distal" site (beyond the point accessible to micropuncture), as does PTH. Although Küntziger *et al.* (1972) have suggested that ECVE enhances phosphate reabsorption in the loop of Henle, they have shown a similar effect of PTX which can be reversed by exogenous cAMP (Küntziger *et al.*, 1974). This, of course, could have happened in the remainder of the proximal tubule and the pars recta. In contrast, Poujeol *et al.* (1976) did not find any significant degree of phosphate reabsorption in the loop during free-flow micropuncture or tracer microinjection, although they did demonstrate that approximately 1% of the filtered phosphate load can be reabsorbed in the distal nephron. In microinjection studies of the rat distal nephron (Greger *et al.*, 1977) and isolated microperfusion of the rabbit cortical collecting duct *in vitro* (Dennis *et al.*, 1977), no evidence of significant phosphate reabsorption could be detected.

Recent clearance studies by Frick and Durasin (1977) have shown that in rats handled in an identical manner to those in Frick's original study (1968), ECVE diminished Tm for phosphate in both intact and acutely PTX rats. This effect was observable provided phosphate infusions were given. In other words, as in the dog (Hebert *et al.*, 1972), an increase in reabsorptive capacity may have taken place because of the acute PTX.

Changes in the response of intact rats to ECVE may also be observed if either calcium or magnesium is given (Frick, 1969; Maesaka *et al.*, 1976). A role for calcium in the regulation of phosphate excretion has been shown to exist in the rat. Popovtzer and his collaborators (1975) examined the effect of hypercalcemia on PTX rats (two days prior to study) during ECVE and PTH infusion. Hypercalcemia consistently blunted the effect of ECVE on phosphate excretion; however, the phosphaturia and the rise in urinary cAMP which occur in response to PTH infusion were not blocked. From these observations, it was suggested that TRP has two components: one, suppressed by ECVE and stimulated by hypercalcemia; the second, suppressed by PTH and not affected by hypercalcemia. This last component also appears to be stimulated by vitamin D (Popovtzer *et al.*, 1975).

3. VOLUME EXPANSION AND PHOSPHATE EXCRETION IN HUMANS

ECVE has also been shown to increase phosphate excretion in normal individuals and in subjects with essential hypertension (Chaimovitz *et al.*, 1975; Steele, 1970). In normal subjects, expansion by infusion of saline equivalent to approximately 10% of ECV raised phosphate excretion in the face of decreasing ultrafilterable serum calcium and magnesium. Superimposition of hypertonic saline did not change calcium and magnesium concentrations further, yet it did cause further rises in phosphate excretion. Calcium infusion, despite a rise in the ultrafilterable fraction, could not rapidly reverse the phosphaturia. These results strongly suggest that in intact humans, as in dogs and rats, the phosphaturia of ECVE is the result of changes in ECV rather than in PTH secretion secondary to hypocalcemia (as a result of dilution). An exaggerated phosphaturic response to ECVE has also been observed in subjects with essential hypertension, a finding which is compatible with the general mechanisms of sodium reabsorption in these subjects and which gives support to the possibility of proximal tubular inhibition of phosphate by ECVE in humans (Chaimovitz *et al.*, 1975). In an interesting study, Epstein and his collaborators (1976) have examined the relationship among PTH, phosphaturia, and ECVE. Unfortunately, the model utilized, water immersion to the neck, produces central hypervolemia by redistribution of blood volume, a change which is different from that of ECVE with saline infusion. Nevertheless, despite a natriuresis which is comparable to acute administration of 2 liters of saline, no phosphaturia occurred. Neither serum calcium nor PTH was altered. Since neck immersion leads to bicarbonaturia, the presumed site of action for the natriuresis is the proximal tubule. The results suggested to the authors that, in humans there is also distal phosphate reabsorption. Because of the complexity of this model and the lack of precise knowledge of the level of natriuresis (maximal fractional sodium excretion was 1.4% in this study) required to affect phosphaturia, it is premature to accept any speculation in reference to "distal" phosphate reabsorption in humans.

4. MECHANISM OF PHOSPHATURIA DURING VOLUME EXPANSION

The mechanism by which ECVE diminishes phosphate reabsorption in the dog was an early source of controversy. Despite the clear demonstration by our group (Suki *et al.*, 1969) and Massry *et al.* (1969) that PTH secretion was unnecessary for the phosphaturia, it was also clear that if PTH were eliminated completely, the phosphaturia was blunted. Schneider and his collaborators (1975) and Knox *et al.* (1974) advanced definitive evidence that in the dog, while decreases in serum ionized calcium resulted in enhanced PTH secretion during ECVE, the phosphaturia which resulted was not dependent on PTH. Furthermore, the alternative possibility that decreases in ionized calcium per se may be responsible for the phosphaturia of ECVE was eliminated by the demonstration that a 25% reduction of this ion by the infusion of EDTA into the renal artery did not have a significant effect on the renal handling of phosphate (Cuche *et al.*, 1976b).

Renal vasodilatation enhances phosphate excretion in the dog (Ahumada and Massry, 1971; Cuche *et al.*, 1976a; Schneider *et al.*, 1973). It is possible that the consequences of renal vasodilatation, diminished filtration fraction with lower peritubular protein concentration and increased peritubular hydrostatic pressure (as in ECVE), account for the phosphaturia. Because under certain circumstances, vasodilatation does not lead to phosphaturia, it has been suggested that some agents may play "endogenous roles" in phosphate regulation. Dopamine, for example, is phosphaturic, whereas isoproterenol is not (Cuche *et al.*, 1976b). The same is true of acetylcholine and PGE_1 (phosphaturic), as compared to low doses of bradykinin or PGE_2 (not phosphaturic) (Schneider *et al.*, 1973). Rather than proposing independent roles in regulation of phosphate metabolism for an array of vasodilators, it must be clarified whether they do or do not interfere with proximal tubular reabsorption (low doses of bradykinin and PGE_2 do not), which appears to be important in the development of phosphaturia in the intact animal. Properties besides their vasodilatory effect may be operative in the phosphaturia. In addition to increased backflux, alterations in the transport kinetics of phosphate may be responsible for the phosphaturia of ECVE (Fig. 1). Whether these changes may result from alterations in cell metabolism or cell permeability characteristics or from changes in the composition of blood and/or filtrate remains undefined.

5. EFFECTS OF DIURETICS ON PHOSPHATE EXCRETION

Until recently, most of the reports on the effects of diuretics on phosphate excretion were fragmentary and inconclusive. Nevertheless, although diuretics have been most profitably utilized in the analysis of the renal handling of other ions, their contribution to our understanding of phosphate handling has been substantial.

The roles of the different groups of diuretic agents can best be con-

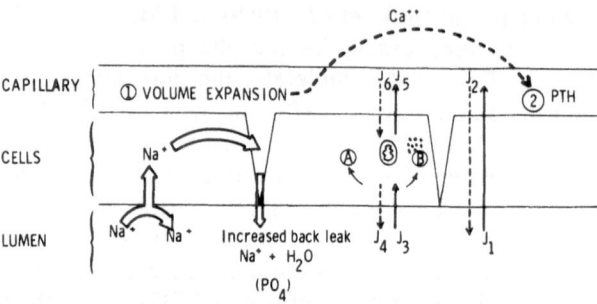

Fig. 1. Diagrammatic representation of possible mechanisms by which ECVE may inhibit phosphate reabsorption. The size or nature (solid, open, dashed) of the arrows does *not* indicate magnitude but rather differences in mechanisms. ECVE may increase backleak of fluid through tight junctions and thus increase intratubular phosphate concentration with subsequent loss in urine. It may diminish movement of sodium from lumen into cell and reduce phosphate reabsorption. Indirectly, it may raise serum PTH by reducing serum ionized calcium (curved, dashed arrow). Either PTH or some consequence of ECVE per se may alter tubular fluxes (J). Net flux ($J_1 > J_2$) or luminal flux ($J_3 > J_4$) may be affected. Alternatively, net efflux at the basolateral membrane ($J_5 > J_6$), achieved by asymmetry of the membrane carrier (A), may be decreased. Decreased metabolic runout (B), with decreased Pi incorporation into organic pools, is another alternative by which ECVE may alter phosphate transport. (From Scriver *et al.*, 1976.)

sidered against a background of the normal renal handling of phosphate (Fig. 2). Details of this process and the sites in the nephron where phosphate is reabsorbed are described in other chapters of this book.

The magnitude of the changes in urinary excretion of phosphate will depend on the tubular sites of action and potency of the diuretics used and on whatever effect the drug has on renal and extrarenal factors affecting phosphate reabsorption (Table 1).

5.1. Osmotic Agents

Mannitol and urea are freely filterable nonionized substances which behave as nonreabsorbable solutes within the tubular lumen. They retard tubular fluid reabsorption and increase urinary flow and sodium excretion. Mannitol, the most commonly utilized osmotic diuretic, significantly inhibits proximal water reabsorption (20%), with only a small decrease in sodium reabsorption at this site (4%). It exerts its major effect on sodium reabsorption in the loop of Henle (Goldberg *et al.*, 1965; Seely and Dirks, 1969).

A number of reports indicate that neither urea nor mannitol increases phosphate excretion (Better *et al.*, 1966; Mudge *et al.*, 1949; Seldin and Tarail, 1949; Wesson, 1962; Wesson and Anslow, 1948). The lack of phos-

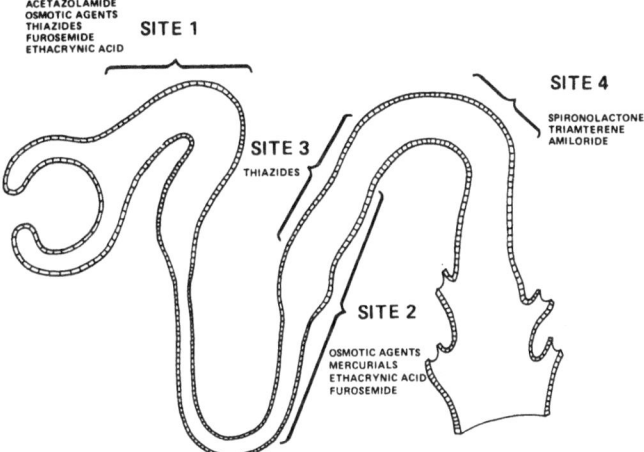

Fig. 2. Diagrammatic representation of the nephron with major sites of action of diuretics.

phaturic effect despite a marked diuresis may be attributed to the fact that mannitol exerts its effect at a site where little phosphate reabsorption occurs (Table 1, Fig. 2). This lack of an observed phosphate diuresis in some of the earlier studies is more likely due to mannitol's interference with phosphate determination when the method of Fisk and Subbarrow is used (Cook and Simmons, 1962). When this technical problem is circumvented, the infusion of mannitol results in an increase in phosphate excretion in the rat (Maesaka *et al.*, 1976). All of these animals developed dilutional hypocalcemia which may have stimulated PTH secretion. This could explain the phosphaturia. When serum calcium and magnesium were maintained constant, the rise in phosphate excretion was blunted. A phosphaturic effect was not obtained in TPTX animals, except during the constant infusion of PTH. Thus, the phosphaturia that occurs with mannitol diuresis seems to be dependent on the presence of PTH.

5.2. Mercurial Diuretics

The major natriuretic effect of these potent diuretics is inhibition of ion transport in the loop of Henle (Hook and Williamson, 1965; Seldin *et al.*, 1966). Several micropuncture studies in the dog have failed to demonstrate a proximal inhibitory effect of these agents (Clapp and Robinson, 1968; Evanson *et al.*, 1972). While the changes in phosphate excretion with mercurial diuresis have been variable (Goldberg, 1973), most of the results available show an increase in phosphate excretion following the administration of several of the organomercurial diuretics (Barber *et*

Table 1. Site of Action in the Nephron,[a] Maximal Fractional Excretion of Sodium and Phosphate, and Relative Carbonic Anhydrase Inhibitory Activity of Diuretics

Diuretic	Proximal tubule	Ascending loop of Henle		Distal tubule	Maximal fractional excretion (%)		Relative carbonic anhydrase inhibitory activity[b]
		Medullary	Cortical		Sodium	Phosphate	
Osmotic agents	+	+++			8	23	—
Mercurials		+++	+	+	20	25	—
Acetazolamide	+++			+	5	30–60	1.0
Thiazides	+		+++		8	30	0.15
Furosemide	+	+++	+		25	20–45	0.02
Ethacrynic acid	+	+++	++		25	25–30	0.000003
Potassium-sparing diuretics				+++	2		—

[a] The relative potency of the inhibitory action at various sites is indicated by + for a minor effect to +++ for a major effect.
[b] Relative to the concentration of acetazolamide required for 50% inhibition of carbonic anhydrase, considered as unity.

al., 1959; Eknoyan *et al.*, 1970; Wesson, 1962). The studies in which no change or an actual decrease in phosphate excretion was reported were conducted in human subjects whose urinary losses were not being replaced (Blumgart *et al.*, 1934; Ford *et al.*, 1958; Keith and Whelan, 1976; Parfitt, 1969; Wesson, 1962). Contraction of ECV induced by these relatively potent diuretics could have easily resulted in an increase in proximal tubular reabsorption of phosphate, which would then mask any effect of the diuretic (Eknoyan *et al.*, 1970). Indeed, in the published studies in which data on fractional urine collection are presented, there is no reduction in phosphate excretion during the first collection periods and a marked reduction during the next two or three timed collections several hours after administration of the agent. In one of these studies in which acetazolamide was also studied, the results are said to show no change in phosphate excretion, whereas, in actuality, both clearance and micropuncture studies (see below) have clearly shown acetazolamide to be a potent inhibitor of phosphate reabsorption. In the study of Wesson (1962), in which an equivocal effect of mercurials on TRP was reported, phosphate excretion increased in four of the seven animals studied. In the three animals that failed to show a phosphaturic effect, phosphate excretion during control periods was very low and actually undetectable in one. Conceivably, these could have been phosphate-depleted dogs and, hence, the inconsistency of the results obtained.

When considered in light of the tubular site of action of mercurials, that is, the loop of Henle, where the reabsorption of phosphate is modest, the marked phosphaturic effect of these agents may be hard to explain. Yet the phosphaturic effect of mercurials is actually more potent than that of the loop diuretics (Eknoyan *et al.*, 1970) and would suggest a site of action beyond the loop where phosphate reabsorption is largely sodium independent and where the mercurials exert an effect (at least on potassium secretion) which is also unrelated in a major way to the natriuresis produced by these agents (Evanson *et al.*, 1972; McBride *et al.*, 1958).

5.3. Carbonic Anhydrase Inhibitors

5.3.1. Acetazolamide

Earlier reports showing little (Freeman and Jacobsen, 1957; Malvin and Lotspeich, 1956) or no (Counihan *et al.*, 1954; Hanley and Platts, 1956) phosphaturic effect of carbonic anhydrase inhibitors notwithstanding, it is now evident that these agents consistently increase the excretion of phosphate to as much as 30–60% of the filtered load of inorganic phosphate (Beck and Goldberg, 1973; Eknoyan *et al.*, 1970; Goldberg, 1973). These are probably the most potent phosphaturic diuretics and have an effect which is equal to that of PTH (Agus *et al.*, 1971, 1973; Beck and Goldberg, 1973).

Inhibition of carbonic anhydrase in the cells of the proximal and distal tubules by acetazolamide inhibits bicarbonate reabsorption at both sites and causes a marked bicarbonaturia but only a modest natriuresis (Beck and Goldberg, 1973; Counihan *et al.*, 1954; Freeman and Jacobsen, 1957; Hanley and Platts, 1956; Malvin and Lotspeich, 1956). Micropuncture studies in the rat have demonstrated that carbonic anhydrase inhibitors also reduce proximal tubular reabsorption of water and chloride (Agus *et al.*, 1973; Kunau, 1972). They exert no direct effect in the loop of Henle (Clapp and Robinson, 1968), although augmented delivery of bicarbonate to the ascending limb represents a nonreabsorbable substrate and interferes with the concentrating mechanism (Rosin *et al.*, 1970).

The effect of bicarbonate diuresis on phosphate excretion is similar to that of carbonic anhydrase inhibition. It has been suggested (Fulop and Brazeau, 1968; Puschett and Goldberg, 1969) that alkalinization of luminal fluid increases the intratubular concentration of the more polar and less transportable divalent phosphate ion (HPO_4^{2-}) over that of the more easily reabsorbed monovalent ion ($H_2PO_4^-$). This results in decreased phosphate reabsorption at its major reabsorptive site within the nephron. This cannot be the explanation, since carbonic anhydrase inhibition results in a fall in proximal tubular pH because of the development of "disequilibrium" pH (Rector *et al.*, 1965). The phosphaturic effect of acetazolamide nevertheless appears to be dependent on the presence of bicarbonate, as suggested by studies on the isolated perfused kidney. In these studies (Besarb *et al.*, 1975), phosphaturia was not observed following acetazolamide when bicarbonate was omitted from the perfusion medium. Thus, in the presence or absence of bicarbonate, fractional excretion of phosphate was 7.2%. It remained unchanged when acetazolamide was added in the absence of bicarbonate but increased sixfold (to 42.9%) following acetazolamide in the presence of bicarbonate. Stop-flow microperfusion experiments in the rat (Cassola and Malnic, 1977) also point to an important role for bicarbonate in modulating phosphate reabsorption. Alteration in the perfusion pH of proximal tubular fluid from a low of 5.5 to a high of 8.2 resulted in alterations in ^{32}P reabsorption. The average half-time of phosphate loss was 31.9 sec during acid and 66 sec during alkaline perfusion. Acetazolamide infusion retarded phosphate absorption from the tubular lumen significantly (77 sec), but only during acid perfusion. The mechanism mediating this observation remains undefined. It could be dependent on the rate of hydrogen ion secretion rather than tubular pH or on changes in cell permeability induced by the drug, the change in pH, or some other as yet unidentified nonspecific effect. The effect of urinary alkalinization on renal handling of phosphate is discussed in Chapter 8.

The effect of acetazolamide is a direct one and not mediated by PTH, since it continues to produce phosphaturia in chronically PTX animals (Eknoyan *et al.*, 1970). In acutely TPTX animals, the phosphaturia is less than that in chronically TPTX and intact dogs (Beck and Goldberg, 1973; Knox *et al.*, 1976). As already mentioned, the effects of acetazolamide on phosphate, bicarbonate, and sodium excretion are similar to those observed following the administration of PTH (Agus *et al.*, 1971, 1973; Beck and Goldberg, 1973). An interaction of carbonic anhydrase inhibitors with the PTH-activated adenyl cyclase system in bone has been demonstrated (Minkin and Jennings, 1972; Waite *et al.*, 1970). Because of this, Rodriguez *et al.* (1974) examined the effect of acetazolamide on the adenyl cyclase system in the kidney. In studies on normal and PTX rats, acetazolamide was shown to increase urinary excretion of cAMP and to increase the generation of cAMP by renal cortical slices *in vitro*. Both of these effects were identical to those obtained with PTH, whereas alkalinization of the urine with bicarbonate infusion failed to result in a change in the excretion of either phosphate or cAMP. These results, however, have not been reproduced in the rat or dog. In humans, the infusion of acetazolamide in patients with hypoparathyroidism or pseudohypoparathyroidism has been shown to result in augmented excretion of phosphate without an increase in urinary cAMP (Sinha *et al.*, 1977). Indirect evidence for a role of the adenyl cyclase system in the phosphaturic effect of acetazolamide has been presented from clearance studies in normal dogs and in dogs treated with lithium, an inhibitor of adenyl cyclase (Arruda *et al.*, 1976). Both normal and lithium-treated animals exhibited natriuresis and bicarbonaturia following acetazolamide administration. On the other hand, while normal dogs exhibited phosphaturia, phosphate excretion did not increase in lithium-treated dogs. Thus, a dissociation exists between the effect of these agents on bicarbonate reabsorption (through their carbonic anhydrase inhibitory activity) and their effect on phosphate reabsorption (through the adenyl cyclase system).

5.3.2. Benzothiadiazines (Thiazides)

The urinary excretion of sodium chloride, bicarbonate, and potassium increases following the administration of the benzothiadiazine drugs (Beyer, 1958; Kahn, 1962). The carbonic anhydrase inhibitory activity of these agents, although less than that of acetazolamide, is nevertheless significant and may account for the reduced bicarbonate reabsorption in the proximal tubule (Beyer, 1958; Holzgreve, 1969; Maren, 1967). A proximal effect for thiazides was suspected from clearance studies (Seldin *et al.*, 1966). Initially, this could not be confirmed by proximal tubular micropuncture studies (Dirks *et al.*, 1966), either because of failure to replace urinary losses or because of the fall in GFR (Clapp *et al.*, 1971) which invariably ensues when thiazides are administered intravenously (Fernandez and Puschett, 1973). In free-flow micropuncture studies, which circumvent the hemodynamically induced fall in GFR, a definite inhibition of proximal reabsorption can be demonstrated (Fernandez and Puschett, 1973; Weinman and Eknoyan, 1975). The major action of thiazides, however, is inhibition of sodium reabsorption in the cortical diluting segment of the ascending limb of the loop of Henle (Clapp and Robinson, 1968; Quamme *et al.*, 1975; Seldin *et al.*, 1966; Suki *et al.*, 1965), which accounts for their natriuretic and chloriuretic effects.

The administration of thiazides results in a significant phosphaturia, with levels of fractional excretion of phosphate close to these attained with acetazolamide (Brickman *et al.*, 1972; Eknoyan *et al.*, 1970; Puschett and Goldberg, 1968; Steinmuller and Puschett, 1972; Suki *et al.*, 1972). This would be expected from their proximal tubular site of action, where a significant portion of the filtered phosphate is reabsorbed. As shown in simultaneous micropuncture and clearance studies, there is a marked decline in the proximal fractional reabsorption of phosphate following the administration of chlorothiazide or metolazone (Fernandez and Puschett, 1973). This has been attributed by some investigators (Puschett and Goldberg, 1968) to their carbonic anhydrase inhibitory activity. However, as discussed above, the phosphaturic effect of acetazolamide seems to be independent of its carbonic anhydrase inhibitory activity. It is possible that the phosphaturic effect of thiazides might also be initiated by the adenyl cyclase system, since thiazides have been shown to inhibit phosphodiesterase, which inactivates cAMP to 5'-monophosphate (Senft *et al.*, 1968). Contrary to the studies with acetazolamide (Rodriguez *et al.*, 1974), a definite correlation between thiazides and activation of the adenyl cyclase system has not been obtained. While such a mechanism must await further confirmation, it is of note that chlorothiazide and acetazolamide differ in their effects on phosphate excretion in acutely PTX animals. Thus, whereas acetazolamide causes a significant phosphaturia in the acutely PTX rat, chlorothiazide fails to do so except during phosphate infusion (Popovtzer, 1977). The failure of chlorothiazide to increase phosphate excretion in the acutely PTX animals might be attributed to the reabsorption of the phosphate distally when this mechanism is unveiled by the PTX or to an increased threshold or tubular reabsorptive capacity (Amiel *et al.*, 1970; Beck and Goldberg, 1973, 1974; Hebert *et al.*, 1972; Wen, 1974a). In chronically PTX animals, the filtered loads of phosphorus are higher than those in the acute animal models, and the phosphaturic response can again be elicited (Eknoyan *et al.*, 1970; Popovtzer, 1977).

5.3.3. Loop Diuretics (Furosemide and Ethacrynic Acid)

These two structurally different diuretics are grouped together because of their common locus of action in the ascending limb of the loop of Henle (Clapp and Robinson, 1968; Dirks and Seely, 1970; Morgan *et al.*, 1970; Seldin *et al.*, 1966; Suki *et al.*, 1965).

Both agents exert some degree of inhibition of proximal tubular reabsorption, as initially suggested from clearance studies and subsequently confirmed by micropuncture studies. This is particularly the case when a fall in glomerular filtration is prevented and the urinary losses are replaced to avoid volume depletion (Clapp *et al.*, 1971; Knox *et al.*, 1969; Morgan *et al.*, 1970; Seldin *et al.*, 1966; Suki *et al.*, 1965).

No effect on the renal excretion of phosphate was detected in earlier studies with furosemide and ethacrynic acid (Demartini *et al.*, 1967; Duarte, 1968; Stein *et al.*, 1968). It was subsequently shown by several investigators that both furosemide and ethacrynic acid increase phosphate excretion when urinary volume losses are replaced and changes in the PTH level obviated (Duarte, 1974; Eknoyan *et al.*, 1970; Haas *et al.*, 1977; Puschett and Goldberg, 1968; Steele, 1971).

The phosphaturic effect of furosemide has been attributed to its inhibition of bicarbonate reabsorption in the proximal tubule (Holzgreve, 1969), perhaps due to its carbonic anhydrase inhibitory activity (Puschett and Goldberg, 1968). This effect is at best a modest one (Table 1) and, from *in vitro* studies, 50 times less potent than that of acetazolamide (Puschett and Goldberg, 1968; Stein *et al.*, 1968). That furosemide might share a common mechanism of action with acetazolamide has been suggested from studies in dogs receiving acetazolamide in which the subsequent administration of furosemide was neither phosphaturic nor bicarbonaturic (Haas *et al.*, 1977). Unlike acetazolamide, however, furosemide has no effect on the urinary excretion of cAMP or on the activity of renal cortical tissue adenyl cyclase (Rodriguez *et al.*, 1974). As suggested by Rodriguez *et al.*, it is possible that the concentrations of furosemide used in their studies may not have been high enough. Similar to the thiazides, large doses of furosemide were noted to inhibit phosphodiesterase in the cortical tissue of the rat kidney (Senft *et al.*, 1968). This would result in increased intracellular cAMP, which could then act as the inhibitor of phosphate reabsorption. This suggestion remains to be examined.

The suggestion has been made (Haas *et al.*, 1977) that the phosphaturia induced by furosemide is dependent on the presence of PTH. In acutely PTX dogs, furosemide failed to augment fractional phosphate excretion except when given during the constant infusion of bovine PTH. The issues involved in such studies during acute PTX have been discussed in Section 5.3.2. An additional problem with this particular study (Haas *et al.*, 1977) was the 40–50% reduction in GFR when furosemide was given alone as compared to a 20–26% drop when it was given with PTH. Since these acutely PTX animals have a lower serum phosphate, the reduction in GFR would result in a significantly reduced load of filtered phosphate at a time when the distal tubular phosphate reabsorption has been unveiled by the PTX. Furthermore, furosemide acts in the distal nephron upon the luminal side because of its active secretion by the proximal tubule (Rector *et al.*, 1967). Reduction in renal function could, therefore, result in decreased delivery of the drug to its site of action (Dirks and Seely, 1970). Moreover, in a similar study to that of Haas *et al.* (1977) with ethacrynic acid and furosemide in non-PTX intact dogs (Duarte, 1974), aortic clamping reduced but did not abolish the phosphaturia. Finally, an inhibitory effect on phosphate reabsorption has been demonstrated in the isolated perfused kidney, obviously in the total absence of PTH (Nizet, 1972).

Bumetamide, a new diuretic with a site of action similar to that of furosemide and ethacrynic acid, has also been shown to cause phosphaturia in humans (Bourke *et al.*, 1973).

5.4. Potassium-Sparing Diuretics

None of the three drugs in this group—aldactone (Ben Ishay *et al.*, 1972), triamterene (Walker *et al.*, 1972), and amiloride (Johny *et al.*, 1969)—has been shown to inhibit phosphate reabsorption.

6. REFERENCES

Agus, Z. S., Puschett, J. B., Senesky, D., and Goldberg, M., 1971, Mode of action of parathyroid hormone and cyclic adenosine 5′-monophosphate on renal tubular phosphate reabsorption in the dog, *J. Clin. Invest.* **50:**617.

Agus, Z. S., Gardner, L. B., Beck, L. H., and Goldberg, M., 1973, Effects of parathyroid hormone on renal tubular reabsorption of calcium, sodium and phosphate, *Am. J. Physiol.* **224:**1143.

Ahumada, J. J., and Massry, S. G., 1971, Renal vasodilatation: Effect on renal handling of phosphate, *Clin. Sci.* **41:**109.

Amiel, C., Küntziger, H., and Richet, G., 1970, Micropuncture study of handling of phosphate by proximal and distal nephron in normal and parathyroidectomized rat. Evidence for distal reabsorption, *Pflügers Arch.* **317:**93.

Arruda, J. A. L., Richardson, J. M., Wolfson, J. A., Nascimento, L., Rademacher, D. R., and Kurtzman, N. A., 1976, Lithium administration and phosphate excretion, *Am. J. Physiol.* **231:**1140.

Barber, E. S., Elkington, J. R., and Clark, J. K., 1959, Studies of the renal excretion of magnesium in man, *J. Clin. Invest.* **38:**1733.

Baumann, K., de Rouffignac, C., Roinel, N., Rumrich, G., and Ullrich, K. J., 1975a, Renal phosphate transport: Inhomogeneity of local proximal transport rates and sodium dependence, *Pflügers Arch.* **356**:287.

Baumann, K., Rumrich, G., Papavassiliou, F., and Kloss, S., 1975b, pH dependence of phosphate reabsorption in the proximal tubule of rat kidney, *Pflügers Arch.* **360**:183.

Beck, L. H., and Goldberg, M., 1973, Effects of acetazolamide and parathyroidectomy on renal transport of sodium, calcium and phosphate, *Am. J. Physiol.* **224**:1136.

Beck, L. H., and Goldberg, M., 1974, Mechanism of the blunted phosphaturia in saline-loaded thyroparathyroidectomized dogs, *Kidney Int.* **6**:18.

Ben Ishay, D., Viskoper, R. J., and Menczel, J., 1972, Effect of spironolactone on urinary calcium excretion, *Isr. J. Med. Sci.* **8**:495.

Besarb, A., Silva, P., Ross, B., and Epstein, F., 1975, Bicarbonate and sodium reabsorption by the isolated perfused kidney, *Am. J. Physiol.* **228**:1525.

Better, O. S., Gonick, O. S., Chapman, L. C., Varrody, P. D., and Kleeman, C. R., 1966, Effect of urea-saline diuresis on renal excretion of calcium, magnesium and inorganic phosphate in man, *Proc. Soc. Exp. Biol. Med.* **121**:592.

Beyer, K. H., 1958, The mechanism of action of chlorothiazide, *Ann. N.Y. Acad. Sci.* **71**:363.

Blumgart, H. L., Gilligan, D. R., Levy, R. C., Brown, M. G., and Volk, M. C., 1934, Action of diuretic drugs. I. Action of diuretics in normal persons, *Arch. Intern. Med.* **54**:40.

Boulpaep, E. L., and Sackin, H., 1977, Role of the paracellular pathway in isotonic fluid movement across the renal tubule, *Yale J. Biol. Med.* **50**:115.

Bourke, E., Asbury, M. J., O'Sullivan, S., and Gatenby, P. B., 1973, The site of action of bumetamide in man, *Eur. J. Pharmacol.* **23**:283.

Brickman, A. S., Massry, S. G., and Coburn, J., 1972, Changes in serum and urinary calcium during treatment with hydrochlorothiazide. Studies on mechanism. *J. Clin. Invest.* **51**:945.

Brunette, M. G., Taleb, L., and Carriere, S., 1973, Effect of parathyroid hormone on phosphate reabsorption along the nephron of the rat, *Am. J. Physio.* **225**:1076.

Cassola, A. C., and Malnic, G., 1977, Phosphate transfer and tubular pH during renal stopped flow microperfusion experiments in the rat, *Pflügers Arch.* **367**:249.

Chaimovitz, C., Spierer, A., Leibowitz, H., Tuma, S., and Better, O. S., 1975, Exaggerated phosphaturic response to volume expansion in patients with essential hypertension, *Clin. Sci. Mol. Med.* **49**:207.

Clapp, J. R., and Robinson, R. R., 1968, Distal sites of action of diuretic drugs in the dog nephron, *Am. J. Physiol.* **215**:225.

Clapp, J. R., Nottebohm, G. A., and Robinson, R. R., 1971, Proximal site of action of ethacrynic acid: Importance of filtration rate, *Am. J. Physiol.* **220**:1355.

Cook, B. S., and Simmons, D. H., 1962, Mannitol interference in phosphate determination: Method of correction, *J. Lab. Clin. Med.* **60**:160.

Counihan, T. B., Evans, B. M., and Milne, M. D., 1954, Observations on the pharmacology of the carbonic anhydrase inhibitor "Diamox" *Clin. Sci.* **13**:585.

Cuche, J. L., Marchand, G. R., Gregor, R. F., Lang, F. C., and Knox, F. G., 1976a, Phosphaturic effect of dopamine in dogs, *J. Clin. Invest.* **58**:71.

Cuche, J. L., Ott, C. E., Marchand, G. R., and Knox, F. G., 1976b, Lack of effect of hypocalcemia on renal phosphate handling, *J. Lab. Clin. Med.* **88**:271.

Demartini, F. E., Briscol, A. M., and Ragan, C., 1967, Effect of ethacrynic acid on calcium and magnesium excretion, *Proc. Soc. Exp. Biol. Med.* **124**:320.

Dennis, V. W., Bello-Reuss, E., and Robinson, R. R., 1977, Response of phosphate transport to parathyroid hormone in segments of rabbit nephron, *Am. J. Physiol.* **233**:F29.

Dirks, J. H., and Seely, J. F., 1970, Effect of saline infusions and furosemide on the dog distal nephron, *Am. J. Physiol.* **219:**114.

Dirks, J. H., Cirksena, W. J., and Berliner, R. W., 1965, The effects of saline infusion on sodium reabsorption by the proximal tubule of the dog, *J. Clin. Invest.* **44:**1160.

Dirks, J. H., Cirksena, W. J., and Berliner, R. W., 1966, Micropuncture study of the effect of various diuretics on sodium reabsorption by the proximal tubules of the dog, *J. Clin. Invest.* **45:**1975.

Duarte, C. G., 1968, Effects of ethacrynic acid and furosemide on urinary calcium, phosphate and magnesium, *Metabolism* **17:**867.

Duarte, C. G., 1974, Effects of ethacrynic acid and furosemide on urinary phosphate in the dog, *Clin. Sci. Mol. Med.* **46:**671.

Eknoyan, G., Suki, W. N., and Martinez-Maldonado, M., 1970, Effect of diuretics on urinary excretion of phosphate, calcium and magnesium in thyroparathyroidectomized dogs, *J. Lab. Clin. Med.* **76:**257.

Epstein, M., Pins, D. S., Silvers, W., Loutzenhiser, R., Canterbury, J. M., and Reiss, E., 1976, Failure of water immersion to influence parathyroid hormone secretion and renal phosphate handling in normal man, *J. Lab. Clin. Med.* **87:**218.

Evanson, R. E., Lockhart, E. A., and Dirks, J. H., 1972, Effect of mercurial diuretics on tubular sodium and potassium transport in the dog, *Am. J. Physiol.* **222:**282.

Fernandez, P. V., and Puschett, J. B., 1973, Proximal tubular actions of metolazone and chlorothiazide, *Am. J. Physiol.* **225:**954.

Ford, R. V., Rochelle, J. B., Handley, C. A., Moyer, J. H., and Spurr, L. C., 1958, Choice of diuretic agent based on pharmacological principles, *J. Am. Med. Assoc.* **166:**129.

Freeman, S., and Jacobsen, A. B., 1957, Acute effects of acetazolamide (Diamox) on plasma and urinary electrolytes of dogs with special reference to calcium, *Am. J. Physiol.* **191:**388.

Frick, A., 1968, Reabsorption of inorganic phosphate in the rat kidney. I. Saturation of transport mechanism. II. Suppression of fractional phosphate reabsorption due to expansion of extracellular fluid volume, *Pflügers Arch.* **304:**351.

Frick, A., 1969, Mechanism of inorganic phosphate diuresis secondary to saline infusions in the rat, *Pflügers Arch.* **313:**106.

Frick, A., 1972, Proximal tubular reabsorption of inorganic phosphate during saline infusion in the rat, *Am. J. Physiol.* **223:**1034.

Frick, A., and Durasin, I., 1977, Effect of expansion of extracellular fluid volume on the maximal reabsorptive capacity for inorganic phosphate in parathyroidectomized and intact rats, *Pflügers Arch.* **370:**115.

Frick, A., Rector, F. C., Jr., and Seldin, D. W., 1967, Vergleich der transtbulären Konzentrationsquotienten für Kaliuum, Calcium[45], Bicarbonat und anorganisches Phosphat im proximalen Tubulus der Rattenniere. *Pflügers Arch. Gesamte Physiol Menschen Tiere* **297:**R8.

Fulop, M., and Brazeau, P., 1968, The phosphaturic effect of sodium bicarbonate and acetazolamide in dogs, *J. Clin. Invest.* **47:**983.

Goldberg, M., 1973, The renal physiology of diuretics, in: *Renal Physiology—Handbook of Physiology* (J. Orloff and R. W. Berliner, eds.), pp. 1003–1031, American Physiological Society, Washington, D.C.

Goldberg, M., McCurdy, D. K., and Ramirez, M. A., 1965, Differences between saline and mannitol diuresis in hydropenic man, *J. Clin. Invest.* **44:**182.

Gradowska, L., Caglar, S., Rutherford, E., Harter, H., and Slatopolsky, E., 1973, On the mechanism of the phosphaturia of extracellular fluid volume expansion in the dog, *Kidney Int.* **3:**230.

Greger, R., Lang, F., Marchand, G., and Knox, F. G., 1977, Site of renal phosphate reabsorption. Micropuncture and microinfusion study, *Pflügers Arch.* **369:**111.

Haas, J. A., Larson, M. V., Marchand, G. R., Lang, F. C., Greger, R. F., and Knox, F. G., 1977, Phosphaturic effect of furosemide: Role of PTH and carbonic anhydrase, *Am. J. Physiol.* **232**:F105.

Hanley, T., and Platts, M. M., 1956, Observations on the metabolic effects of the carbonic anhydrase inhibitor Diamox: Mode and rate of recovery from the drug's action, *J. Clin. Invest.* **35**:20.

Harris, C. A., Baer, P. G., Chirito, E., and Dirks, J. H., 1974, Composition of mammalian glomerular filtrate, *Am. J. Physiol.* **227**:972.

Hebert, C. S., Rouse, D., Eknoyan, G., Martinez-Maldonado, M., and Suki, W. N., 1972, Decreased phosphate reabsorption by volume expansion in the dog, *Kidney Int.* **2**:247.

Holzgreve, H., 1969, The pattern of inhibition of proximal tubular reabsorption by diuretics, in: *Renal Transport and Diuretics* (K. Thurau and H. Jahrmarker, eds.), pp. 229–234, Springer, Heidelberg.

Hook, J. B., and Williamson, H. E., 1965, Effect of chlormerodrin on medullary sodium transport, *Pharmacologist* **7**:167.

Jacobson, H. R., and Seldin, D. W., 1977, Proximal tubular reabsorption and its regulation, in: *Annual Review of Pharmacology and Toxicology*, Vol. 17 (H. W. Elliott, ed.), pp. 623–646, Annual Reviews, Palo Alto, Calif.

Johny, K. V., Lawrence, J. R., and O'Halloran, W., 1969, Amiloride hydrochloride, a hypercalciuric diuretic, *Aust. Ann. Med.* **18**:267.

Kahn, M., 1962, The effect of chlorothiazide on electrolyte excretion in intact and adrenalectomized rats, *Am. J. Physiol.* **202**:1141.

Keith, N. M., and Whelan, M., 1976, A study of the action of ammonium chloride and organic mercury compounds, *J. Clin. Invest.* **3**:149.

Knox, F. G., and Lechêne, C., 1975, Distal site of action of parathyroid hormone and phosphate reabsorption, *Am. J. Physiol.* **229**:1556.

Knox, F. G., Wright, F. S., Howard, S. S., and Berliner, R. W., 1969, Effect of furosemide on sodium reabsorption by the proximal tubule in the dog, *Am. J. Physiol.* **217**:192.

Knox, F. G., Schneider, E. G., Willis, L. R., Strandhoy, J. W., and Ott, C. E., 1973, Site and control of phosphate reabsorption by the kidney, *Kidney Int.* **3**:347.

Knox, F. G., Schneider, E. G., Willis, L. R., Strandhoy, J. W., Ott, C. E., Cuche, J. L., Goldsmith, R. S., and Arnaud, C. D., 1974, Proximal tubule reabsorption after hyperoncotic albumin infusion, *J. Clin. Invest.* **53**:501.

Knox, F., Haas, J., and Lechêne, C., 1976, Effect of parathyroid hormone on phosphate reabsorption in the presence of acetazalomide, *Kidney Int.* **10**:216.

Knox, F. G., Osswald, H., Marchand, G. R., Spielman, W. S., Haas, J. A., Berndt, T., and Youngberg, S. P., 1977, Phosphate transport along the nephron, *Am. J. Physiol.* **233**:F261.

Kunau, R. T., 1972, The influence of the carbonic anhydrase inhibitor, Benzolamide (Cl-11, 366) on the reabsorption of chloride, sodium and bicarbonate in the proximal tubule of the rat, *J. Clin. Invest.* **51**:294.

Küntziger, H., Amiel, C., and Gaudebout, C., 1972, Phosphate handling by the rat nephron during saline diuresis, *Kidney Int.* **2**:318.

Küntziger, H., Amiel, C., Roinel, N., and Morel, F., 1974, Effects of parathyroidectomy and cyclic AMP on renal transport of phosphate, calcium and magnesium, *Am. J. Physiol.* **227**:905.

Maesaka, J. K., Levitt, M. F., and Abramson, R. G., 1973, Effect of saline infusion on phosphate transport in intact and thyroparathyroidectomized rats, *Am. J. Physiol.* **225**:1421.

Maesaka, J. K., Berger, M. L., Bornia, M. E., Abramson, R. G., and Levitt, M. F., 1976, Effect of mannitol on phosphate transport in intact and acutely thyroparathyroidectomized rats, *J. Lab. Clin. Med.* **87**:680.

Malvin, R. L., and Lotspeich, W. D., 1956, Relation between the tubular transport of inorganic phosphate and bicarbonate in the dog, *Am. J. Physiol.* **187**:51.

Maren, T. H., 1967, Carbonic anhydrase: Chemistry, physiology and inhibition, *Physiol. Rev.* **47**:597.

Martinez-Maldonado, M., Eknoyan, G., and Suki, W. N., 1971, Natriuretic effects of vasopressin and cyclic AMP: Possible site of action in the nephron, *Am. J. Physiol.* **220**:2013.

Massry, S. G., Coburn, J. W., and Kleeman, C. R., 1969, The influence of extracellular volume expansion on renal phosphate reabsorption in the dog, *J. Clin. Invest.* **48**:1237.

McBride, W. O., Weiner, I. M., and Mudge, G. H., 1958, Inhibition of potassium secretion by mercurial diuretics, *Fed. Proc. Fed. Am. Soc. Exp. Biol.* **17**:107.

Minkin, C., and Jennings, J. M., 1972, Carbonic anhydrase and bone remodeling: Sulfonamide inhibition of bone reabsorption in organ culture, *Science* **176**:1031.

Morgan, T., Tadokoro, M., Martin, D., and Berliner, R. W., 1970, Effect of furosemide on Na^+ and K^+ transport studied by microperfusion of the rat nephron, *Am. J. Physiol.* **218**:292.

Mudge, G. H., Foulks, J., and Gilman, A., 1949, Effect of urea diuresis on renal excretion of electrolytes, *Am. J. Physiol.* **158**:218.

Nizet, A., 1972, Excretion and tubular reabsorption of sodium, glucose and phosphate by isolated dog kidneys. Influence of blood dilution, *Pflügers Arch.* **332**:248.

Parfitt, A. M., 1969, The acute effects of mersalyl, chlorothiazide and mannitol on the renal excretion of calcium and other ions in man, *Clin. Sci.* **36**:267.

Pitts, R. F., and Alexander, R. S., 1944, The renal reabsorption mechanism for inorganic phosphate in normal and acidotic dogs, *Am. J. Physiol.* **142**:648.

Popovtzer, M. M., 1977, Renal response to phosphaturic agents in acutely and chronically parathyroidectomized rats, *Proc. Soc. Exp. Biol. Med.* **154**:522.

Popovtzer, M. M., Robinette, J. B., McDonald, K. M., and Kuruvila, C. K., 1975, Effect of Ca^{++} on renal handling of PO_4^{3-}: Evidence for two reabsorptive mechanisms, *Am. J. Physiol.* **229**:901.

Poujeol, P., Chabardès, D., Roinel, N., and de Rouffignac, C., 1976, Influence of extracellular fluid volume expansion on magnesium, calcium and phosphate handling along the rat nephron, *Pflügers Arch.* **365**:203.

Puschett, J. B., and Goldberg, M., 1968, The acute effects of furosemide on acid and electrolyte excretion in man, *J. Lab. Clin. Med.* **71**:666.

Puschett, J. B., and Goldberg, M., 1969, The relationship between the renal handling of phosphate and bicarbonate in man, *J. Lab. Clin. Med.* **73**:956.

Puschett, J. B., Agus, Z. S., Senesky, D., and Goldberg, M., 1972, Effects of saline loading and aortic obstruction on proximal phosphate transport, *Am. J. Physiol.* **223**:851.

Quamme, G. A., Wong, N. M. L., Sutton, R. A. L., and Dirks, J. H., 1975, Interrelationship of chlorothiazide and parathyroid hormone: A micropuncture study, *Am. J. Physiol.* **229**:200.

Rector, F. C., Carter, N. W., and Seldin, D. W., 1965, The mechanism of bicarbonate reabsorption in the proximal and distal tubule of the kidney, *J. Clin. Invest.* **44**:278.

Rector, F. C., Jr., Sellman, J. C., Martinez-Maldonado, M., and Seldin, D. W., 1967, The mechanism of suppression of proximal tubular reabsorption by saline infusions, *J. Clin. Invest.* **46**:47.

Rodriguez, H. J., Walls, J., Yates, J., and Klahr, S., 1974, Effect of acetazolamide on the urinary excretion of cyclic AMP and on the activity of renal adenyl cyclase, *J. Clin. Invest.* **53**:122.

Rosin, J. M., Katz, M. A., Rector, F. C., and Seldin, D. W., 1970, Acetazolamide in studying sodium reabsorption in diluting segment, *Am. J. Physiol.* **219**:731.

Schneider, E. G., Strandhoy, J. W., Willis, L. R., and Knox, F. G., 1973, Relationship between proximal sodium reabsorption and excretion of calcium, magnesium and phosphate, *Kidney Int.* **4:**369.

Schneider, E. G., Goldsmith, R. S., Arnaud, C. D., and Knox, F. G., 1975, Role of parathyroid hormone in the phosphaturia of extracellular fluid volume expansion, *Kidney Int.* **7:**317.

Scriver, C. R., Stacey, T. E., Tenenhouse, H. S., and MacDonald, W. A., 1976, Transepithelial transport of phosphate anion in kidney. Potential mechanisms for hypophosphatemia, in: *Phosphate Metabolism* (S. G. Massry and E. Ritz, eds.), pp. 55–70, Plenum Press, New York.

Seely, J. F., and Dirks, J. H., 1969, Micropuncture study of hypertonic mannitol diuresis in the proximal and distal tubule of the dog kidney, *J. Clin. Invest.* **48:**2330.

Seldin, D. W., and Tarail, R., 1949, Effect of hypertonic solutions on metabolism and excretion of electrolytes, *Am. J. Physiol.* **159:**160.

Seldin, D. W., Eknoyan, G., Suki, W. N., and Rector, F. C., 1966, Localization of diuretic action from the pattern of water and electrolyte excretion, *Ann. N.Y. Acad. Sci.* **139:**328.

Senft, G., Munske, K., Schultz, G., and Hoffman, M., 1968, Der Einfluss von Hydrochlorothiazide und anderen sulfonamidierten Diuretica auf die 3′,5′ AMP phosphodiesterase—Activität in der Rattenniere, *Arch. Exp. Pathol. Pharmakol.* **259:**344.

Sinha, P. K., Allen, D. O., Cleaner, S. F., and Bell, N. H., 1977, Effect of acetazolamide on the renal excretion in hypoparathyroidism and pseudohypoparathyroidism, *J. Lab. Clin. Med.* **89:**1188.

Staum, B. B., Hamburger, R. J., and Goldberg, M., 1972, Tracer micro-injection study of renal tubular phosphate reabsorption in the rat, *J. Clin. Invest.* **51:**2271.

Steele, T. H., 1970, Increased urinary phosphate excretion following volume expansion in normal man, *Metabolism* **19:**129.

Steele, T. H., 1971, Dual effect of potent diuretics on renal handling of phosphate in man, *Metabolism* **20:**749.

Stein, J., Wilson, C., and Kirkendall, W., 1968, Differences in the acute effects of furosemide and ethacrynic acid, *J. Lab. Clin. Med.* **71:**654.

Steinmuller, S. R., and Puschett, J. B., 1972, Effects on metolazone in man: Comparison with chlorothiazide, *Kidney Int.* **1:**169.

Suki, W. N., Rector, F. C., and Seldin, D. W., 1965, The site of action of furosemide and other sulfonamide diuretics in the dog, *J. Clin. Invest.* **44:**1458.

Suki, W. N., Martinez-Maldonado, M., Rouse, D., and Terry, A., 1969, Effect of expansion of extracellular fluid volume on renal phosphate handling, *J. Clin. Invest.* **48:**1888.

Suki, W. N., Dawoud, F., Eknoyan, G., and Martinez-Maldonado, M., 1972, Effects of metolazone on renal function in normal man, *J. Pharmacol. Exp. Ther.* **180:**6.

Waite, L. C., Volkert, W. A., and Kenney, A. D., 1970, Inhibition of bone resorption by acetazolamide in the rat, *Endocrinology* **87:**1129.

Walker, B. R., Hoppe, R. C., and Alexander, F., 1972, Effect of triamterene on the renal clearance of calcium, magnesium, phosphate and uric acid in man, *Clin. Pharmacol. Ther.* **13:**245.

Weinman, E. J., and Eknoyan, G., 1975, Chronic effects of chlorothiazide on reabsorption by the proximal tubule of the rat, *Clin. Sci. Mol. Med.* **49:**107.

Wen, S. F., 1974a, Micropuncture studies of phosphate transport in the proximal tubule of the dog, *J. Clin. Invest.* **53:**143.

Wen, S. F., 1974b, The effect of vasopressin on phosphate transport in the proximal tubule of the dog, *J. Clin. Invest.* **53:**660.

Wesson, L. G., 1962, Organic mercurial effects on renal tubular reabsorption of calcium and magnesium and on phosphate excretion in the dog, *J. Lab. Clin. Med.* **59:**630.

Wesson, L. G., and Anslow, W. P., 1948, Excretion of sodium and water during osmotic diuresis in the dog, *Am. J. Physiol.* **153:**465.

Influence of Calcium on Renal Handling of Phosphate

ROBERT A. PERAINO and WADI N. SUKI

1. INTRODUCTION

The renal handling of phosphate is homeostatically controlled by a number of hormonal and nonhormonal stimuli—acting directly upon the renal tubule or indirectly by altering the metabolism of this ion elsewhere in the body—which influence its excretion by the kidney. This chapter deals only with the effects of calcium, by direct or indirect means, to induce changes in inorganic phosphate excretion by the kidney independent of changes in phosphate metabolism by other organs.

2. PHYSIOLOGIC STUDIES

Calcium administration can effect changes in phosphate handling by four currently known actions; (1) alterations in serum inorganic phosphate concentration and its ultrafilterable fraction, (2) changes in renal hemodynamics, (3) a direct action upon the renal tubule, and (4) inhibition of hormone secretion by the parathyroid glands. The effect of alteration in parathyroid gland activity on renal handling of phosphate is discussed in detail in Chapter 5.

2.1. Effect of Calcium Infusion on the Serum Inorganic Phosphate Concentration and Its Filtration Characteristics

In mammals, inorganic phosphate exists in blood in a freely filterable form without binding to plasma proteins, as demonstrated *in vitro* by Grollman in 1927 and confirmed by Hopkins *et al.* (1952) using artificial membranes. The measurement of serum inorganic phosphate ultrafilter-ability *in vitro* with modern artificial membranes is valid, as elegantly demonstrated by Le Grimellec *et al.* (1975). These investigators compared the inorganic phosphate concentration of rat glomerular filtrate obtained by micropuncture with the filterable moiety measured *in vitro* and found an excellent correlation (Fig. 1). The addition of calcium to serum or plasma *in vitro* renders phosphate less filterable, most likely by forming soluble calcium–phosphate–protein complexes (Grollman, 1927; Hopkins *et al.*, 1952). This effect of calcium to diminish the filterability of phos-phate has also been demonstrated *in vivo*. Cuche *et al.* (1976a) illustrated an inverse linear relationship between the percentage ultrafilterability of serum inorganic phosphate and the serum calcium–phosphate product during calcium infusion into thyroparathyroidectomized (TPTX) dogs re-ceiving an infusion of parathyroid hormone (PTH). Figure 2 shows our observations before and during calcium infusion into TPTX dogs with and without exogenous PTH, which concur with the conclusion of others that calcium infusion diminishes the ultrafilterability of serum inorganic phos-phate.

The second effect of systemic calcium administration on serum in-organic phosphate is to cause an increase in its concentration, which may be due to exodus of organic phosphate from red blood cells (Chen and Neuman, 1955). The hyperphosphatemic effect of calcium infusion in TPTX dogs studied in our laboratories is illustrated in Fig. 3 and confirms the earlier reports of many investigators (Baylor *et al.*, 1950; Chambers *et al.*, 1956; Chen and Neuman, 1955; Cuche *et al.*, 1976a; Goldman and Bassett, 1954; Hiatt and Thompson, 1957; Howard *et al.*, 1953; Kyle *et al.*, 1954; Nordin and Fraser, 1954; Salvesen *et al.*, 1924; Wallach and Carter, 1961). The effect of calcium is also independent of PTH and cal-

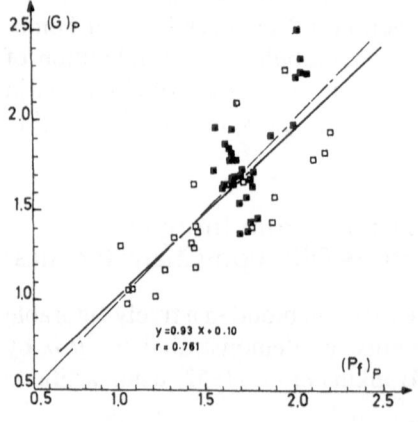

Fig. 1. Absolute concentrations of phos-phorus in artificial and glomerular ultra-filtrate samples. Phosphorus concentra-tions in capsular fluid and plasma ultrafiltrates were measured by electron probe analysis. Abscissa: $(P_f)_P$; phospho-rus concentrations in plasma ultrafiltrates (mM/liter). Ordinate: $(G)_P$, phosphorus concentrations in capsular fluid (mM/liter). Open symbols correspond to female rats and filled symbols to male rats. (From Le Grimellec *et al.*, 1975. Reprinted with per-mission.)

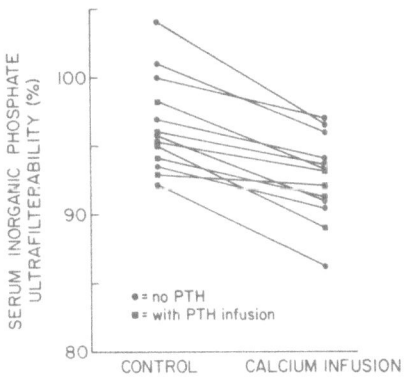

Fig. 2. Effect of calcium infusion on serum inorganic phosphate ultrafilterability in TPTX dogs. Abscissa: control, periods without calcium infusion; calcium infusion, periods during calcium infusion. Ordinate: serum inorganic phosphate ultrafilterability expressed as a percentage of total serum inorganic phosphate concentration. ●, Infusion without exogenous PTH. ■, Infusion of exogenous PTH throughout the experiment and commencing prior to the control periods.

citonin, as the rise in serum inorganic phosphate concentration seen with calcium infused intravenously occurs in TPTX humans and dogs (Anderson and Talmage, 1973; Chambers *et al.*, 1956; Goldman and Bassett, 1954; Hausmann, 1970; Hiatt and Thompson, 1957; Howard *et al.*, 1953).

Thus, calcium infusion may indirectly influence the renal excretion of phosphate. Large increases in serum inorganic phosphate concentration induced by calcium infusion may also be accompanied by an augmented ultrafilterable phosphate concentration and its filtered load, despite a fall in the ultrafilterability of this anion. Depending on the transport characteristics of the renal tubule (see below), the rise in filtered load of phosphate produced by calcium infusion may cause an increase, decrease, or no change in urinary phosphate excretion. Table 1 illustrates the effect of raising the serum calcium concentration from normal to high and from low to normal values by calcium infusion on the serum total and ultrafilterable phosphate concentration and its filtered load in TPTX dogs.

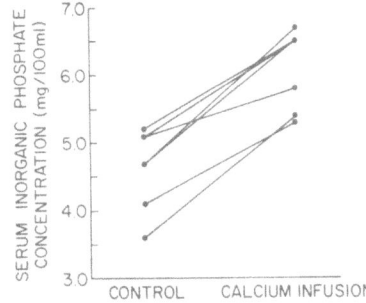

Fig. 3. Effect of calcium infusion on serum inorganic phosphate concentration in TPTX dogs.

Table 1. Effect of Calcium Infusion on Serum Inorganic Phosphate
Concentration and Its Filtered Load in TPTX Dogs[a]

	SCa (mg/100 ml)		SPO₄ (mg/100 ml)		SufPO₄ (mg/100 ml)		FufPO₄ (mg/min)	
	C	I	C	I	C	I	C	I
			A. *Hypercalcemia*					
	8.1	12.2	6.8	8.6	6.1	7.0	6.45	6.57
	8.0	10.3	7.4	8.3	6.6	7.1	3.32	3.51
	7.1	12.2	6.9	8.6	5.8	6.6	2.35	2.88
	7.3	12.9	6.9	7.6	6.3	6.5	2.55	2.74
	9.7	11.2	9.0	8.8	8.9	8.2	7.56	7.76
	7.9	11.6	6.8	8.7	6.6	8.1	2.74	3.15
	9.5	12.5	7.9	9.4	7.9	8.8	5.28	6.12
Mean	8.2	11.8	7.4	8.6	6.9	7.5	4.32	4.68
SE	±0.4	±0.3	±0.3	±0.2	±0.4	±0.3	±0.79	±0.78
p	<0.001		<0.01		NS		<0.02	
			B. *Normocalcemia*					
	6.0	8.3	7.8	8.4	7.1	7.5	2.79	3.15
	6.4	9.2	7.4	8.2	7.2	7.6	2.47	2.48
	6.4	8.8	6.5	6.6	5.8	6.0	2.80	3.63
	7.4	9.9	5.3	6.4	5.0	5.7	2.16	2.30
	4.5	9.1	8.0	9.7	8.4	9.5	3.81	4.04
	6.3	8.6	6.2	7.2	6.2	7.2	6.23	7.63
	5.4	9.4	9.5	9.4	9.5	8.8	5.48	5.67
	5.5	9.2	6.8	7.2	6.8	6.8	2.74	3.15
Mean	6.0	9.1	7.2	7.9	7.0	7.4	3.56	4.01
SE	±0.3	±0.2	±0.5	±0.4	±0.5	±0.5	±0.53	±0.64
p	<0.001		<0.01		NS		<0.05	

[a] Abbreviations: C, control; I, calcium infusion; S, serum concentration; uf, ultrafilterable; F, filtered load; NS, not significant.

2.2. Influence of Calcium on Renal Hemodynamics

The acute intravenous infusion of calcium salts to increase the serum calcium concentration to levels in excess of 15 mg/100 ml has been reported by several investigators to cause reductions in the glomerular filtration rate (GFR) (Chen and Neuman, 1955; Chomdej et al., 1977; Lavender and Pullman, 1963; Wallach and Carter, 1961). In addition, Wallach and Carter (1961) and Lavender and Pullman (1963) reported decreased renal plasma flow as measured by *para*-aminohippurate clearance, and Chomdej et al. (1977) noted decreased renal blood flow (RBF), measured by a flow meter placed around the renal artery, with extreme levels of hypercalcemia. Similar reductions of RBF by aortic obstruction or renal artery clamping have been shown to result in augmented phosphate absorption by the kidney (Cuche et al., 1976a; Puschett et al., 1972). Thus, the attainment of very high levels of serum calcium concentration by the infusion of calcium salts can alter phosphate absorption by the kidney either by reducing the filtered load of phosphate or by increasing the filtration fraction by a disproportionate decrement in the renal plasma flow, a factor known generally to increase solute reabsorption by the proximal tubule. However, Chomdej et al. (1977) noted maintenance of autoregulation by the kidney exposed to hypercalcemia and that the filtration fraction was unchanged by acute calcium infusion. Similar results were reported by Humes et al. (1978). These investigators extended observations on the mechanism of the decline in GFR with hypercalcemia and demonstrated that acute elevation of serum calcium concentration also results in a decline in the glomerular ultrafiltration coefficient (K_f), the latter decline being the major mechanism responsible for the fall in GFR with calcium infusion. In addition, they found that PTH was required as a cofactor for the reduction in GFR produced by acute hypercalcemia. Thus, these most recent results (Humes et al., 1978) would further support a role for altered renal hemodynamics as a mechanism whereby acute calcium infusion might augment phosphate absorption by the kidney.

2.3. Effect of Calcium Infusion on the Absorption of Phosphate by the Renal Tubule

2.3.1. Human Studies

One of the major controlling factors in the renal handling of phosphate is PTH; increased levels of this hormone inhibit phosphate absorption by the kidney, while its absence virtually excludes phosphate from the urine. The concentration of ionized calcium in the blood dictates the response of the parathyroid glands. Thus, the infusion of calcium would be expected to inhibit parathyroid gland secretion and, consequently, decrease the renal excretion of phosphate. In studies in humans with an intact parathyroid–renal axis, intravenous calcium infusion uniformly decreases the excretion of phosphate by the kidney (Baylor et al., 1950; Chambers et al., 1956; Hiatt and Thompson, 1957; Howard et al., 1953; Kyle et al., 1954; Nordin and Fraser, 1954). This effect of calcium infusion to diminish phosphate excretion is reversed by the administration of exogenous PTH, suggesting that calcium infusion into the parathyroid-intact subject reduces phosphate excretion by inhibiting hormone secretion (Hiatt and Thompson, 1957; Kyle et al., 1962). This fact is further supported by some studies in hypoparathyroid individuals in which calcium infusion failed to decrease phosphate excretion by the kidney (Eisenberg, 1965; Goldman and Bassett, 1954; Hiatt and Thompson, 1957; Howard et al., 1953; Nordin and Fraser, 1954).

When the influence of the parathyroid glands on renal phosphate handling is excluded, the effect of calcium on inorganic phosphate excretion is less well defined. In humans, several investigators have reported that intravenous calcium administration to both postsurgical and idiopathic hypoparathyroid patients results in an increase in both absolute and fractional phosphate excretion (Eisenberg, 1965; Goldman and Bassett, 1954; Hiatt and Thompson, 1957; Howard *et al.*, 1953; Nordin and Fraser, 1954). One possible mechanism for the increased phosphate excretion in response to elevation of the serum calcium concentration is the rise in serum inorganic phosphate concentration, and thus the filtered load of phosphate, which accompanied calcium infusion in four of the five studies cited above. However, the patients of Eisenberg (1965) did not manifest a rise in serum phosphate concentration, and thus this mechanism alone cannot account for the observed results in hypoparathyroid patients.

In contrast, two other reports, those of Kyle *et al.* (1954) and Chambers *et al.* (1956), demonstrated variable responses to calcium infusion in their hypoparathyroid patients. The former group of investigators reported a decline in phosphate excretion with calcium infusion in a case of idiopathic hypoparathyroidism in whom serum calcium concentration was elevated from 6 to 8 mg/100 ml without any changes in an already quite elevated serum phosphate concentration (9 mg/100 ml) and an increase in phosphate excretion in a case of postsurgical hypoparathyroidism in whom serum calcium concentration was increased from 4 to 8 mg/100 ml and serum phosphate concentration was unchanged. Similarly, the latter group of researchers reported a fall in phosphate excretion in seven and a rise in five hypoparathyroid patients with highly variable baseline serum phosphate concentrations and also variable increments in this parameter with calcium infusion. Nonetheless, these results remain unexplained buy may be related to disordered vitamin D metabolism, which is known to affect calcium and phosphate handling by the kidney, and/or differences in dietary phosphate balance, subjects discussed in other chapters of this book.

2.3.2. Animal Studies

In animal studies, calcium infusion has been reported to both increase and decrease phosphate excretion independent of PTH. In clearance studies performed in parathyroid ectomized (PTX) rats, Popovtzer *et al.* (1975) demonstrated that the induction of hypercalcemia blunted the phosphaturic effect of volume expansion without changes in serum phosphate concentration, suggesting that calcium infusion directly enhances phosphate absorption by the renal tubule. Amiel *et al.* (1976) also reported that elevation of serum calcium concentration within the hypocalcemic range in PTX rats augmented phosphate absorption by the proximal tubule, loop of Henle, and distal nephron without changes in serum phosphate concentration, again supporting a direct action of calcium on the renal tubule to increase phosphate absorption. Contrasting results were reported by DiBona (1971) in the rat and Edwards *et al.* (1974) in the dog. These investigators and their co-workers demonstrated reduced phosphate absorption by the proximal tubule in response to acute hypercalcemia. Since phosphate handling by the proximal tubule parallels that of sodium in given circumstances (Schneider *et al.*, 1973; Wen, 1974), such may be another mechanism whereby calcium infusion increases phosphate excretion in the absence of PTH. In support of DiBona (1971) and Edwards *et al.* (1974), Goldfarb *et al.* (1978) showed directly that acute hypercalcemia reduced fractional phosphate absorption by the proximal tubule. However, the increased delivery of phosphate from the proximal tubule demonstrated by Goldfarb *et al.* (1978) in response to acute hypercalcemia did not result in augmentation of whole-kidney fractional phosphate excretion, indicating distal absorption of this anion.

In the parathyroid-intact dog, Lavender and Pullman (1963) reported that calcium infusion into the renal artery decreased phosphate excretion to a much greater degree on the infused side. In contrast, Cuche *et al.* (1976a) showed that calcium infusion increased both absolute and fractional phosphate excretion in TPTX dogs with and without an infusion of PTH, suggesting that calcium does not exert a direct effect on the renal tubule to increase phosphate absorption, but rather decreases it. Our observations on calcium infusion into normocalcemic, acute TPTX, and hypocalcemic TPTX dogs support the findings of Cuche *et al.* (1976a). In acutely TPTX dogs, calcium infusion raises serum concentrations of total and ultrafilterable calcium and phosphate, increases the filtered load of phosphate, and increases phosphate absorption (Table 2). In TPTX dogs in which serum phosphate concentration is raised and maintained by prior phosphate infusion, calcium infusion fails to change phosphate absorption by the kidney (Table 3). These results may best be explained by recalling that phosphate absorption by the renal tubule is Tm limited (Pitts and Alexander, 1944; Thompson and Hiatt, 1957). Thus, at normal plasma phosphate levels, increasing the serum calcium concentration, which, in turn, increases serum phosphate concentration and filtered load, results in augmented phosphate absorption due to a mechanism operating below its transport capacity. Increasing phosphate absorption by infusing phosphate so as to saturate the absorptive mechanism results in no change in phosphate absorption with calcium infusion.

Table 2. Effect of Calcium Infusion on Renal Absorption of Phosphate at Endogenous Serum Phosphate Concentrations in TPTX Dogs[a]

SCa (mg/100 ml)		SPO$_4$ (mg/100 ml)		SufPO$_4$ (mg/100 ml)		FufPO$_4$ (mg/min)		RufPO$_4$ (mg/min)		GFR (ml/min)	
C	I	C	I	C	I	C	I	C	I	C	I
8.3	11.7	4.7	6.7	4.7	6.5	3.36	4.21	3.35	4.10	71.4	65.1
9.5	12.8	5.1	5.8	5.0	5.5	3.14	3.68	2.77	3.43	63.4	67.5
8.8	13.1	4.7	6.5	4.4	5.9	3.87	5.69	3.84	5.55	87.9	96.4
9.2	11.7	4.1	5.3	4.3	5.3	2.78	2.90	2.77	2.64	65.2	56.4
8.7	11.5	5.1	6.5	5.2	6.2	3.38	3.92	3.37	3.90	65.4	63.0
8.8	11.7	5.2	6.5	4.8	5.6	1.87	2.42	1.73	2.11	39.1	43.0
7.8	11.2	3.6	5.4	3.5	4.9	1.66	2.47	1.66	2.41	48.7	50.3
Mean 8.7	11.9	4.6	6.1	4.6	5.7	2.86	3.61	2.78	3.45	63.0	63.1
SE ±0.2	±0.3	±0.2	±0.2	±0.2	±0.02	±0.31	±0.44	±0.31	±0.45	±5.9	±6.4
p <0.001		<0.001		<0.001		<0.01		<0.02		NS	

[a] Abbreviations: C, control; I, calcium infusion; S, serum concentration; uf, ultrafilterable; F, filtered load; R, reabsorbed; NS, not significant.

Table 3. Effect of Calcium Infusion on Renal Absorption of Phosphate during Phosphate Infusion in TPTX Dogs[a]

	SCa (mg/100 ml)		SPO$_4$ (mg/100 ml)		SufPO$_4$ (mg/100 ml)		FufPO$_4$ (mg/min)		RufPO$_4$ (mg/min)		GFR (ml/min)	
	C	I	C	I	C	I	C	I	C	I	C	I
	8.1	12.2	6.8	8.6	6.1	7.0	6.45	6.57	3.54	4.06	105.8	93.2
	8.0	10.3	7.4	8.3	6.6	7.1	3.32	3.51	2.58	2.50	50.4	49.8
	7.1	12.2	6.9	8.6	5.8	6.6	2.35	2.88	1.82	1.77	40.8	45.5
	7.3	12.9	6.9	7.6	6.3	6.5	2.55	2.74	1.61	1.69	40.5	42.2
	9.7	11.2	9.0	8.8	8.9	8.2	7.56	7.76	6.57	6.49	85.4	95.0
	7.9	11.6	6.8	8.7	6.6	8.1	2.74	3.15	2.50	2.71	41.9	39.1
	9.5	12.5	7.9	9.4	7.9	8.8	5.28	6.12	5.22	6.10	67.2	72.1
Mean	8.2	11.8	7.4	8.6	6.9	7.5	4.32	4.68	3.41	3.62	61.7	62.4
SE	±0.4	±0.3	±0.3	±0.2	±0.4	±0.3	±0.79	±0.78	±0.70	±0.75	±9.7	±9.1
p	<0.001		<0.01		NS		<0.02		NS		NS	

[a] Abbreviations: C, control; I, calcium infusion; S, serum concentration; uf, ultrafilterable; F, filtered load; R, reabsorbed; NS, not significant.

2.4. Studies during Hypocalcemia

Further evidence for a direct effect of calcium on the transport of phosphate by the renal tubule has been gleaned from studies in which serum calcium concentration was acutely reduced by the infusion of either EDTA or ethylene(bis)oxyethylene-nitrilotetraacetate (EGTA). Estep *et al.* (1965) reported that acute hypocalcemia induced by EDTA infusion increased phosphate clearance in normal human subjects but decreased it in 9 of 11 hyperparathyroid and 5 hypoparathyroid patients. They speculated that calcium and PTH have opposing effects on the kidney with respect to phosphate handling and that the net result of a change in serum calcium concentration depended upon the relative predominance of either of these vectors in a given set of clinical or experimental conditions. In TPTX rats, Rasmussen *et al.* (1967) reported that EGTA, a specific chelator of calcium, resulted in phosphaturia solely as a result of hypocalcemia. In contrast, Cuche *et al.* (1976b) demonstrated that with control of PTH by a constant infusion into TPTX dogs, EDTA failed to elicit a phosphaturia, but when the chelator was given to parathyroid-intact animals, increased fractional phosphate excretion resulted. Unpublished observations from our laboratory demonstrate that EGTA infusion into TPTX dogs causes an increase in fractional phosphate excretion, suggesting that changes in serum calcium concentration per se exert a direct effect on renal phosphate handling (Table 4.)

2.5. Summary of Physiologic Studies

To summarize, it is clear that acute calcium infusion increases serum phosphate concentration, diminishes its filterability, and effects changes in renal hemodynamics, but the delineation of a direct action upon the renal tubule to augment phosphate absorption and reduce urinary phosphate excretion must await further investigation into the relative roles of other modulators of renal phosphate handling such as vitamin D sterols, calcitonin, and dietary phosphate balance.

3. PATHOLOGIC STUDIES

3.1. Introduction

Certain human disorders are characterized by or manifest abnormalities in phosphate homeostasis. Disordered calcium metabolism is frequently but not unequivocally an accompanying feature. Because of the association of calcium with phosphate in bone metabolism and its ex-

Table 4. Effects of EGTA in TPTX Dogs[a]

Experimental period	GFR (ml/min)	RBF (ml/min)	C_{PO_4}/GFR (%)	SCa (mg/100 ml)	$SiCa^{2+}$ (mg/100 ml)	SPO_4 (mg/100 ml)
C						
Mean	31.0	155	12.1	7.8	2.9	5.4
SE	±4.8	±31	±3.2	±0.5	±0.3	±0.9
E						
Mean	30.3	138	18.7	6.5	2.2	5.1
SE	±5.3	±40	±3.9	±0.6	±0.3	±0.7
p	NS	NS	<0.01	<0.005	<0.005	NS

[a] Abbreviations: S, serum concentration; iCa^{2+}, ionized calcium; C_{PO_4}/GFR, fractional excretion; C, control; E, EGTA; NS, not significant.

panding role in cellular and subcellular function, the effects of calcium administration on phosphate homeostasis have been explored in efforts to discover the etiology of human diseases in which abnormalities in the metabolism of this anion are present. Having discussed the physiologic influence of calcium, we will look at the effects of calcium in conditions characterized by abnormal renal phosphate handling.

3.2. Renal Glomerular Insufficiency

The effect of renal insufficiency on the renal handling of phosphate and the role of serum calcium in these disturbances are discussed in detail by Massry and Brautbar in Chapter 12.

3.3. Primary Hyperparathyroidism

Primary hyperparathyroidism is a disorder characterized by autonomous secretion of PTH by adenomatous or hyperplastic gland(s) without regard for the serum ionized calcium concentration. The usual criteria by which the clinical diagnosis can be made are based on the known actions of PTH: Hypercalcemia, hypophosphatemia, and increased phosphate excretion in the urine with a decrease in the tubular absorption of phosphate in the absence of secondary causes of hyperparathyroidism. However, these biochemical parameters are not always readily apparent, prompting investigators to search for more definitive criteria to confirm the diagnosis of primary hyperparathyroidism prior to surgical exploration of the neck. The studies of Pronove and Bartter (1961) demonstrated that phosphate excretion in normal subjects and patients with primary hyperparathyroidism is dependent upon phosphate intake and may be low, average, or high in either group (Fig. 4). Since calcium infusion into parathyroid-intact subjects is known to decrease phosphate excretion by inhibiting PTH secretion, this test has been proposed as a method of distinguishing primary from secondary hyperparathyroidism by Kyle *et al.* (1962). In primary hyperparathyroidism, calcium infusion would not affect the autonomous secretion by the glands, and thus no effect on phosphate excretion woold be discerned. But, as with most diagnostic tests, false-negative responses have been reported (McGeown, 1963; Mosekilde and Anderson, 1973; Pronove and Bartter, 1961). Pronove and Bartter (1961) showed that calcium infusion into normal subjects causes a fall in phosphate excretion followed by a rebound on the day following the infusion, with phosphate excretion higher than on the control days before infusion, whereas patients with hyperparathyroidism exhibit no such rebound (Fig. 5). These investigators emphasized that during testing for hyperparathyroidism, the effect of calcium infusion on phosphate excretion must there-

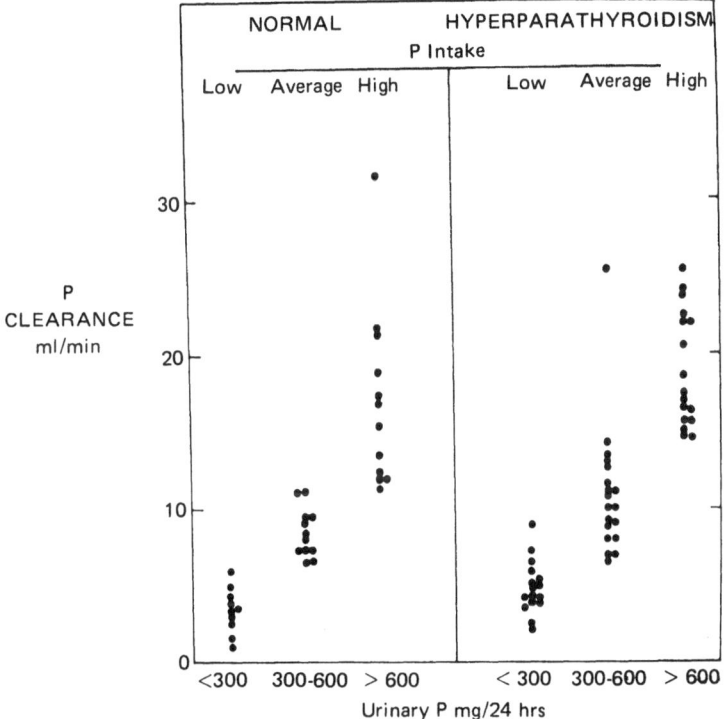

Fig. 4. Effect of low, average, and high phosphate (P) intake on P clearance in 16 normal subjects and in 20 patients with hyperparathyroidism. The data are plotted according to 24-hr urinary P excretion. (From Pronove and Bartter, 1961. Reprinted with permission.)

fore include determinations of phosphate excretion before, the day of, and the day after calcium infusion. Potts *et al.* (1971) reported that serum immunoreactive PTH fell in some patients with proven primary hyper-parathyroidism in response to calcium infusion. Reiss and Canterbury (1971) demonstrated that serum immunoreactive PTH levels declined in response to calcium infusion in patients with chief-cell hyperplasia as the cause of hyperparathyroidism, but hormone concentrations were un-changed with calcium infusion into those patients with parathyroid ad-enoma(ta). The latter findings may explain the earlier reports of a false-negative calcium infusion test with respect to phosphate excretion in pa-tients with surgically proven hyperparathyroidism, those who exhibited a decline in phosphate excretion with calcium infusion having chief-cell hyperplasia, whereas those without a decline in phosphate excretion hav-ing autonomous adenoma(ta).

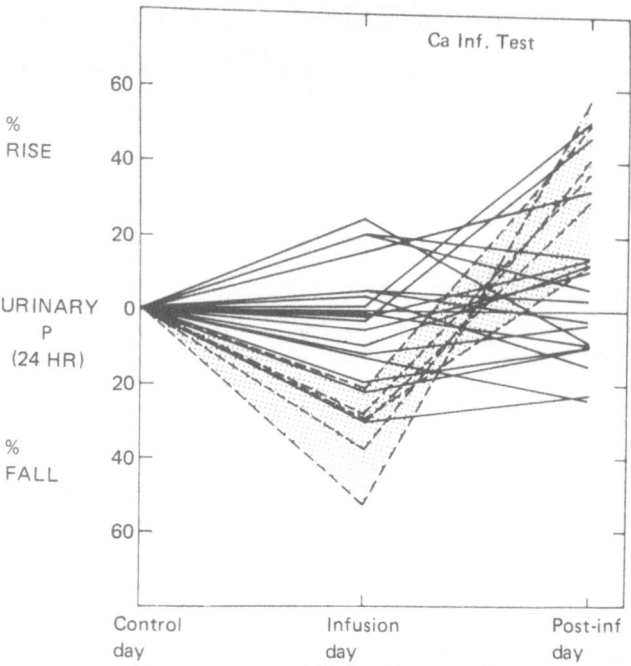

Fig. 5. Effect of calcium infusion (15 mg/kg) on the 24-hr urinary phosphate (P) excretion in 6 normal subjects and in 18 patients with hyperparathyroidism. The data from the infusion and postinfusion days are plotted as percentage deviation from the control day. Dashed lines indicate normal persons; continuous lines indicate hyperparathyroid patients. (From Pronove and Bartter, 1961. Reprinted with permission.)

3.4. Vitamin-D-Resistant Rickets with Hypophosphatemia

This disease is discussed in detail in Chapter 13. Vitamin-D-resistant rickets is a genetic disorder characterized by normocalcemia, hypophosphatemia with inappropriately high phosphate excretion, and rickets resistant to physiological doses of vitamin D. The bone disease, however, may respond to high doses of vitamin D (Winters *et al.*, 1958). The pathogenesis of this disorder is not clear, but several hypotheses have been advanced, including defective intestinal calcium absorption with seconary hyperparathyroidism and a primary defect in phosphate absorption by the renal tubule. In support of the former argument, several investigators have reported an increased serum immunoreactive PTH concentration in untreated patients (Hahn *et al.*, 1975; Lewy *et al.*, 1972; Reitz and Weinstein, 1973) and an increase in renal phosphate absorption with calcium infusion into these patients as evidence for hypersecretion of PTH by the parathyroid glands (Falls *et al.*, 1968; Field and Reiss, 1960; Lamy *et al.*, 1958) (Fig. 6). Although phosphate absorption by the kidney increased in response to calcium infusion into these patients, it did not return to normal in all, suggesting that other factors may be playing a role in the inappropriately high phosphate excretion (Field and Reiss, 1960). Arnaud *et al.* (1971) measured serum immunoreactive PTH in male patients with vitamin-D-resistant rickets and found the concentrations to be in the normal range as compared to a group of control subjects. Only when dietary phosphate was increased were serum PTH levels increased in their patients (Fig. 7). They therefore concluded that a defect in phosphate absorption by the renal tubule was the primary event and that secondary hyperparathyroidism was not the etiology of the hypophosphatemia and elevated phosphate excretion. In support of a primary defect involving the renal tubule, Glorieux and Scriver (1972) reported that calcium infusion enhanced phosphate absorption in patients with D-resistant rickets, but an infusion of bovine PTH did not increase phosphate excretion, suggesting two components of phosphate transport by the renal tubule. Since their patients were already excreting phosphate at a maximum rate at endogenous phosphate levels and did not respond to exogenous PTH, they concluded that the primary defect in X-linked hypophosphatemia was the loss of a PTH-sensitive component of phosphate transport but that the calcium-sensitive phosphate transport system along the nephron was intact. These results, they reasoned, would account for the effect of large doses of vitamin D via increasing positive calcium balance to augment phosphate absorption by the calcium-sensitive transport system. The studies of Popovtzer *et al.* (1975) and Amiel *et al.* (1976) demonstrating increased phosphate absorption in response to calcium infusion into rats would lend support to the hypothesis of Glorieux and Scriver (1972).

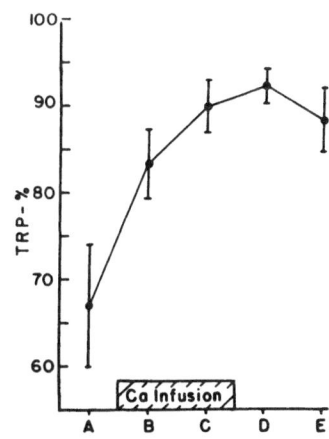

Fig. 6. Effect of calcium infusion on tubular phosphate reabsorption (TRP) in 8 rachitic subjects (mean ± SE). "A" was a 4-hr control period; all other clearance periods extended over 2 hr; 15 mg of calcium/kg of body weight was infused at a constant rate over 4 hr. (From Field and Reiss, 1960. Reprinted with permission.)

In contrast, Short *et al.* (1976) demonstrated an exaggerated phosphaturic response to exogenous PTH in patients with familial X-linked hypophosphatemia when their serum calcium concentrations were normalized by prior calcium infusion. These investigators concluded, therefore, that the expression of this disorder, that is, hypophosphatemia and phosphaturia, requires the presence of PTH and is manifest at normal serum PTH concentrations. Lewy *et al.* (1972) also suggested that the renal defect in D-resistant rickets might involve increased sensitivity of the tubule to the phosphaturic effect of PTH.

3.5. Hypoparathyroidism

Hypoparathyroidism is characterized by absence of hormone secretion by the parathyroid glands, the etiology of which is due to either idiopathic hypofunction of the glands or prior surgery for hyperparathyroidism or thyroid disorders. Clinically, hypocalcemia, hyperphosphatemia, and low urinary phosphate excretion are found. This clinical situation offers a unique opportunity to study the effects of calcium in humans in the absence of PTH. Thompson and Hiatt (1957) studied one

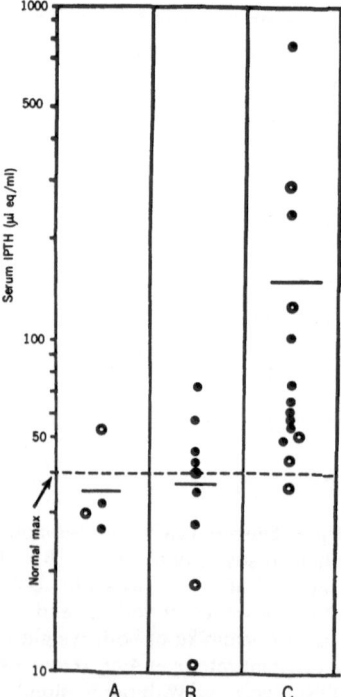

Fig. 7. Serum PTH in patients with X-linked hypophosphatemic rickets. Column A, no treatment; column B, treatment with large doses of vitamin D_2 alone (about 100,000 U/day); column C, treatment with phosphate supplement by mouth (3 g/day as orthophosphate) and vitamin D_2 (up to 100,000 U/day). ○, female patients; ●, male patients. All patients have bone disease. (From Arnaud et al., 1971. Copyright 1971 by the American Association for the Advancement of Science. Reprinted with permission.)

patient with postthyroidectomy hypoparathyroidism in whom the Tm for phosphate was measured during phosphate infusion on varying oral calcium intakes. They found that the Tm for phosphate increased on a low-phosphate diet when calcium intake was increased. Hiatt and Thompson (1957) studied the response of another group of patients with hypoparathyroidism to acute calcium infusion during ingestion of a low-calcium, low-phosphate diet. Phosphate excretion increased in all, but there was also an increase in phosphate absorption by the kidney, most likely as a result of the increase in filtered load of phosphate as determined by these investigators. When some of their hypoparathyroid patients were given exogenous PTH prior to and on the day of the calcium infusion, an increase in phosphate excretion was still observed (Hiatt and Thompson, 1957). In this part of the study, however, only two of four patients given PTH experienced a rise in serum phosphate concentration, suggesting that raising the serum calcium concentration directly augmented phosphate excretion by the renal tubule independent of changes in the filtered load. In support of this argument are the studies of Eisenberg (1965) in which raising the serum calcium concentration from 6 to 12 mg/100 ml by calcium infusion increased phosphate excretion in six hypoparathyroid patients (five postsurgical and one idiopathic) with a slight fall in serum phosphate concentration. Other investigators have also reported an increase in phosphate excretion with calcium infusion into hypoparathyroid patients with minimal or no change in serum phosphate concentration (Goldman and Bassett, 1954; Howard et al., 1953; Kyle et al., 1954; Nordin and Fraser, 1954). Since calcitonin has been reported to be hypophosphatemic and phosphaturic in hypoparathyroid patients (Ardaillou et al., 1969; Singer et al., 1969), a role for this hormone in increasing phosphate excretion during calcium infusion into hypoparathyroid patients has not been ruled out. In contrast, Chambers et al. (1956) reported that calcium infusion decreased phosphate excretion in seven of twelve patients with hypoparathyroidism.

In summary, then, taken with the studies cited above on the effect of calcium on phosphate excretion in TPTX animals, studies in hypoparathyroid humans do not clear the issue as to whether calcium influences the renal tubule directly to either increase or decrease phosphate excretion.

4. REFERENCES

Amiel, C., Küntziger, H., Couette, S., Coureau, C., and Bergounioux, N., 1976, Evidence for a parathyroid hormone-independent calcium modulation of phosphate transport along the nephron, J. Clin. Invest. 57:256.
Anderson, J. B. B., and Talmage, R. V., 1973, The effect of calcium infusion and calcitonin

on plasma phosphate in sham-operated and thyroparathyroidectomized dogs, *Endocrinology* **93**:1222.

Ardaillou, R., Fillastre, J. P., Milhaud, G., Rousselet, F., Delaunay, F., and Richet, G., 1969, Renal excretion of phosphate, calcium and sodium during and after a prolonged thyrocalcitonin infusion in man, *Proc. Soc. Exp. Biol. Med.* **131**:56.

Arnaud, C., Glorieux, F., and Scriver, C., 1971, Serum parathyroid hormone in X-linked hypophosphatemia, *Science* **173**:845.

Baylor, C. H., Van Alstine, H. E. Keutman, E. H., and Bassett, S. H., 1950, The fate of intravenously administered calcium. Effect on urinary calcium and phosphorus, fecal calcium and calcium–phosphorus balance, *J. Clin. Invest.* **29**:1167.

Chambers, E. L., Jr., Gordan, G. S., Goldman, L., and Reifenstein, E. C., 1956, Tests for hyperparathyroidism: Tubular reabsorption of phosphate, phosphate deprivation, and calcium infusion, *J. Clin. Endocrinol. Metab.* **16**:1507.

Chen, P. S., Jr., and Neuman, W. F., 1955, Renal excretion of calcium by the dog, *Am. J. Physio.* **180**:623.

Chomdej, B., Bell, P. D., and Navar, L. G., 1977, Renal hemodynamics and autoregulatory responses to acute hypercalcemia, *Am. J. Physiol.* **232**:490.

Cuche, J. L., Ott, C. E., Marchand, G. R., Diaz-Buxo, J. A., and Knox, F. G., 1976a, Intrarenal calcium in phosphate handling, *Am. J. Physiol.* **230**:790.

Cuche, J. L., Ott, C. E., Marchand, G. R., and Knox, F. G., 1976b, Lack of effect of hypocalcemia on renal phosphate handling, *J. Lab. Clin. Med.* **88**:271.

DiBona, G. F., 1971, Effect of hypercalcemia on renal tubular sodium handling in the rat, *Am. J. Physiol.* **220**:49.

Edwards, B. R., Sutton, R. A. L., and Dirks, J. H., 1974, Effect of calcium infusion on renal tubular reabsorption in the dog, *Am. J. Physiol.* **227**:13.

Eisenberg, E., 1965, Effects of serum calcium level and parathyroid extracts on phosphate and calcium excretion in hypoparathyroid patients, *J. Clin. Invest.* **44**:942.

Estep, H. L., Gardner, C. T., Jr., Taylor, J. P., Minott, A., and Tucker, H. St.G., Jr., 1965, Phosphate excretion patterns following intravenous injection of ethylenediaminetetraacetate (EDTA), *J. Clin. Endocrinol. Metab.* **25**:1385.

Falls, W. F., Jr., Carter, N. W., Rector, F. C., Jr., and Seldin, D. W., 1968, Familial vitamin D-resistant rickets, *Ann. Intern. Med.* **68**:553.

Field, M. H., and Reiss, E., 1960, Vitamin D-resistant rickets: The effect of calcium infusion on phosphate reabsorption, *J. Clin. Invest.* **39**:1807.

Glorieux, F., and Scriver, C. R., 1972, Loss of a parathyroid hormone-sensitive component of phosphate transport in X-linked hypophosphatemia, *Science* **175**:997.

Goldfarb, S., Bosanac, P., Goldberg, M., and Agus, Z. S., 1978, Effects of calcium on renal tubular phosphate reabsorption, *Am. J. Physiol.* **234**:22.

Goldman, R., and Bassett, S. H., 1954, Effect of intravenous calcium gluconate upon the excretion of calcium and phosphorus in patients with idiopathic hypoparathyroidism, *J. Clin. Endocrinol. Metab.* **14**:278.

Grollman, A., 1927, The condition of the inorganic phosphorus of the blood with special reference to the calcium concentration, *J. Biol. Chem.* **72**:565.

Hahn, T. J., Scharp, C. R., Halstead, L. R., Haddad, J. G., Karl, D. M., and Avioli, L. V., 1975, Parathyroid hormone status and renal responsiveness in familial hypophosphatemic rickets, *J. Clin. Endocrinol. Metab.* **41**:926.

Hausmann, E., 1970, Change in plasma phosphate concentration on infusion of calcium gluconate or Na_2EDTA, *Proc. Soc. Exp. Biol. Med.* **134**:182.

Hiatt, H. H., and Thompson, D. D., 1957, Some effects of intravenously administered calcium on inorganic phosphate metabolism, *J. Clin. Invest.* **36**:573.

Hopkins, T., Howard, J. E., and Eisenberg, E., 1952, Ultrafiltration studies on calcium and phosphorus in human serum, *Bull. Johns Hopkins Hosp.* **91**:1.

Howard, J. E., Hopkins, T. R., and Connor, T. B., 1953, On certain physiologic responses to intravenous injection of calcium salts into normal, hyperparathyroid and hypoparathyroid persons, *J. Clin. Endocrinol. Metab.* **13**:1.

Humes, H. D., Ichikawa, I., Troy, J. L., and Brenner, B. M., 1978, Evidence for a parathyroid hormone dependent influence of calcium on the glomerular ultrafiltration coefficient, *J. Clin. Invest.* **61**:32.

Kalu, D. N., Miyasaki, B. C., and Foster, G. V., 1974, Effects of ethylenediaminetetraacetate (EDTA) on urinary excretion of hydroxyproline, calcium, and phosphorus in the rat, *Calcif. Tissue Res.* **16**:1.

Kyle, L. H., Schaaf, M., and Erdman, L. A., 1954, The metabolic effects of intravenous administration of calcium, *J. Lab. Clin. Med.* **43**:123.

Kyle, L. H., Canary, J. J., Mintz, D. H., and de Leon, A., 1962, Inhibitory effects of induced hypercalcemia on secretion of parathyroid hormone, *J. Clin. Endocrinol. Metab.* **22**:52.

Lamy, M., Royer, P., Frézal, J., and Lestradet, H., 1958, Le rachitisme vitamine-résistant familial hypophosphatémique primitif, *Arch. Fr. Pédiatr.* **15**:1.

Lavender, A. R., and Pullman, T. N., 1963, Changes in inorganic phosphate excretion induced by renal arterial infusion of calcium, *Am. J. Physiol.* **205**:1025.

Le Grimellec, C., Poujeol, P., and de Rouffignac, C., 1975, ^{3}H-inulin and electrolyte concentrations in Bowman's capsule in rat kidney. Comparison with artificial ultrafiltration, *Pflügers Arch.* **354**:117.

Lewy, J. E., Cabana, E. C., Repetto, H. A., Canterbury, J. M., and Reiss, E., 1972, Serum parathyroid hormone in hypophosphatemic vitamin D-resistant rickets, *J. Pediatr.* **81**:294.

McGeown, M. G., 1963, Tests of parathyroid function in the human subject, in: *Hormones and the Kidney* (P. C. Williams, ed.), pp. 149–163, Academic Press, New York.

Mosekilde, L., and Andersen, P., 1973, The calcium infusion test in primary hyperparathyroidism, *Acta. Med. Scand.* **193**:331.

Nordin, B. E. C., and Fraser, R., 1954, The effect of intravenous calcium on phosphate excretion, *Clin. Sci.* **13**:477.

Pitts, R. F., and Alexander, R. S., 1944, The renal reabsorptive mechanism for inorganic phosphate in normal and acidotic dogs, *Am. J. Physiol.* **142**:648.

Popovtzer, M. M., Robinette, J. B., McDonald, K. M., and Kuruvila, C. K., 1975, Effect of Ca^{++} on renal handling of PO$_4^{3-}$: Evidence for two reabsorptive mechanisms, *Am. J. Physiol.* **229**:901.

Potts, J. J., Jr., Murray, T. M., Peacock, M., Niall, H. D., Tregear, G. W., Keutmann, H. T., Powell, D., and Deftos, L. J., 1971, Parathyroid hormone: Sequence, synthesis, immunoassay studies, *Am. J. Med.* **50**:639.

Pronove, P., and Bartter, F. C., 1961, Diagnosis of hyperparathyroidism, *Metabolism* **10**:349.

Puschett, J. B., Agus, Z. S., Senesky, D., and Goldberg, M., 1972, Effects of saline loading and aortic obstruction on proximal phosphate transport, *Am. J. Physiol.* **223**:851.

Rasmussen, H., Anast, C., and Arnaud, C., 1967, Thyrocalcitonin, EGTA, and urinary electrolyte excretion, *J. Clin. Invest.* **46**:746.

Reiss, E., and Canterbury, J. M., 1971, Genesis of hyperparathyroidism, *Am. J. Med.* **50**:679.

Reitz, R. E., and Weinstein, R. L., 1973, Parathyroid hormone secretion in familial vitamin D-resistant rickets, *N. Engl. J. Med.* **289**:941.

Salvesen, H. A., Hastings, A. B., and McIntosh, J. F., 1924, The effect of the administration of calcium salts on the inorganic composition of the blood, *J. Biol. Chem.* **60**:327.

Schneider, E. G., Strandhoy, J. W., Willis, L. R., and Knox, F. G., 1973, Relationship between proximal sodium reabsorption and excretion of calcium, magnesium, and phosphate, *Kidney Int.* **4**:369.

Short, E., Morris, R. C., Jr., Sebastian, A., and Spencer, M., 1976, Exaggerated phosphaturic response to circulating parathyroid hormone in patients with familial X-linked hypophosphatemic rickets, *J. Clin. Invest.* **58**:152.

Singer, F. R., Woodhouse, N. J. Y., Parkinson, D. K., and Joplin, G. F., 1969, Some acute effects of administered porcine calcitonin in man, *Clin. Sci.* **37**:181.

Thompson, D. D., and Hiatt, H. H., 1957, Renal reabsorption of phosphate in normal human subjects and in patients with parathyroid disease, *J. Clin. Invest.* **36**:550.

Wallach, S., and Carter, A. C., 1961, Metabolic and renal effects of acute hypercalcemia in dogs, *Am. J. Physiol.* **200**:359.

Wen, S.-F., 1974, Micropuncture studies of phosphate transport in the proximal tubule of the dog, *J. Clin. Invest.* **53**:143.

Winters, R. W., Graham, J. B., Williams, T. F., McFalls, V. W., and Burnett, C. H., 1958, A genetic study of familial hypophosphatemia and vitamin D resistant rickets with a review of the literature, *Medicine* **37**:97.

Renal Handling of Phosphate in Renal Failure

SHAUL G. MASSRY and NACHMAN BRAUTBAR

1. INTRODUCTION

The renal handling of phosphate in patients with renal failure has received considerable attention. Goldman and Bassett (1954) found that tubular reabsorption of phosphate (TRP) decreases as renal failure progresses. They concluded that this phenomenon is responsible for the maintenance of the concentration of inorganic phosphorus in blood until the glomerular filtration rate (GFR) decreases to 20–30% of normal. Similar observations have been reported by Better et al. (1967), Kleeman et al. (1967), Coburn et al. (1969), and Popovtzer et al. (1970b) (Fig. 1).

2. FACTORS AFFECTING RENAL HANDLING OF PHOSPHATE IN RENAL FAILURE

Since parathyroid hormone (PTH) decreases the renal TRP (Agus et al., 1971; Bernstein et al., 1962; Hiatt and Thompson, 1957), and since elevation in the blood levels of PTH occurs early in the course of renal failure (Arnaud, 1973; Reiss et al., 1968), it was reasonable to suggest that the alteration in the renal handling of phosphate in renal failure is largely dependent on the state of secondary hyperparathyroidism. Indeed, Slatopolsky et al. (1966, 1968) have demonstrated the importance of the elevated blood levels of PTH in increasing the fractional excretion of phosphate in dogs and humans with renal failure. They showed that the suppression of parathyroid gland activity by prolonged elevation of serum calcium (Slatopolsky et al., 1968) or removal of the parathyroid glands

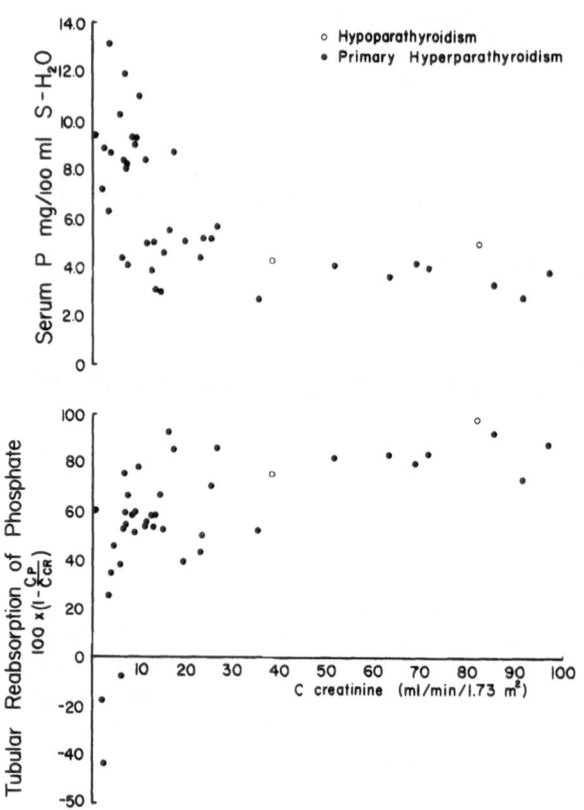

Fig. 1. The relationship between the degree of renal insufficiency and the concentration of serum phosphorus (upper panel) and TRP (lower panel). Each data point represents one patient. (From Kleeman et al., 1967. Reprinted with permission.)

reversed the augmented fractional excretion of phosphate (Slatopolsky et al., 1972).

The effect of PTH on renal handling of phosphate appears to be critical for the maintenance of body phosphate homeostasis and normal concentrations of serum phosphorus during the progressive decline of GFR from normal to 25% of normal. However, in advanced renal failure, the number of functioning nephrons is small, and the effect of PTH on the TRP by the nephron is maximal, and, therefore, further elevation in blood levels of PTH is no longer effective in maintaining body phosphate balance. Hyperphosphatemia then ensues.

Indeed, Goldman and Bassett (1954) and Slatopolsky et al. (1968) reported that the administration of parathyroid extract did not affect TRP in patients with advanced renal failure. Their data are consistent with either a refractory state of the renal tubules to PTH or the existence of a maximal phosphaturic effect on the tubule due to preexisting markedly elevated levels of PTH in such patients. Massry *et al.* (1973) evaluated the renal handling of phosphate during the infusion of parathyroid extract into a large number of patients with varying degrees of renal failure (Fig. 2). In patients with moderate and advanced renal failure, fractional excretion of phosphate $[(C_{PO_4}/C_{cr}) \times 100]$ was significantly greater than in normals. Only in normal subjects and in patients with moderate renal failure (GFR 87–27 ml/min) did $(C_{PO_4}/C_{cr}) \times 100$ increase significantly during the infusion of parathyroid extract. In patients with advanced renal failure $(C_{PO_4}/C_{cr}) \times 100$ increased in only 7 of 22 patients; these observations are in agreement with those of Goldman and Bassett (1954) and Slatopolsky *et al.* (1968). Levels of endogenous PTH show considerable variation among individual patients with chronic renal failure (Massry *et al.*, 1972), and it is possible that the patients who had a phosphaturic

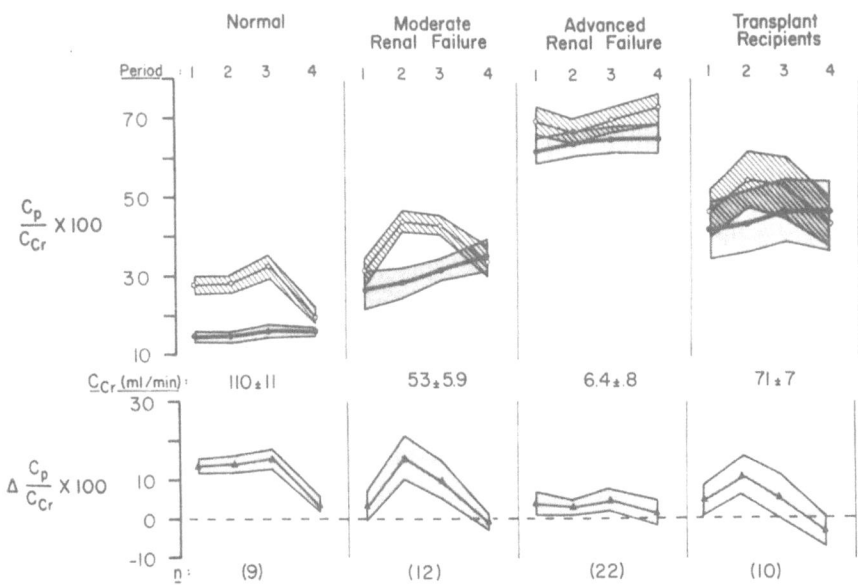

Fig. 2. The percentages of filtered phosphate excreted in the urine $[(C_p/C_{Cr}) \times 100]$ on the control day (solid circles and shaded areas) and the day of infusion of parathyroid extract (open circles and crosshatched areas) are depicted in the upper panel. The lower panel (solid triangles) shows the changes in $(C_p/C_{Cr}) \times 100$ produced by the infusion. Data are shown as mean ± SE. Periods 1, 2, and 3 represent successive urine collections at 4-hr intervals from 8 A.M. to 8 P.M. and period 4, collection from 8 P.M. to 8 A.M. the next morning. C_{Cr} indicates endogenous creatinine clearance. (From Massry *et al.*, 1973. Reprinted with permission.)

response to exogenous parathyroid extract were those with lower levels of endogenous hormone.

Since a rise in serum calcium inhibits the activity of the parathyroid glands, the effects of acute and chronic elevation in serum calcium on tubular transport of phosphate were studied. Slatopolsky *et al.* (1968) found that an increase in the concentration of blood calcium produced by calcium supplementation and vitamin D administration and sustained for two to three weeks was associated with a fall in $(C_{PO_4}/C_{cr}) \times 100$ toward normal. In four patients who did not display a decrease in $(C_{PO_4}/C_{cr}) \times 100$, the parathyroid glands were very large, and $(C_{PO_4}/C_{cr}) \times 100$ fell after parathyroidectomy (PTX). Massry *et al.* (1968) also observed three uremic patients with severe hyperparathyroidism in whom calcium infusion failed to suppress $(C_{PO_4}/C_{cr}) \times 100$ before subtotal PTX; however, when the test was repeated after surgery, reduction of $(C_{PO_4}/C_{cr}) \times 100$ occurred in all three patients. The weight of the parathyroid glands of these patients ranged between 2.0 and 4.5 g.

Popovtzer *et al.* (1970a) studied the effect of calcium infusion on TRP in normal subjects and in patients with various degrees of renal failure (Fig. 3). They found that in patients with mild renal failure ($C_{cr} > 40$ ml/min), $(C_{PO_4}/C_{cr}) \times 100$ decreased by 50–90% during calcium infusion, and this change was similar to that seen in normal subjects. In contrast, calcium infusion failed to produce a significant decrease in $(C_{PO_4}/C_{cr}) \times 100$ in patients with advanced renal failure ($C_{cr} < 8$ ml/min). These observations and those of Slatopolsky *et al.* (1968) and Massry *et al.* (1969) suggest that the effect of a rise in serum calcium on $(C_{PO_4}/C_{cr}) \times 100$ in patients with renal failure is influenced by the size of the parathyroid glands and the degree of renal failure and, as such, is related to the magnitude of the elevation in blood levels of PTH.

Reiss *et al.* (1968), Genuth *et al.* (1970), and Massry *et al.* (1972) found that acute hypercalcemia produced by calcium infusion lowered the blood levels of PTH, but in almost all patients, all levels of the hormone were still above normal (Fig. 4). The data of Massry *et al.* (1972) also demonstrated that the blood levels of PTH after a calcium infusion are a function of the hormone levels before the infusion (Fig. 5). It is evident, therefore, that those patients in whom the blood levels of PTH are very high would still have hormone levels adequate to maintain maximal $(C_{PO_4}/C_{cr}) \times 100$ after calcium infusion and, hence, the failure of hypercalcemia to reduce $(C_{PO_4}/C_{cr}) \times 100$. The data of Gill *et al.* (1969) provide further support for this notion. They measured blood levels of PTH and $(C_{PO_4}/C_{cr}) \times 100$ before and during calcium infusion. Although the blood levels of PTH were reduced, they were still high enough to maintain the high $(C_{PO_4}/C_{cr}) \times 100$.

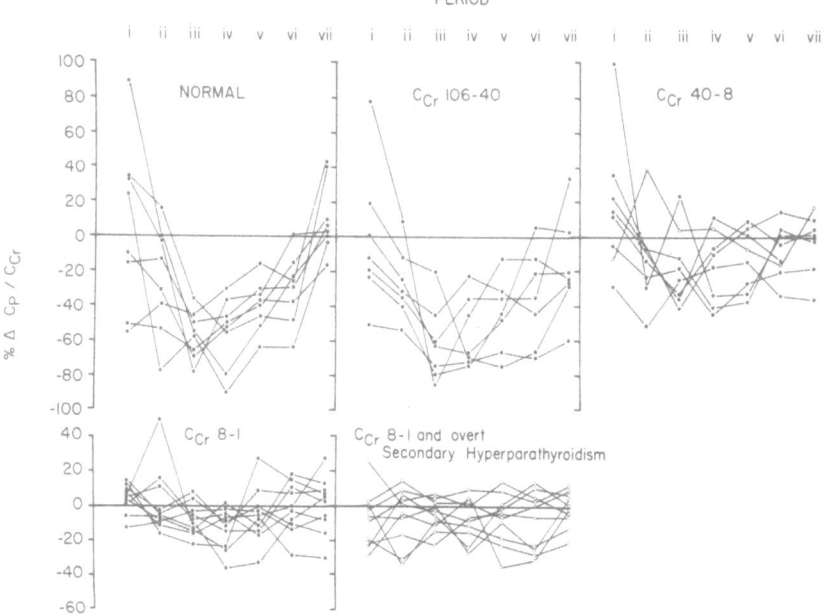

Fig. 3. The changes in fractional excretion of phosphorus observed after calcium infusion into both normal subjects and patients with renal failure. The data are expressed as percentage change from the control value measured on the day preceding the infusion. C_{Cr}, endogenous creatinine clearance; C_P/C_{Cr}, fractional excretion of phosphorus; $\%\Delta C_P/C_{Cr}$, (preinfusion C_P/C_{Cr} − postinfusion C_P/C_{Cr})/preinfusion C_P/C_{Cr}. The period numbers indicate the times of urine collection after the calcium infusion: i, between 8 P.M. and midnight (calcium infusion is given during this period); ii, between midnight and 8 A.M.; iii, between 8 A.M. and noon; iv, between noon and 4 P.M.; v, between 4 P.M. and 8 P.M.; vi, between 8 P.M. and midnight (20 hr after infusion); vii, between midnight and 8 A.M. (28 hr after infusion). (From Popovtzer et al., 1970a. Reprinted with permission.)

Bank et al. (1978) utilized micropuncture techniques to evaluate the renal handling of phosphate in rats with chronic uremia of three to four weeks duration. They found that (1) filtered phosphate per nephron was increased, mainly due to a high single-nephron GFR, (2) proximal tubular fluid to plasma ratios for phosphate were greater than 1.0, (3) fractional reabsorption of phosphate was reduced, and (4) urinary phosphate was greater than that in superficial distal nephron. The latter finding suggests either secretion of phosphate in the collecting duct or a larger contribution of the deep nephrons to urinary phosphate. Removal of the parathyroid glands in the uremic rats corrected the suppression of the proximal TRP as well as the differences between urinary and distal tubular fluid phos-

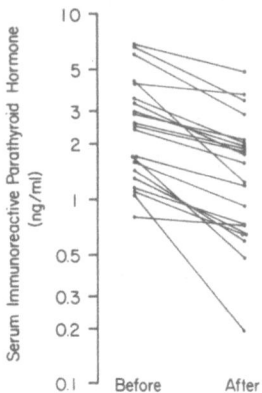

Fig. 4. Levels of immunoreactive PTH in sera of 21 uremic patients before and after a calcium infusion supplying 20 or 30 mg of Ca^{2+}/kg over a 4-hr period. (From Massry et al., 1972. Reprinted with permission.)

phate. These observations underscore the important role of PTH in modulating the tubular transport of phosphate in renal failure.

Wen et al. (1976) studied the effect of extracellular fluid volume expansion (ECVE) on renal phosphate transport in intact and thyroparathyroidectomized (TPTX) dogs. Their data are consistent with PTH playing a major role in decreased phosphate reabsorption in uremia. However, in the absence of PTH, ECVE may also be contributory. Furthermore, Purkerson et al. (1976) reported that in uremic rats, the remaining nephron exhibited increased sensitivity to the phosphaturic response to PTH.

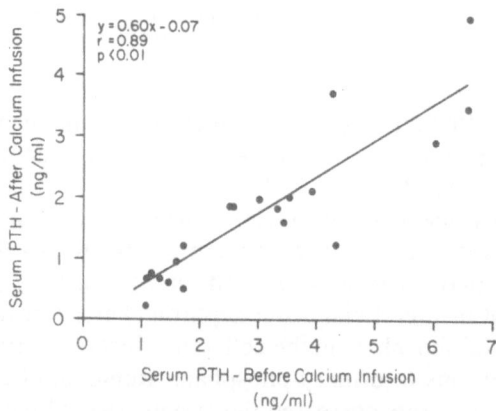

Fig. 5. The relationship between the serum levels of immunoreactive PTH observed in the same patient before and at the end of calcium infusion.

3. ROLE OF SERUM PHOSPHORUS

Since the concentration of serum phosphorus is elevated and single-nephron GFR is usually increased in renal failure, it is possible that an increase in the filtered load of phosphate per nephron may contribute to the augmented $(C_{PO_4}/C_{cr}) \times 100$. The data of Bank *et al.* (1978) provide support for this postulate. The effect of a reduction in serum inorganic phosphorus on $(C_{PO_4}/C_{cr}) \times 100$ may depend on the degree of renal failure. Popovtzer *et al.* (1969) found that a fall in the concentration of serum phosphorus in four patients with C_{cr} of 37–55 ml/min was followed by a significant decrement in $(C_{PO_4}/C_{cr}) \times 100$. Fotino (1977) studied the effect of two to seven weeks of dietary phosphate restriction on $(C_{PO_4}/C_{cr}) \times$ 100 in patients with C_{cr} of 22–63 ml/min. He found that this maneuver was associated with a significant reduction in $(C_{PO_4}/C_{cr}) \times$ 100. Similar observations were reported by Friis *et al.* (1968).

Popovtzer *et al.* (1969) evaluated the effect of variations in serum phosphorus concentration on $(C_{PO_4}/C_{cr}) \times 100$ in 42 patients with advanced renal failure and C_{cr} of 10 ml/min. They found that there was no correlation between the concentration of serum phosphorus and the fraction of filtered phosphate excreted (Fig. 6). In 11 of these 42 patients, serum phosphorus levels were reduced from 9.24 ± 0.76 to 5.11 ± 0.43 mg/100 ml ± SE by feeding the patients low-phosphate diet and giving them aluminum hydroxide gel. Despite the fall in serum phosphorus levels, $(C_{PO_4}/C_{cr}) \times 100$ did not decrease. In contrast, Slatopolsky *et al.*

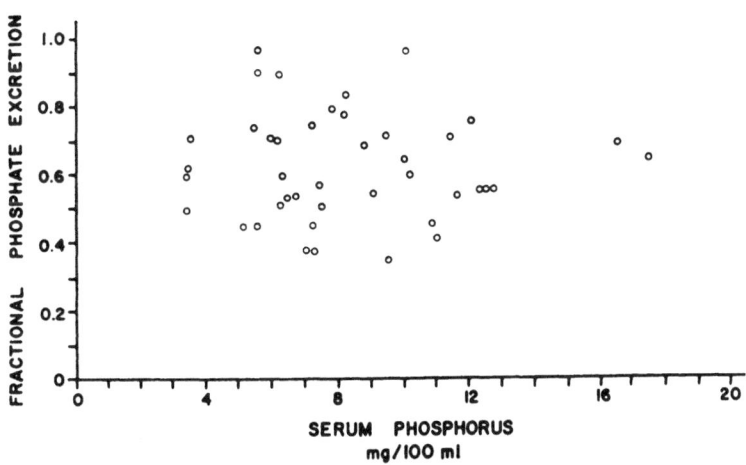

Fig. 6. The relationship between serum inorganic phosphorus and fractional phosphate excretion in patients with advanced renal failure. (From Popovtzer *et al.*, 1969. Reprinted with permission.)

(1968) found that a marked decrement in serum phosphorus from 8.18 $\pm$ 0.30 to 2.38 $\pm$ 0.20 mg/100 ml $\pm$ SE was associated with a modest reduction in $(C_{PO_4}/C_{cr}) \times 100$ from 85 to 53%. These data indicate that variations in the concentration of serum phosphorus in patients with advanced renal failure are not a major detriment to fractional phosphate excretion.

Certain data challenge the concept that the state of secondary hyperparathyroidism and the elevated levels of PTH in renal failure are the paramount factors responsible for the adaptive and progressive decrements in the TRP.

Swensen et al. (1975) studied the effect of renal failure on phosphate homeostasis in TPTX dogs. They found that when the blood concentration of serum calcium was maintained at normal levels with vitamin D supplementation, the fraction of filtered phosphate excreted increased and the concentration of phosphorus in the blood remained normal despite progressive renal failure. Their data are consistent with the postulate that phosphate homeostasis can be maintained in dogs with renal failure even in the absence of parathyroid glands. Further support for this concept is provided by the work of Loreau et al. (1977). They immunized rats against tubular basement membrane and abolished the effect of PTH on renal adenylcyclase. Interstitial nephritis and renal failure developed in the animals as well. Fractional excretion of phosphate increased substantially despite the lack of renal effect of PTH.

Popovtzer et al. (1969) reported that even after total PTX in a patient with advanced renal failure, $(C_{PO_4}/C_{cr}) \times 100$ remained elevated. Fotino (1977) found that the decrement in $(C_{PO_4}/C_{cr}) \times 100$ during phosphate restriction in patients with moderate renal failure occurred despite the presence of markedly elevated blood levels of PTH. Finally, Christensen et al. (1977) found that treatment of patients with renal failure with 1α-hydroxyvitamin D produced a marked reduction (60%) in blood PTH levels and normalization of the hormone levels in five patients. Despite the fall in blood PTH levels, fractional excretion of phosphate increased. All of these data suggest that factors other than PTH may be involved in the control of TRP in renal failure.

Detailed discussions in other chapters of this book indicate that the renal handling of phosphate may be affected by the state of body stores of phosphate, extracellular fluid volume, vitamin D and its metabolites, serum calcium concentration, and hormones other than PTH. Since renal failure may be associated with alterations in these factors, it is not surprising that experimental and clinical data point to factors other than PTH that may be responsible for the modulation of renal tubular transport of phosphate in uremia.

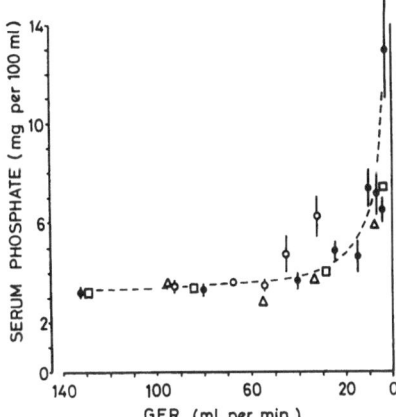

Fig. 7. The relationship between serum phosphorus (mean ± SE) and GFR in normal subjects and in patients with chronic renal disease. Adapted from data by Goldman and Bassett (1954) (□), Lichtwitz et al. (1960) (○), Friis et al. (1968) (△), and Popovtzer et al. (1970b) (●). (From Morgan, 1973. Reprinted with permission.)

The analysis of the available data on urinary phosphate in patients with renal failure in terms of Tm_{PO_4}/GFR, as recommended by Bijvoet (1969), and not in terms of %TRP may provide better understanding of the renal handling of phosphate in renal failure. Using this concept, Morgan (1973) calculated the predicted levels of serum phosphorus and %TRP in patients with impaired renal function assuming that Tm_{PO_4}/GFR remains constant, that is, without factors that decrease Tm_{PO_4}/GFR such as PTH. He concluded that a fall in GFR to 50 ml/min causes little change in serum phosphorus levels or %TRP, but a further decrease in GFR causes a large increase in serum phosphorus levels and a decrease in %TRP. These predictions are similar to actual data reported by various investigators (Friis et al., 1968; Goldman and Bassett, 1954; Lichtwitz et al., 1960; Popovtzer et al., 1972; Slatopolsky et al., 1968)(Figs. 7 and 8). Thus, it

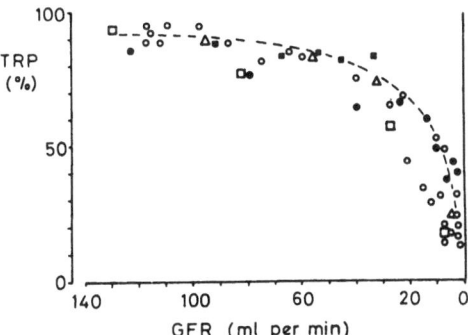

Fig. 8. The relationship between %TRP and GFR in normal persons and in patients with chronic renal disease. Adapted from data by Goldman and Bassett (1954) (□), Lichtwitz et al. (1960) (○), Friis et al. (1968) (△), Slatopolsky et al. (1968) (■), and Popovtzer et al. (1970b) (●). (From Morgan, 1973. Reprinted with permission.)

appears that the change in serum inorganic phosphorus levels and %TRP can be explained by the fall in GFR per se, without the need to involve factors that decrease Tm_{PO_4}/GFR. This does not occur in patients with renal failure. Calculation of Tm_{PO_4}/GFR from the few short-term clearance studies available in the literature (Friis *et al.*, 1968; Goldman and Bassett, 1954; Slatopolsky *et al.*, 1968) shows that a small reduction in Tm_{PO_4}/GFR is present in early renal insufficiency, but a considerable decrease in Tm_{PO_4}/GFR occurs in advanced renal failure (Fig. 9).

4. RENAL HANDLING OF PHOSPHATE AFTER RENAL TRANSPLANTATION

Several investigators have reported reduced TRP in renal allograft recipients during the first two months after renal transplantation despite good function of the graft (Alfrey *et al.*, 1968; Massry *et al.*, 1973; Schwartz *et al.*, 1970). Alfrey *et al.* (1968) found that %TRP was normal in only two of ten patients evaluated 30–320 days after transplantation. Massry *et al.* (1973) found low values of %TRP in nine of ten renal transplant recipients studied 1–48 months following transplantation. Several factors may be responsible for the phosphaturia in these patients. Since hyperplasia of the parathyroid glands usually exists before renal transplantation, and since renal function is rarely restored to normal, it is likely that the secretion of PTH remains elevated, accounting for the high values of $(C_{PO_4}/C_{cr}) \times 100$ during the first few months after renal transplantation. Schwartz *et al.* (1970) found elevated levels of PTH associated with a reduced %TRP in most patients during the first few weeks after transplantation; however, two patients had reduced values of %TRP despite normal blood levels of the hormone. Chatterjee *et al.* (1976) reported that the blood levels of PTH were elevated in many transplant recipients followed for up to six years. Ward *et al.* (1977) reported that the degree of

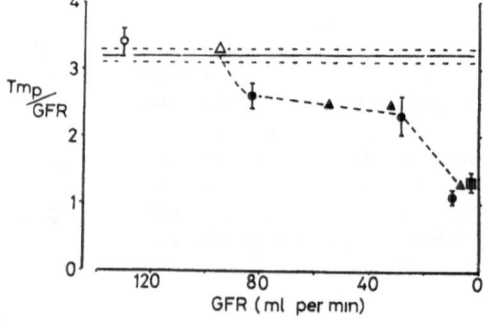

Fig. 9. The relationship between Tmp/GFR (mean ± SE) and GFR in normal subjects (○ and △) and in patients with chronic renal disease. Adapted from data of short clearance studies reported by Goldman and Bassett (1954) (●), Friis *et al.* (1968) (▲), and Slatopolsky *et al.* (1968) (■). (From Morgan, 1973. Reprinted with permission.)

secondary hyperparathyroidism after renal transplantation reflected the renal function of the allograft and a positive correlation between blood levels of PTH and GFR in their patients. In contrast, Roof *et al.* (1971) reported that blood levels of PTH generally fell to normal within three weeks after renal transplantation. Although these observations indicate that persistently high levels of PTH may contribute to the phosphaturia observed after renal transplantation, they suggest that other factors may also be operative. Glucocorticoids can cause phosphaturia (Ingbar *et al.*, 1951), and continued therapy of these patients with prednisone may account, in part, for increased phosphate excretion. It is not infrequent that, even with good renal function, some patients will require chronic diuretic therapy for hypervolemia and/or hypertension. Both hypervolemia and diuretic therapy can contribute to increased urinary losses of phosphate. Theoretically, a primary defect in the TRP could also exist in some renal transplant recipients secondary to immunological attack on the graft (Wilson and Siddiqui, 1973). Rosenbaum *et al.* (1978) reported evidence for primary phosphate leak in six renal transplant receipients. These patients had phosphaturia, hypophosphatemia, and normal blood levels of PTH, and calcium infusion did not affect their renal excretion of phosphate.

5. REFERENCES

Agus, Z. S., Puschett, J. B., Senesky, D., and Goldberg, M., 1971, Mode of action of parathyroid hormone and cyclic adenosine 3'5'-monophosphate on renal tubular phosphate reabsorption in kidney, *J. Clin. Invest.* **50:**617.

Alfrey, A. C., Jenkins, D., and Groth, C. G., 1968, Resolution of hyperparathyroidism, renal osteodystrophy and metastatic calcification after renal homotransplantation, *N. Engl. J. Med.* **279:**1349.

Arnaud, C. D., 1973, Hyperparathyroidism and chronic renal failure, *Kidney Int.* **4:**89.

Bank, N., Wei-Shing, S., and Synedjian, H. S., 1978, A micropuncture study of renal phosphate transport in rats with chronic renal failure and secondary hyperparathyroidism, *J. Clin. Invest.* **61:**884.

Bernstein, D., Kleeman, C. R., Rockney, R., Dowling, J. T., and Maxwell, M. H., 1962, Studies on the renal clearance of phosphate and the role of parathyroid glands in its regulation, *J. Clin. Endocrinol. Metab.* **22:**641.

Better, O. S., Kleeman, C. R., Gonick, H. C., Varady, P. D., and Maxwell, M. H., 1967, Renal handling of calcium, magnesium, and inorganic phosphate in chronic renal failure, *Isr. J. Med Sci.* **3:**60.

Bijvoet, O. L. M., 1969, Relation of plasma phosphate concentration to the renal tubular reabsorption of phosphate, *Clin. Sci.* **37:**23.

Chatterjee, S. N., Friedler, R. M., Berne, T. V., Olomham, S. G., Singer, F. R., and Massry, S. G., 1976, Persistent hypercalcemia after successful renal transplantation, *Nephron.* **17:**1.

Christensen, M. S., Bröchner-Mortensen, J., Tougaard, L., Sornsen, E., and Rödbro, P., 1977, Minor influence of parathyroid hormone on fractional tubular reabsorption of phosphate in chronic renal failure, in: *Phosphate Metabolism* (S. G. Massry and E. Ritz, eds.), pp. 131–139, Plenum Press, New York.

Coburn, J. W., Popovtzer, M. M., Massry, S. G., and Kleeman, C. R., 1969, The physicochemical state and renal handling of divalent ions in chronic renal failure, *Arch. Intern. Med.* **124**:301.

Fotino, S., 1977, Phosphate excretion in chronic renal failure: Evidence for a mechanism other than circulatory parathyroid hormone, *Clin. Nephrol.* **8**:499.

Friis, T., Hahnema, S., and Weeke, E., 1968, Serum calcium and serum phosphorus in uremia during administration of sodium phytate and aluminum hydroxide, *Acta Med. Scand.* **183**:497.

Genuth, S. M., Sherwood, L. M., Vertes, V., and Leonard, J. R., 1970, Plasma parathyroid hormone, calcium and phosphorus in patients with renal osteodystrophy undergoing chronic hemodialysis, *J. Clin. Endocrinol. Metab.* **30**:15.

Gill, G., Pallota, J., Kashgarian, M., Kessner, D., and Epstein, F. H., 1969, Physiologic studies in renal osteodystrophy treated by subtotal parathyroidectomy, *Am. J. Med.* **46**:930.

Goldman, R., and Bassett, S. H., 1954, Phosphate excretion in renal failure. *J. Clin. Invest.* **33**:1623.

Hiatt, H. H., and Thompson, D. D., 1957, The effects of parathyroid extract on renal function in man, *J. Clin. Invest.* **36**:557.

Ingbar, S. H., Kass, E. H., and Burnett, C. H., 1951, Effect of ACTH and cortisone on renal tubular transport of uric acid, phosphorus and electrolytes in patients with normal renal and adrenal functions, *J. Lab. Clin. Med.* **38**:533.

Kleeman, C. R., Better, O., Massry, S. G., and Maxwell, M. H., 1967, Divalent ion metabolism and osteodystrophy in chronic renal failure, *Yale J. Biol. Med.* **40**:1.

Lichtwitz, A., Deseze, S., Parlier, R., Hioco, D., and Bordier, P., 1960, Le hypocalciurie glomérulaire, *Bull. Soc. Méd. Hôp. Paris* **76**:98.

Loreau, N., Cosyns, J. P., Lepreuz, C., and Ardaillou, R., 1977, Renal adenylate calcitonin receptors and phosphate excretion in rats immunized against tubular basement membrane, in: *Phosphate Metabolism* (S. G. Massry, and E. Ritz, eds.), pp. 71–75, Plenum Press, New York.

Massry, S. G., Coburn, J. W., Popovtzer, M. M., Shinaberger, J. H., Maxwell, M. H., and Kleeman, C. R., 1969, Secondary hyperparathyroidism in chronic renal failure. The clinical spectrum in uremia, during hemodialysis, and after renal transplantation, *Arch. Intern. Med.* **124**:431.

Massry, S. G., Coburn, J. W., Peacock, M., and Kleeman, C. R., 1972, Turnover of endogenous parathyroid hormone in uremic patients and those undergoing hemodialysis, *Trans. Am. Soc. Artif. Intern. Organs* **18**:416.

Massry, S. G., Coburn, J. W., Lee, D. N. B., Jowsey, J., and Kleeman, C. R., 1973, Skeletal resistance to parathyroid hormone in renal failure. Study in 105 human subjects, *Ann. Intern. Med.* **78**:357.

Morgan, B., 1973, *Osteomalacia, Renal Osteodystrophy and Osteoporosis*, Charles C. Thomas, Springfield, Ill.

Popovtzer, M. M., Massry, S. G., Makoff, D. L., Maxwell, M. H., and Kleeman, C. R., 1969, Renal handling of phosphate in patients with chronic renal failure, *Isr. J. Med. Sci.* **5**:1018.

Popovtzer, M. M., Massry, S. G., Coburn, J. W., Kopel, M. H., Dirnkard, J. J., and Kleeman, C. R., 1970a, Calcium infusion test in renal failure, *Nephron* **7**:400.

Popovtzer, M. M., Schainack, L. I., Massry, S. G., and Kleeman, C. R., 1970b, Divalent ion excretion in chronic kidney disease: Relation to degree of renal insufficiency, *Clin. Sci.* **38**:297.

Popovtzer, M. M., Penggera, W. F., Hutt, M. P., Robinette, J., Halgrimson, C. G., and Starzl, T. E., 1972, Serum parathyroid hormone levels and renal handling of phosphorus in patients with chronic renal diseases, *J. Clin. Endocrinol. Metab.* **35**:213.

Purkerson, M. L., Rolf, D., Miller, S., Slatopolsky, E., and Klahr, S., 1976, Increased nephron sensitivity to parathyroid hormone (PTH) as renal mass is decreased, *Proc. Am. Soc. Nephrol.* **9**:6.

Reiss, E., Canterbury, J. M., and Egdahl, R. H., 1968, Experience with a radioimmunoassay of parathyroid hormone in human sera, *Trans. Assoc. Am. Physicians* **81**:104.

Roof, B. S., Rames, L., and Carpenter, B., 1971, The myth of tertiary hyperparathyroidism, *Clin. Res.* **19**:196.

Rosenbaum, R. W., Hruska, K. A., and Slatopolsky, E., 1978, Evidence for parathyroid hormone (PTH)–calcium independent phosphate leak in renal transplant patients, in: *Proceedings of the 5th International Congress of Nephrology*, Montreal, p. E-15.

Schwartz, G. H., David, D. S., Rigo, R. R., Savhlte, P. D., Whitsell, J. C., Stenzel, K. H., and Rubin, A. L., 1970, Hypercalcemia after renal transplantation, *Am. J. Med.* **49**:42.

Slatopolsky, E., Gradowska, L., Kashemsant, C., Keltner, R., Manley, C., and Bricker, N. S., 1966, The control of phosphate excretion in uremia *J. Clin. Invest.* **45**:672.

Slatopolsky, E., Robson, M., Elkan, I., and Bricker, N. S., 1968, Control of phosphate excretion in uremic man, *J. Clin. Invest.* **47**:1865.

Slatopolsky, E., Rutherford, E., Hoffsten, P. E., Elkan, I. O., Batcher, H. R., and Bricker, N. S., 1972, Nonsuppressible secondary hyperparathyroidism in chronic progressive renal disease, *Kidney Int.* **1**:38.

Swensen, R. S., Weisinger, J. R., Rubberi, J. L., and Rearen, G. M., 1975, Evidence that parathyroid hormone is not required for phosphate homeostasis in renal failure, *Metabolism* **24**:199.

Ward, H. N., Pabico, R. C., McKenna, B. A., and Freeman, R. B., 1977, The renal handling of phosphate by renal transplant patients: Correlation with serum parathyroid hormone (S_{PTH}), cyclic 3',5'-adenosine monophosphate (cAMP) urinary excretion, and allograft function, in: *Phosphate Metabolism* (S. G. Massry and E. Ritz, eds.), pp. 173–181, Plenum Press, New York.

Wen, S. F., Boynar, J. W., and Stoll, R. W., 1976, Effect of volume expansion on phosphate transport in uremic dogs, *Proc. Am. Soc. Nephrol.* **9**:7.

Wilson, D. R., and Siddiqui, A., 1973, Renal tubular acidosis after renal transplantation, *Ann. Intern. Med.* **79**:352.

Tubular Defects in Phosphate Reabsorption in Clinical Medicine

RUSSELL W. CHESNEY

1. INTRODUCTION

Renal tubular reabsorption of phosphorus requires that the phosphate anion traverse two membranes in order to proceed from the lumen to the interstitial fluid contiguous with the peritubular surface. The actual transport mechanisms for many solutes and ions, including phosphate, differ at each of these membrane surfaces. In humans, it is difficult to dissect out the relative contributions of the two opposing membrane surfaces to the overall net transepithelial transport process (Scriver *et al.*, 1976). It is obvious that reabsorption of any substance, including inorganic orthophosphate, requires a vectorial process favoring movement out of the tubular lumen. Nonetheless, the precise membrane surface involved in human inborn errors of renal tubular transport is not known and can only be the subject of inferential speculation (Scriver *et al.*, 1976). Several recent reviews have described those disease states which perturb the net reabsorption of calcium, phosphate, and various solutes, including glucose and amino acids (Massry *et al.*, 1973; Morris *et al.*, 1976; Rosenberg, 1969; Scriver, 1974; Scriver and Bergeron, 1974; Scriver *et al.*, 1976), but none of these has focused on the entire spectrum of human disorders of tubular phosphate transport. The explosion of knowledge concerning the renal handling of phosphate has been outlined in great detail in preceding chapters which point out that phosphate reabsorption is a complex process occurring at more than one nephron site and is strongly influenced by extracellular volume status, vitamin D and its metabolites, parathyroid hormone (PTH) and calcitonin, cyclic nucleotides, and by both plasma and intracellular levels of calcium and phosphorus. This chapter will discuss the major clinical disorders of the renal tubular reabsorption of phosphorus and, where appropriate, will examine some of the animal models of these disorders.

Disorders of phosphate transport may involve (1) the absence of a plasma membrane transport protein from mutation (Scriver *et al.*, 1976); (2) the absence of an effector hormone or failure of the transport process to respond to normal levels of this hormone (Albright *et al.*, 1942; Steele, 1976); (3) an exaggerated response to a hormone (Grose and Scriver, 1968; Short *et al.*, 1976); (4) the absence of or defects in intracellular enzymes important in the transport process (Chase *et al.*, 1969); or, finally, (5) the alteration of energy-producing processes within tubular epithelium (Morris *et al.*, 1971). These disorders fit into two major subgroups: hypophosphatemia and hyperphosphatemia. Hypophosphatemia is usually the result of decreased net tubular reabsorption of phosphate or a renal phosphate "leak." Increased phosphate excretion, under unusual circumstances such as phosphate loading, may also represent net tubular secretion of this anion (Glorieux and Scriver, 1972; Scriver, 1974; Scriver and Bergeron, 1974; Scriver *et al.*, 1976). Hyperphosphatemia, in contrast, represents increased reabsorption. The defect in transport or in hormonal response which results in hypo- or hyperphosphatemia may not only be confined to the renal tubule, but may involve other epithelial surfaces, including the intestine, where there may be a transport defect in patients with hypophosphatemic rickets (Short *et al.*, 1973), or the skeleton, where PTH fails to act to increase serum calcium levels in pseudohypoparathyroidism (Potts, 1972).

Despite the caution in a 1924 textbook of genetics (Osman, 1924) that "heredity is not a conspicuous feature of those forms of renal disease that occur with any frequency," an inherited mode of transmission is obvious for nearly all of the disorders of phosphate tubular transport. Familial hypophosphatemic rickets is ordinarily inherited as an X-linked dominant (Winters *et al.*, 1958), but both autosomal dominant (Harrison *et al.*, 1966) and autosomal recessive (Stamp and Baker, 1976) modes have been documented. In pseudohypoparathyroidism, an autosomal recessive, X-linked dominant, or sex-influenced autosomal mode can be evident (Potts, 1972). As further evidence of heterogeneity in inheritance of these disorders, nearly all of the diseases associated with the Fanconi syndrome are transmitted as an autosomal recessive trait (Schneider and Seegmiller, 1972), but some of the idiopathic forms may have autosomal dominant inheritance (Hunt *et al.*, 1966), and Lowe's syndrome is an X-linked recessive disorder (Schneider and Seegmiller, 1972; Scriver *et al.*, 1976).

In addition to the disorders in which there is a primary leak of phosphate at the renal tubule, enhanced urinary excretion may be secondary to other influences. In these states, the loss of a transport protein cannot be invoked, and phosphaturia is related to excess hormonal secretion (Fraser *et al.*, 1967) or to increased tissue stores of several metabolites, including cystine (Schneider and Seegmiller, 1972), fructose-1-phosphate (Kranhold *et al.*, 1969), galactose (Segal, 1972), and tyrosine (Fritzell *et al.*, 1964). At present, the direct role of these hormones or metabolites in phosphate leak is not known (Morris *et al.*, 1976). Exogenous compounds, including copper (Walshe, 1972), other heavy metals (Clarkson and Kench, 1962), and tetracycline oxidation products (Gross, 1963), will also inhibit normal tubular phosphate reabsorption as part of the Fanconi syndrome.

At present, the precise nephron location of any of these human disorders of phosphate transport is unknown; however, by inference, the site of phosphate leak in the Fanconi syndrome is felt to be the proximal tubule (Schneider and Seegmiller, 1972). Excess phosphate excretion from one of many sites in the nephron is possible, since the proximal convoluted tubule is not the only location for phosphate recovery (Knox *et al.*, 1977), and this anion can be recovered from more distal nephron sites, including proximal tubular pars recta, late distal tubule, and in the arcades connecting the distal tubules of deep nephrons to the collecting duct (Poujeol *et al.*, 1976). Since PTH leads to cyclic nucleotide production in these same terminal nephron sites (Chabardès *et al.*, 1975), disorders of reduced PTH response and renal phosphate excretion, such as pseudohypoparathyroidism, might involve distal sites just as reasonably as a proximal tubular location.

I will now focus my attention on those disorders of the renal tubule involving phosphate loss (Table 1) and later turn to those involving phosphate retention (Table 2).

2. DISEASES MANIFESTED BY A TUBULAR PHOSPHATE LEAK

2.1. Primary Renal Tubular Phosphate Hyperexcretion

2.1.1. Primary Hypophosphatemic Rickets

Primary hypophosphatemic rickets is a well-characterized disorder in which there is increased renal clearance of phosphate despite profound hypophosphatemia, normocalcemia, and, during childhood, rickets nonresponsive to treatment with vitamin D doses that cure simple vitamin D deficiency (Williams *et al.*, 1972). Several names for this disorder are in common usage: vitamin-D-resistant rickets (Albright *et al.*, 1937; Walton, 1976); familial vitamin-D-resistant rickets with hypophosphatemia (Williams *et al.*, 1972); X-linked hypophosphatemic rickets (Fraser and

Table 1. Clinical Disorders of Renal Tubular Phosphate Transepithelial Transport Involving Excessive Phosphate Excretion or Leak

A. Primary tubular wasting
  1. Familial primary hypophosphatemic rickets
  2. Oncogenous phosphaturia with rickets
  3. Adult sporadic hypophosphatemic osteomalacia
  4. Hypophosphatemic bone disease without rickets
  5. Phosphate leak with idiopathic hypercalciuria
B. Secondary PTH-induced hyperphosphaturia
  1. Vitamin D deficiency
    a. Lack of calciferol
    b. Lack of 25-hydroxycholecalciferol
    c. Lack of 1α,25-dihydroxycholecalciferol
C. Part of a complex renal tubulopathy
  1. Fanconi syndrome
    a. Cystinosis
    b. Other acquired causes
    c. Idiopathic
  2. Lowe's X-linked oculocerebrorenal syndrome
  3. Luder–Sheldon syndrome
  4. Hypophosphatemia with glucosuria, glycinuria, and glycylprolinuria
  5. Glycine loss with adult sporadic hypophosphatemic, osteomalacia

Scriver, 1976); familial X-linked hypophosphatemic rickets (Short *et al.*, 1976); familial hypophosphatemic rickets (Hahn *et al.*, 1975); primary hypophosphatemic rickets (Harrison and Harrison, 1975); renal phosphate diabetes (Kistler *et al.*, 1976); and familial hypophosphatemia (Royer *et al.*, 1974). The term "primary hypophosphatemic rickets" is most preferable, since not all forms are familial and since the X-linked dominant mode of transmission, although the most common, is not the

Table 2. Clinical Disorders of Renal Tubular Phosphate Transepithelial Transport Involving Tubular Phosphate Retention with Hyperphosphatemia

A. Hypoparathyroidism
  1. Surgical
  2. Idiopathic
  3. Familial idiopathic
  4. *Candida* endocrinology syndrome
  5. DiGeorge syndrome (absence of third and fourth pharyngeal pouches)
  6. Magnesium deficiency
  7. Chromosomal abnormalities
B. Pseudohypoparathyroidism
  1. With typical somatic phenotypic features
  2. Other variants
C. Phosphate depletion syndrome
D. Growth hormone excess

only identified genetic mechanism. Other inheritance patterns, including autosomal dominant (Bianchine *et al.*, 1971; Harrison *et al.*, 1966), autosomal recessive (Stamp and Baker, 1976), and sporadic cases (Kistler *et al.*, 1976; Kleerekoper *et al.*, 1977), have been reported.

Clinical and Laboratory Features. This disorder was first described by Albright *et al.* (1937) in a carefully documented report in which the authors proved that vitamin D resistance is not related to vitamin malabsorption but that 150,000–1,500,000 IU of vitamin D₂ daily corrected hypophosphatemia and healed rickets. The usual patient with hypophosphatemic rickets develops rickets upon assumption of an erect posture. Growth retardation and rickets are mainly manifested in the lower segment (Scriver, 1974), and changes include coxa vara, genu valgum, bowed legs, and pelvic deformities. Teeth erupt on time with normal enamel, but the dentin is defective. Early craniostenosis, resulting in a protuberant forehead and enlarged bridge of the nose, is frequent (Albright *et al.*, 1937). Patients have all signs of rickets except myopathy (Table 3). Males universally manifest the disease, but females are variably affected. In the X-linked form of this disorder, affected females are heterozygotes and males are hemizygotes by definition. Although males are invariably hypophosphatemic and demonstrate bone disease, hypophosphatemia and bone disease are less certain in females. The milder disease found in female heterozygotes may explain their better response to therapy. Indeed, female subjects may have a normal height, minimal bowing, and mild reduction of serum phosphorus levels demonstrable only in the fasting state (R. W. Chesney, personal observation). Untreated patients remain short, achieving an adult height of 140–155 cm (Winters *et al.*, 1958). Older patients often have joint pains, join degeneration, and other rheumatic manifestations (Moses and Fessel, 1974).

The radiologic appearance of affected bones shows two typical lesions: rickets in the region of the epiphysis and metaphysis and widening of bone shafts with a loose reticular pattern of trabeculae. Evidence of hyperparathyroidism is not present, and Looser–Milkman striae are rare. Young adults may have osteosclerosis, greater than normal bone tissue, and increased bone calcium as determined by *in vivo* neutron activation analysis (Harrison *et al.*, 1976). Bone biopsy specimens show the typical features of rickets but may also demonstrate irregular orientation of collagen fibers, abnormal deposition of bone mineral, irregular cement lines, and increased low-density bone around osteocytic lacunae (Parfitt, 1972; Witmer and Balsan, 1968).

The universal biochemical feature of this disorder is severe depression of the serum phosphate concentration to the range of 1.0–2.4 mg/dl (0.13–0.32 mM/liter). Serum calcium levels are normal or slightly reduced, and serum alkaline phosphatase activity is only mildly elevated. Urinary

Table 3. Clinical Features of the Forms of Hypophosphatemic Bone Disorders Related to Phosphaturia[a]

	Vitamin-D-deficiency rickets	Primary hypophosphatemic rickets	Vitamin-D-dependency rickets	Hypophosphatemic bone disease
Bone disease	Rickets Bowing	Rickets Bowing	Rickets Bowing	Increased trabeculation No bowing
Muscle weakness	Yes	No	Yes	No
Age of onset	9–12 mo	12–18 mo	3–6 mo	Variable
Serum calcium	↓	Normal	↓	Normal
Serum phosphate	↓	↓	↓	↓
Serum alkaline phosphatase	↑	↑	↑	↑
Serum immunoreactive PTH	↑	Normal or minimal ↑	↑	Normal
Increased aminoaciduria	Yes	No	Yes	No
Tm$_{PO_4}$ at endogenous [PO$_4$]	↓	↓	↓	Normal
Urinary phosphate at Endogenous levels	↑	↑	↑	Normal
Loaded levels	↑	↑	↑	Normal
Intestinal calcium absorption	↓	↓	↓	↑ ?

Genetics	None	X-linked dominant Autosomal dominant Autosomal recessive	Autosomal recessive	X-linked Autosomal dominant
Response to 10 μg vitamin D_3/day	Curative	None	None	None
Response to 2 μg 1,25(OH)$_2$D$_3$/day	Curative	None	Curative	Possible curative
Response to 1 mg vitamin D_3/day	Curative	Rickets partially healed	Curative	Bone disease partially healed Hypophosphatemia
Oral phosphate supplementation	Hypercalcemia	Hypophosphatemia persists Heals rickets Increased growth		Increases serum phosphate

^{a} Compiled from Scriver *et al.* (1974, 1977); Walton (1976); and Frymoyer and Hodgkin (1977).

calcium excretion is low, but phosphate clearance is markedly increased, particularly for the level of reduction in serum phosphate (Arnstein and Hansen, 1969; Hahn et al., 1975; Steendijk, 1960). As initially reported by Albright et al. (1937), increased fecal excretion of calcium and phosphate is found. The circulating levels of PTH in patients not treated with oral phosphate are either normal (Arnaud et al., 1971; Fanconi et al., 1974; Roof et al., 1972; Short et al., 1976) or only slightly elevated (Glorieux and Scriver, 1974; Hahn et al., 1975; Lewy et al., 1972; Reitz and Weinstein, 1973). Patients receiving the large doses of oral phosphate used in therapy of this disorder have increased PTH levels (Arnaud et al., 1971; Fanconi and Fischer, 1976) and may demonstrate radiologic evidence of secondary hyperparathyroidism. Aminoaciduria does not occur in the absence of secondary hyperparathyroidism.

    Pathogenesis. Essentially all studies of patients with X-linked or primary hypophosphatemic rickets have demonstrated that the net tubular reabsorption and fractional reabsorption of phosphate are decreased (Arnstein and Hansen, 1969; Glorieux and Scriver, 1972, 1973; Hahn et al., 1975; Scriver, 1974; Short et al., 1976; Steendijk, 1960; Wilson et al., 1965). Fractional excretion of phosphate is further increased by the ingestion of additional phosphate (Glorieux and Scriver, 1973; Steendijk, 1960; Wilson et al., 1965), and phosphate deprivation results in a rise in the fractional reabsorption of phosphate.

    Two completely opposing theories of the pathogenesis of this hyperphosphaturia have arisen since 1937. The first states that the primary defect is diminished intestinal calcium and phosphate absorption, presumably related to an abnormality of vitamin D metabolism. Albright (Albright et al., 1937), the author of this hypothesis, further ascribed hypophosphatemia and augmented phosphate excretion to the secondary hyperparathyroidism from decreased intestinal calcium absorption. Since recent evidence suggests no abnormalities of vitamin D metabolism (Balsan and Garabedian, 1972; Haddad et al., 1973), the impaired reclamation of phosphate may result from "hypersensitivity" of the renal tubule to PTH action (Arnstein and Hansen, 1969; Glorieux and Scriver, 1972; Hahn et al., 1975). This alternative corollary is necessary, since there are normal or only slightly raised PTH levels in untreated patients (Lewy et al., 1972) and since Albright's original proposal (Albright et al., 1937) is probably invalid. The second major thesis relates hypophosphatemia directly to defective transport of phosphate in the proximal tubule and intestine because of the absence of a transport protein specific for phosphate at these epithelial surfaces. This hypothesis was first proposed by Robertson et al. (1942) and later by Fanconi (Fanconi, 1956; Fanconi and Girardot, 1952). Glorieux and Scriver have found that the PTH-responsive component of phosphate transport appears to be missing, so that it does not respond to provision of exogenous hormone (Arnaud *et al.*, 1971; Glorieux and Scriver, 1972). In this second hypothesis, a selective defect in the transepithelial movement of phosphate at the level of the gut and tubule ultimately results in undermineralization of the growing surface of bone and rickets (Arnaud *et al.*, 1971; Glorieux and Scriver, 1973; Glorieux *et al.*, 1972). The evidence for and arguments against both of these theories will now be discussed in more detail.

As stated above, Albright (Albright *et al.*, 1937) proposed more than 40 years ago that hypocalcemia from defective vitamin D metabolism and inadequate gut absorption of this divalent cation led to hyperparathyroidism and hyperphosphaturia. In that his original patient had demonstrable parathyroid adenomas, this hypothesis (at first) seemed tenable. Early support for this idea came from two separate lines of evidence. First, using radioisotope-labeled vitamin D_3, an abnormality in vitamin D metabolism was found in a few patients with either sporadic or X-linked hypophosphatemic rickets (Avioli *et al.*, 1967; DeLuca *et al.*, 1967). Second, evidence of mild secondary hyperparathyroidism has been reported (Blackard *et al.*, 1962; Falls *et al.*, 1968; Field and Reiss, 1960; Nigrin *et al.*, 1962), and phosphaturia will diminish after the administration of intravenous calcium sufficient to suppress endogenous PTH secretion. However, Albright's theory will not explain the need for oral phosphorus supplementation at a dose of 1–4 g daily in order to reverse hypophosphatemia (Glorieux and Scriver, 1973; Glorieux *et al.*, 1972; Harrison *et al.*, 1966; McEnery *et al.*, 1972; Teitelbaum *et al.*, 1976; West *et al.*, 1964; Wilson *et al.*, 1965), the requirement for massive vitamin D doses to reverse rickets (Stickler *et al.*, 1971), and the finding that these large doses of vitamin D, at best, correct serum phosphate levels to the low-normal or subnormal range. Vitamin D, given at a dose of 150,000–1,500,000 IU daily, will not correct growth failure and hypophosphatemia (Glorieux *et al.*, 1972; McEnery *et al.*, 1972) despite leading to hypercalcemia and nephrocalcinosis (Stickler *et al.*, 1971). With the recent finding that serum concentrations of 25-hydroxyvitamin D_3 (25OHD$_3$) (Balsan and Garabedian, 1972; Haddad *et al.*, 1973) and 1,25-dihydroxyvitamin D_3 [1,25(OH)$_2$D$_3$] (Haussler *et al.*, 1976) are normal, vitamin D metabolism is probably normal. In addition, PTH levels are either normal (Arnaud *et al.*, 1971) or so slightly elevated (Lewy *et al.*, 1972) that Albright's basic pathogenic sequence today seems untenable.

As mentioned above, PTH might play a pathogenic role if the renal tubule in patients with this disorder were hypersensitive to the phosphaturic effect of this hormone. Augmented phosphate excretion after stimulation by normal or minimally elevated circulating active PTH could both explain the reduced tubular reabsorption of phosphate (TRP) (Harrison, 1959) and the increased percentage of TRP that follows the induction of hypercalcemia in these patients (Falls *et al.*, 1968; Field and Reiss, 1960; Glorieux and Scriver, 1972). This proposal was first put forward about 15 years ago (Arnstein and Hansen, 1969; Harrison, 1959), but most recently has been espoused by Hahn *et al.* (1975) and Short *et al.* (1976). Hahn and his colleagues (1975) found that PTH levels in untreated hypophosphatemic subjects were elevated to 11.4 versus 5.1 ng/ml in control subjects and that urinary cyclic AMP (cAMP) excretion was also augmented twofold. cAMP excretion was further increased in response to PTH infusion, and an additional decrease in the percentage of TRP was noted. Calcium infusion suppressed PTH release and cAMP excretion; nonetheless, the percentage of TRP remained inappropriately low for the serum phosphate level. The authors interpreted these results to suggest that mild hyperparathyroidism might be important in the pathogenesis of the hyperphosphatemia in their patients.

Short and her associates found completely normal circulating PTH concentrations and normal urinary cAMP levels (Short *et al.*, 1976). Calcium infusion sufficient to achieve serum levels of 13–15 mg/dl resulted in reduced serum PTH and urinary cAMP excretion. PTH infusion at increasing doses led to phosphate excretion rates strikingly higher than those found in control subjects or in the patients prior to PTH infusion. Since cAMP levels were the same in hemizygotes and in control subjects, only the phosphaturic response to exogenous PTH was exaggerated, suggesting that the hyperphosphaturia in these patients is dependent on circulating levels of PTH.

The alternative proposal relates to a primary defect in transepithelial transport of the phosphate anion. The major criticism leveled at this thesis is that it cannot explain the finding that calcium infusion increases the percentage of TRP and the uniform finding of decreased gut calcium absorption (Albright *et al.*, 1937). Proponents of this second thesis, including Glorieux and Scriver (1972, 1973, 1974), have argued that although calcium infusion may lead to suppression of PTH secretion, it could also indicate that calcium ions directly influence phosphate reabsorption at the renal tubular level, as has been shown in the animal experiments of Lavender and Pullman (1963). In addition, increased gut phosphate might be expected to increase fecal calcium wastage. The major positive support for the phosphate transport defect theory comes from the observation that patients with primary hypophosphatemia have no hypocalcemia and minimal or no increase in circulating PTH levels and from the fact that renal phosphaturia is an isolated finding, without associated net decreased reclamation of amino acids, bicarbonate, uric acid, and glucose which would be expected were the tubule hyperresponsive to PTH action (Scriver, 1974; Scriver *et al.*, 1976). In contrast to the studies reported previously, Glorieux and Scriver found no augmented phosphaturia after PTH infusion (1972, 1974) and no increased cAMP excretion (1973, 1974). They also found transient enhancement of phosphate reabsorption following calcium infusion. The net tubular secretion of phosphorus found in some patients after phosphate infusion has led Scriver (1974, 1976), Glorieux and Scriver (1972) to postulate that the transport defect may be augmented backflux across the luminal membrane into the tubular lumen once initial brush-border uptake has occurred. Selective phosphate backflux across the apical pole of the renal epithelial cell could result in hyperphosphaturia. Some of the data leading Scriver to hypothesize a backflux leak will be summarized later when the animal model is discussed.

The intestinal block in phosphate uptake and absorption, initially found by Albright (Albright *et al.*, 1937), has been substantiated *in vivo* (Condon *et al.*, 1971) and using intestinal biopsy specimens *in vitro* (Short *et al.*, 1973), but it is not a uniform finding (Gerbaux-Balsan, 1965; Glorieux *et al.*, 1976). The differences among studies of phosphate absorption across the gut may represent clinical heterogeneity among patients, but all of the patients studied in these four reports demonstrated the X-linked dominant mode of inheritance of hypophosphatemia. Another explanation is that there were considerable differences among the techniques used by these investigators. In a more recent study, Walton (1976) has observed reduced jejunal phosphate transport, which can be shown by the use of a triple lumen tube, and, in the absence of phosphate in the perfusion solution, decreased calcium uptake, possibly indicating that calcium malabsorption may be unrelated to the block in phosphate transport.

Despite the presence of normal levels of the vitamin D metabolites 25OHD$_3$ (Balsan and Garabedian, 1972; Haddad *et al.*, 1973) and 1,25(OH)$_2$D$_3$ (Haussler *et al.*, 1976), the finding of decreased intestinal calcium absorption (Albright *et al.*, 1937; Walton, 1976) makes tempting the idea that an abnormality in vitamin D metabolism may be of pathogenic significance. Decreased levels of 1,25(OH)$_2$D$_3$ could account for reduced gut calcium and phosphate absorption (DeLuca, 1976), and hypophosphatemia will stimulate intestinal calcium and phosphorus absorption after the administration of this vitamin D analogue (Rizzoli *et al.*, 1977). Furthermore, hypophosphatemia normally enhances intestinal calcium uptake in the presence of normal dietary vitamin D intake (Lotz *et al.*, 1968); however, the luminal Ca × PO$_4$ activity ratio may be critical in determining the magnitude of this uptake (Scriver, 1976). Patients have undergone therapeutic trials with 25OHD$_3$ (Balsan and Garabedian, 1972; Earp *et al.*, 1970; Pak *et al.*, 1972; Rosen and Finberg, 1972), 1α-hydroxyvitamin D$_3$ (1αOHD$_3$) (Peacock *et al.*, 1977), and 1,25(OH)$_2$D$_3$ (Brickman *et al.*, 1973; Glorieux *et al.*, 1973; Russell *et al.*, 1975; Walton, 1976) in an effort to correct hypophosphatemia. Each of these vitamin D metabolites increases intestinal calcium absorption, often strikingly (Walton,

1976), and sometimes produces transient elevations of serum phosphate levels. Nonetheless, prolonged administration has not produced sustained phosphate concentrations in the normal range, has failed to increase the percentage of TRP, and has not healed rickets.

Rasmussen and his colleagues have suggested that the renal tubule is maladapted in these patients in that it may lack the ability both to reclaim filtered orthophosphate and to 1α-hydroxylate circulating $25OHD_3$ from a blunted response to the signal of intracellular hypophosphatemia (Rasmussen and Anast, 1978; Rasmussen et al., 1976). Further, the fact that these hypophosphatemic patients do not actually have elevated circulating $1,25(OH)_2D_3$ levels, as found in animals with hypophosphatemia, may indicate impaired 1α-hydroxylase activity in renal tissue (Haussler and McCain, 1977). However, this hypothesis would require at least two genetic defects, one influencing renal phosphate reabsorption and the other being the failure of 1α-hydroxylase activity, since therapy with $1,25(OH)_2D_3$ will not alter renal phosphaturia. Finding two mutant alleles on the X chromosome in some cases and on autosomal chromosomes in other cases seems highly improbable. Further, the hypocalcemia, elevated PTH levels, and aminoaciduria that would be predicted if 1α-hydroxylase activity were reduced have not been found (Scriver, 1974, 1976).

Although Albright (Albright et al., 1937) found a parathyroid adenoma in the first case of hypophosphatemic rickets, and although some patients develop parathyroid hyperplasia as a complication of phosphate therapy, primary hyperparathyroidism in association with hypophosphatemia is uncommon. Only ten patients with hyperparathyroidism and hypercalcemia unrelated to vitamin D toxicity have been described (Kleerekoper et al., 1977), and many of these patients have sporadic hypophosphatemic osteomalacia (see below). In two patients with X-linked hypophosphatemia (Glorieux et al., 1972; Tarwalkar et al., 1974), the renal tubular phosphate leak was unaltered both by the development of hyperparathyroidism and after the surgical excision of at least three-and-one-half parathyroid glands. Albright's (Albright et al., 1937) original patient had improved phosphate reabsorption but not total correction of phosphaturia by partial parathyroidectomy (PTX). In a single patient, renal transplantation following a three-and-one-half-gland PTX did not correct hyperphosphaturia (Morgan et al., 1973). This patient, however, received a renal allograft from his HLA-identical sister for whom no fasting phosphate concentration was obtained prior to her donor nephrectomy. After nephrectomy, she had a percentage of TRP of 73 at a serum phosphate level of 3.2 mg/dl, which could indicate mild hyperphosphaturia; nonetheless, the transplant recipient had marked hypophosphatemia and a percentage of TRP of 30 on numerous occasions. To date, no patient with familial hypophosphatemia and a total PTX has been described.

Since orthophosphate reabsorption is impaired in kidney and possibly in intestine (Condon *et al.*, 1971; Glorieux and Scriver, 1972; Walton, 1976), phosphate transport has been examined in other tissues. No evidence for increased salivary phosphate clearance was found in 14 patients with primary hypophosphatemia (Hahn *et al.*, 1975). Changes in phosphate-dependent metabolism within erythrocytes of hypophosphatemic patients have been reported (Cartier *et al.*, 1970; Glorieux *et al.*, 1972), but probably can be attributed to reduced phosphate availability. However, no defect in the facilitated diffusion of phosphate into erythrocytes has been found (Scriver *et al.*, 1974; Tenenhouse and Scriver, 1975).

The discovery of an X-linked dominant mutation in the laboratory mouse resulting in hypophosphatemia, rickets, and short stature offers promise in unraveling the basic pathogenic defect in this disorder. Since both the murine and human diseases are inherited as an X-linked dominant, and since genes coded on the X chromosome are well preserved among various mammalian species, it is highly probable that the same gene has undergone mutation in both species. These mice have, in addition, diminished bone ash and high urinary fractional excretion of phosphate, and their rickets can be ameliorated by oral phosphate therapy (Eicher *et al.*, 1976). Significantly decreased intestinal phosphate uptake was found in mutant mice as compared to controls, but intestinal calcium uptake was similar (O'Doherty *et al.*, 1976). The hypophosphatemic mice also exhibited the slight reduction in serum calcium levels that has been reported for humans (Albright *et al.*, 1937; Glorieux *et al.*, 1972). Provision of $1,25(OH)_2D_3$ has not increased intestinal phosphate uptake but has augmented calcium uptake. Total PTX in these mice did not alter the degree of renal hyperphosphaturia, suggesting that the primary defect is a failure of normal intestinal and renal epithelial transport of orthophosphate (Cowgill *et al.*, 1977). Tenenhouse *et al.* (1977) have found identical tissue inorganic phosphorus content in renal cortical slices from mice and similar rates of uptake across the basolateral membrane, the membrane surface exposed by the slice technique (Scriver *et al.*, 1976). Uptake by the arsenate-sensitive sodium-activated component of phosphate transport in isolated brush-border (luminal) membranes from these mice is impaired, suggesting that the transport defect is located in the apical luminal membrane (Tenenhouse *et al.*, 1977). Since brush-border vesicles could be either inside out or right side out, the theory of an augmented backflux of phosphate from cell into lumen previously suggested by Scriver *et al.* (1974, 1976) cannot be tested. Some sizable differences in hormone-sensitive adenyl cyclase activity along various nephron sites have been found between normal and hypophosphatemic mice in one study (Brunette *et al.*, 1977), but the physiological significance of these differences is not known (Butlen and Jard, 1972). Hopefully, more extensive use of this serendipitous discovery of an animal model of hypophosphatemia will be made in the future.

Therapy. Vitamin D in sufficient doses will heal rachitic lesions (Williams *et al.*, 1958), but serum phosphate levels remain subnormal and serum alkaline phosphatase activity falls only slightly. Although the rachitic growth plate becomes normal, the coarse trabecular pattern of patients' long bones is unchanged (Harrison *et al.*, 1976). The dose of vitamin D required to heal rickets is often toxic (Stickler *et al.*, 1971; Winters *et al.*, 1958), and the dwarfism prevalent in these patients' remains unaltered.

Although early studies did not seem to substantiate a role for oral phosphate supplementation in the treatment of hypophosphatemia and rickets (Frame *et al.*, 1963; Stickler *et al.*, 1965), these patients probably did not receive the frequent and large doses of phosphate required to maintain normophosphatemia. Later, the observation that intravenous phosphate could heal rickets (Scriver *et al.*, 1964) led others to administer this anion by mouth and achieve positive calcium and phosphate balance (Gerbaux-Balsan, 1965; West *et al.*, 1964). Long-term studies of the daily provision of 1–4 g of inorganic phosphate given every 4–5 hr indicate that healing of rickets and increased growth velocity can occur (Glorieux *et al.*, 1972; Harrison *et al.*, 1966; McEnery *et al.*, 1972). Catch-up growth has been demonstrated, and, if started early, reasonable height can be achieved and maintained (Fraser and Scriver, 1976; Harrison *et al.*, 1966). After an oral phosphorus dose, the serum level peaks at 90–120 min and returns to pretherapeutic levels in approximately 4 hr (Glorieux *et al.*, 1972).

Oral phosphate administration leads to decreased calcium absorption, which, in turn, raises serum immunoreactive PTH to levels that may lead to hyperparathyroid bone disease (Glorieux *et al.*, 1972). The use of vitamin D_2 in large doses and oral calcium has proved useful in preventing this secondary hyperparathyroidism (Glorieux *et al.*, 1972; Harrison *et al.*, 1966; McEnery *et al.*, 1972; Teitelbaum *et al.*, 1976), well outlined elsewhere (Glorieux *et al.*, 1972).

Summary. Although a thorough study of the X-linked hypophosphatemic mouse may ultimately demonstrate which pathogenic theory is correct, many discrepancies remain unresolved. Despite persistence of hyperphosphaturia after subtotal PTX in hypophosphatemic rachitic humans (Glorieux *et al.*, 1972; Tarwalker *et al.*, 1974; Williams *et al.*, 1972), no patients have been described after total removal of the parathyroids. Thus, even in the presence of minimal levels of PTH, hyperresponsiveness to the phosphaturic action of this hormone is possible. Although serum levels of vitamin D metabolites appear to be normal, more data relating serum

$1,25(OH)_2D_3$ concentrations to serum phosphate concentrations are needed.

The finding of mild hyperparathyroidism reported by some (Hahn *et al.*, 1975) may possibly be explained by the 1200-mg phosphate diet given patients in the control period, an amount equivalent to the therapeutic levels used in some hypophosphatemic children (Glorieux *et al.*, 1972; Stamp, 1971). In addition, the hyperresponsiveness to PTH administration found in the patients described by Short *et al.* (1976) may be the result of PTH action on a site distal to the proximal tubule (Knox *et al.*, 1977). Alternatively, the administration of phosphate to these same patients prior to PTH administration may have uncovered the phosphate secretion reported by others (Glorieux *et al.*, 1972; Scriver *et al.*, 1964).

The patients reported with either autosomal dominant (Harrison *et al.*, 1966; Wilson *et al.*, 1965) or recessive (Stamp and Baker, 1976) modes of inheritance and the sporadic cases described in adults (Dent and Stamp, 1971) have not been as fully evaluated. The pathogenic mechanisms for these forms of hypophosphatemia remain unknown but appear to require oral phosphate therapy in addition to large doses of vitamin D.

2.1.2. Oncogenous Rickets

In some patients, hypophosphatemia may be associated with tumors of soft tissues or bone (Harrison, 1973; Prader *et al.*, 1959) or with some generalized disorders such as fibrous dysplasia (Dent and Gertner, 1976), neurofibromatosis (Falkson and Frame, 1958), or the epidermal nevus syndrome (Aschinberg *et al.*, 1977). The hypophosphatemia in these instances appears to be related to some substance(s) elaborated by the tumor or fibrous tissue, since it regresses when the tumor of fibroma is removed—hence, the name "ocogenous rickets." In a review of 14 cases of hypophosphatemic osteomalacia or rickets associated with mesenchymal tumors of either bone or soft tissue, improvement or cure was noted in nine cases after tumor excision (Dent and Gertner, 1976). Failure of this therapy to reverse hypophosphatemia indicated malignancy with metastatic spread. The removal of osteotic fibrous dyspastic bone lesions (Dent and Gertner, 1976) or the fibroangiomas in the epidermal nevus syndrome (Falkson and Frame, 1958) reversed hypophosphatemia and rickets.

The demonstration of a rise in the percentage of TRP from very low to normal levels after removal of tumor (Dent and Gertner, 1976; Falkson and Frame, 1958; Pollack *et al.*, 1973) suggested that the neoplastic tissue might elaborate a humoral substance which inhibited normal transepithelial phosphate reabsorption. The lack of hypercalcemia and of elevated immunoreactive PTH levels and the absence of hyperaminoaciduria, which would be anticipated were PTH elaborated from these "nonendocrine" tumors (Falkson and Frame, 1958; Wyman *et al.*, 1977), tend to militate against PTH or a block in vitamin D metabolism as a pathogenic mechanism. Further, the hypocalcemia that would be expected were calcitonin secretion or an inhibitor of vitamin D metabolism a likely mechanism has not been found. In those metastatic diseases in which PTH-like substances, not immunologically identical to PTH, have been elaborated, hypercalcemia has been a prominent feature, but it has not been present in patients with oncogenous rickets (O'Regan *et al.*, 1977; Singer *et al.*, 1973); Tashjian *et al.*, 1964. The most likely explanation is that whatever is produced by these tumors of pleomorphic mesenchymal origin appears to directly influence TRP. Urinary cAMP excretion has not been measured in these patients, and most of these studies have not excluded a PTH-like substance working only in phosphate transport. Aschinberg *et al.* (1977) have homogenized excised fibroangioma tissue from one patient and injected the supernatant into a young puppy. This extract, which was not PTH or calcitonin by immunoassay technique, led to marked phosphaturia and, within 2 hr, a fall in the percentage of TRP from 81 to 12.

Recently, a patient with a giant-cell tumor of bone and biopsy-proven osteomalacia, hypophosphatemia, and reduced intestinal calcium and phosphorus absorption was shown to have normal serum concentrations of $25OHD_3$ but significant reduction in $1,25(OH)_2D_3$ levels (Drezner and Feinglos, 1977). Treatment with 3 μg daily of $1,25(OH)_2D_3$ led to normalization of osteomalacic changes. Whether tumor-induced inhibition of vitamin D metabolism is the pathogenic mechanism of the phosphate leak in other patients with oncogenous rickets remains to be shown. The time course of the phosphaturic response found in the puppy receiving tumor extract (Aschinberg *et al.*, 1977) suggests that not all tumors act to inhibit $1,25(OH)_2D_3$ formation.

Although tumor removal whenever feasible is the optional mode of treatment, some patients have responded to high-dose vitamin D and oral phosphate therapy (Dent and Gertner, 1976; Peacock *et al.*, 1977; Pollack *et al.*, 1973). Other patients have not had a satisfactory response to even massive doses of these agents (Aschinberg *et al.*, 1977; Prader *et al.*, 1959; Wyman *et al.*, 1977). Rheumatic symptoms, reported in adults with oncogenous hypophosphatemia, have improved following oral phosphate therapy (Moser and Fessel, 1974). Myopathy, found in these patients in contrast to patients with primary hypophosphatemia, may also respond to oral phosphate. Depression of growth during hypophosphatemic periods, with acceleration of growth velocity after oral phosphate supplementation, has been documented (Pollack *et al.*, 1973). These patients may also require vitamin D therapy to prevent the development of secondary hyperparathyroidism. Obviously, in any patient in whom hypophosphatemia is detected, a search for a mesenchymal tumor should be made, since excision may be curative and a sizable proportion of these tumors are malignant.

2.1.3. Hypophosphatemic Nonrachitic Bone Disease

Patients have been described having decreased renal tubular reabsorption of phosphorus, phosphopenic bone disease, and hypophosphatemia, but absolutely no evidence of rickets (Frymoyer and Hodgkin, 1977; Scriver et al., 1977). These patients have selective phosphaturia with normal immunoreactive PTH levels. The percentage of TRP is in the "normal" range (usually 82–90) at the reduced endogenous serum phosphate levels, but following phosphate infusion sufficient to raise serum levels, a phosphate leak is evident, and the theoretical renal phosphate threshhold (Walton and Bijvoet, 1975) is subnormal. Phosphate and cAMP excretion is markedly enhanced following rapid infusion of PTH, in contrast to the finding in some patients with X-linked hypophosphatemia (Glorieux et al., 1972; Scriver et al., 1977), but the maximal response is found at a time later than that found in normal subjects. At similar serum phosphate concentrations, the percentage of TRP is significantly lower in patients with X-linked hypophosphatemia than in patients with hypophosphatemic bone disease.

An X-linked mode of inheritance was evident in one family of 133 members in whom hypophosphatemia was found in 37 (Frymoyer and Hodgkin, 1977). In this kindred extending over seven generations, no instance of a father-to-son transmission could be found. Either an autosomal dominant or indeterminate mode of inheritance was reported in five other patients with this disorder (Scriver et al., 1977).

Bone alterations consist of femoral bowing, internal femoral and tibial torsion, elbow flexion contractures, and radiologic evidence of increased bone density, coarse trabeculation, and sclerosis. Rickets were not apparent in the 42 hypophosphatemic individuals reported. These bone abnormalities occur at serum phosphate levels comparable to those found in primary hypophosphatemic rickets but are obviously of less severity. In one report, bone changes were more manifest during adulthood, with relative sparing of children (Frymoyer and Hodgkin, 1977). Dwarfing and short stature are mild, particularly in comparison to the finding in primary hypophosphatemia (Scriver et al., 1977).

Two patients with the autosomal dominant inheritance pattern appeared to have increased serum phosphate concentrations and percentage of TRP following therapy with $1\alpha OHD_3$. Long-term oral phosphate supplementation may improve the growth pattern. As more of these patients are described, the major differences between this disorder and primary hypophosphatemic rickets may become apparent; nonetheless, the absence of rickets in these patients makes them readily identifiable.

2.1.4. Adult Sporadic Hypophosphatemic Osteomalacia

An interesting type of patient has been characterized (Dent and Stamp, 1971; Parfitt, 1972) who develops hypophosphatemic osteomalacia between the ages of 15 and 60 years. Age peaks in onset are found during the third and fourth decades and then again at age 50. These infrequent cases are entirely sporadic, without previous history of rickets, short stature, or bone pain, and have a homogeneous presentation and clinical pattern (Segar *et al.*, 1956). These patients appear initially with debilitating bone pain, Looser zones, and a rather prominent myopathy, and, in addition to hypophosphatemia, may commonly have isolated hyperglycinuria and, less often, glucosuria (glycosuria). Often, the interval between the onset of bone pain and diagnosis is long. Typical osteomalacic features are seen on bone biopsy, and, in contrast to the situation in X-linked hypophosphatemia, the spine is especially afflicted. Compression fractures of the spine with considerable loss of height (up to 6 cm) may be prominent.

Radiologic changes are distinct, with no evidence of the osteosclerosis reported in primary hypophosphatemia. Bone disease is characterized by markedly diminished bone density, reduced cortical thickness, and, with long-standing disease, marked angulation of bones, collapsed codfish vertebrae, kyphosis, and scoliosis. Tibial and femoral bowing and shortening of the lower segment are absent.

Laboratory findings include normal calcium levels, hypophosphatemia in the range of 2–2.5 mg/dl (seldom as reduced as the values found in X-linked hypophosphatemia), mild increase in serum alkaline phosphatase activity, and the aforementioned glycinuria. This hyperglycinuria has also been occasionally seen in oncogenous hypophosphatemia (Harrison, 1973; Pollack *et al.*, 1973) but never in the X-linked form. The percentage of TRP and the theoretical renal phosphate threshhold are reduced, and a biochemical feature in common with nonrachitic hypophosphatemic bone disease in the finding of "normal" urinary phosphate excretion at endogenous serum phosphate levels but marked hyperphosphaturia after phosphate loading (Dent and Stamp, 1971).

The pathogenesis is unclear, but, in most cases, hyperparathyroidism appears to play no role. Phosphaturia persists despite high-dose vitamin D and oral phosphate therapy. Immunoreactive PTH and 25OHD$_3$ concentrations are normal (Offerman *et al.*, 1976), and in those patients with hyperparathyroidism, subtotal PTX does not alter phosphaturia and hypophosphatemia (Kistler *et al.*, 1976; Kleerekoper *et al.*, 1977; Thomas and Fry, 1970). Several instances of the association of adult sporadic hypophosphatemic osteomalacia with parathyroid adenomas have been reported (Dent and Stamp, 1971; Kistler *et al.*, 1976; Kleerekoper *et al.*, 1977; Thomas and Fry, 1970), and nearly all cases in which parathyroid adenomas are found are the sporadic rather than familial forms (Parfitt, 1972). The reduced intestinal calcium absorption and negative calcium balances shown by Dent and Stamp (1971) in careful balance studies may lead to the stimulation of the parathyroid glands, with adenoma formation following years of chronic hyperplasia (Thomas and Fry, 1970). Again, unlike the situation in familial forms, hypercalcemia may be present in the sporadic form (Glanville and Bloom, 1965; Henneman *et al.*, 1962; Kistler *et al.*, 1976). The reason for hyperglycinuria is not obvious. Although hyperglycinuria has been ascribed to the action of PTH on bone, the generalized aminoaciduria seen after secondary hyperparathyroidism in D-deficiency rickets is of the usual urinary amino acid pattern (Scriver, 1974; Scriver *et al.*, 1976).

Treatment with oral phosphate and large doses of vitamin D is universally advocated (Dent and Stamp, 1971; Kistler *et al.*, 1976; Parfitt, 1972; Scriver, 1976; Wilson *et al.*, 1965). Calcium balance becomes positive, and gut absorption of calcium and phosphorus is improved. Both radiologic and histologic evidence of bone healing is found, and, with rare exceptions (Dent and Friedman, 1964), phosphate and vitamin D administration must continue for life to avoid recurrence. Because of the overlap in findings between these patients and those with oncogenous rickets, a thorough search for a tumor is indicated.

2.1.5. Phosphate Leak in Idiopathic Hypercalciuria

Recently, it has been suggested that a renal tubular phosphate leak, not related to overt hyperparathyroidism, may be important in the pathogenesis of excessive urinary calcium excretion in some patients wtih idiopathic hypercalciuria (Bordier *et al.*, 1977). Hypercalciuria with numerous renal calculi occurring in families in a typical autosomal dominant fashion is the picture in this disorder. Patients usually fall into three clinical patterns: (1) absorptive hypercalciuria, wherein increased intestinal calcium absorption ultimately leads to excess urinary excretion; (2) a renal tubular defect in calcium reabsorption, known as renal hypercalciuria (Nordin *et al.*, 1972); and (3) hypercalciuria due to hyperparathyroidism with normal serum calcium levels, which is usually termed "normocalcemic primary hyperparathyroidism" (Broadus *et al.*, 1977; Willis *et al.*, 1969). The classical clinical and laboratory characteristics of normocalcemia, mild hypophosphatemia, hypercalciuria, and recurrent calcium phosphate and calcium oxalate lithiasis were first described by Fuller Albright and his colleagues (Albright *et al.*, 1953). The suggestion has surfaced for some patients with hypercalciuria that phosphate depletion resulting from a primary renal tubular phosphate leak may stimulate the synthesis of $1,25(OH)_2D_3$. With higher $1,25(OH)_2D_3$ levels, intestinal calcium absorption would appear (DeLuca, 1976), and hypercalciuria would ensue (Bordier *et al.*, 1977). In these patients, immunoreactive PTH levels are normal, and the renal phosphaturia would be the primary event. Bordier *et al.* (1977) explain the absence of rickets or osteomalacia in these patients by the suggestion that the site of phosphate leak in these patients differs from the nephron location perturbed in primary hypophosphatemic rickets. The elevated levels of $1,25(OH)_2D_3$ predicted on the basis of hypophosphatemia have been found in one study (Gray *et al.*, 1977). The proportion of patients with this disorder who have primary renal tubular phosphate reabsorptive defects remains to be clarified, but this leak appears to be milder than those found in the disorders previously discussed.

2.2. Secondary Renal Tubular Phosphate Hyperexcretion

Scriver has classified those forms of rickets or osteomalacia which impair primarily the availability of calcium and only secondarily the availability of phosphorus for the mineralization of bone matrix as "calciopenic" (Scriver, 1974). Calciopenic rickets includes those disorders which occur because the supply of the active form of vitamin D, $1,25(OH)_2D_3$, is decreased and its normal action on the intestine in terms of calcium absorption is inadequate (DeLuca, 1976). Reduced intestinal calcium absorption leads to decreased serum ionized calcium levels and elevation of immunoreactive PTH concentrations, thereby resulting in secondary hyperphosphaturia (Fraser *et al.*, 1967; Scriver, 1974). Both vitamin D deficiency and vitamin D dependency are clinical examples of this secondary renal tubular phosphate leak. Excessive PTH secretion also results in aminoaciduria and renal bicarbonate wasting by poorly understood mechanisms (Morris *et al.*, 1976); hence, phosphaturia is not an isolated event in these disorders as it is in the states of primary renal phosphate leak.

2.2.1. Vitamin D Deficiency

Calciopenic rickets almost invariably results from decreased vitamin D availability, since only bizarre circumstances would result in a calcium-free diet (Kooh *et al.*, 1977; Maltz *et al.*, 1970). Rarely an individual receiving total parenteral nutrition may be given a calcium-free and vitamin-D-deficient alimentation mixture (Gutcher and Chesney, 1978). Nutritional vitamin D deficiency, once the scourge of major urban industrialized areas of western Europe, the United Kingdom, and North America (Park, 1923), has all but disappeared with our knowledge of the value of vitamin-D-fortified foods. Malabsorption of vitamin D secondary to steatorrhea, gluten-induced enteropathy, biliary cirrhosis, and extrahepatic biliary atresia are predictable forms of vitamin D deficiency (Avioli and Haddad, 1973). Hepatic disease may also result in decreased 25-hydroxylase activity (Daum et al., 1975). D deficiency in pregnant women leads to decreased circulating 25OHD$_3$ [and presumably 1,25(OH)$_2$D$_3$ in offspring] (Moncrieff and Fadahunsi, 1974). Subnormal levels of 25OHD$_3$ are well described in patients on chronic anticonvulsant therapy, particularly in those patients with long-term drug exposure, marginal vitamin D intake, and scant exposure to sunshine (Silver et al., 1974). The combination of diphenylhydantoin and phenobarbital is felt to induce hepatic microsomal enzymes, which further convert 25OHD$_3$ into inactive metabolites by glucuronidation (Hahn et al., 1972).

There are disorders in which serum 1,25(OH)$_2$D$_3$ levels are decreased, but 25OHD$_3$ levels are normal or elevated. This would imply impaired renal 1α-hydroxylation. Three such disorders are uremia (Chesney et al., 1978), hypoparathyroidism (Chesney et al., 1977), and vitamin-D-dependency rickets (Fraser et al., 1973). In uremia, with reduced phosphate glomerular filtration, and in hypoparathyroidism, with absent PTH, one finds phosphate retention and hyperphosphatemia that can impair 1,25(OH)$_2$D$_3$ synthesis (Fig. 1).

The resultant hypocalcemia from any of these causes of vitamin D deficiency leads to increased PTH secretion (stage I rickets), which acts on bone to restore the serum calcium concentration to normal (stage II rickets) (Rasmussen and Bordier, 1974). Phosphate released from increased osteoclastic activity and bone dissolution is lost in the urine by virtue of the phosphaturic action of PTH (Knox et al., 1977; Butlen and Jard, 1972). As bone becomes resistant to PTH action, both serum calcium and phosphate levels are reduced (Jowsey, 1972) (stage III rickets as described in Scriver, 1974, and Fraser et al., 1967). The combination of PTH elevation and reduction of calcium and phosphate concentrations in both serum and cells may be important in the modulation or alteration of renal tubular function (Morris et al., 1976). The hyperexcretion of many solutes, including phosphate, bicarbonate, uric acid, amino acids, glucose, and sodium, may complicate stage III rickets and is sometimes readily reversible by provision of vitamin D (Chesney and Harrison, 1975) (Fig. 2). In addition, the phosphaturic effect of PTH is enhanced by hypocalcemia (Beck et al., 1974), possibly since ionized calcium is a recognized modulator of renal cortical adenyl cyclase activity (Marcus and

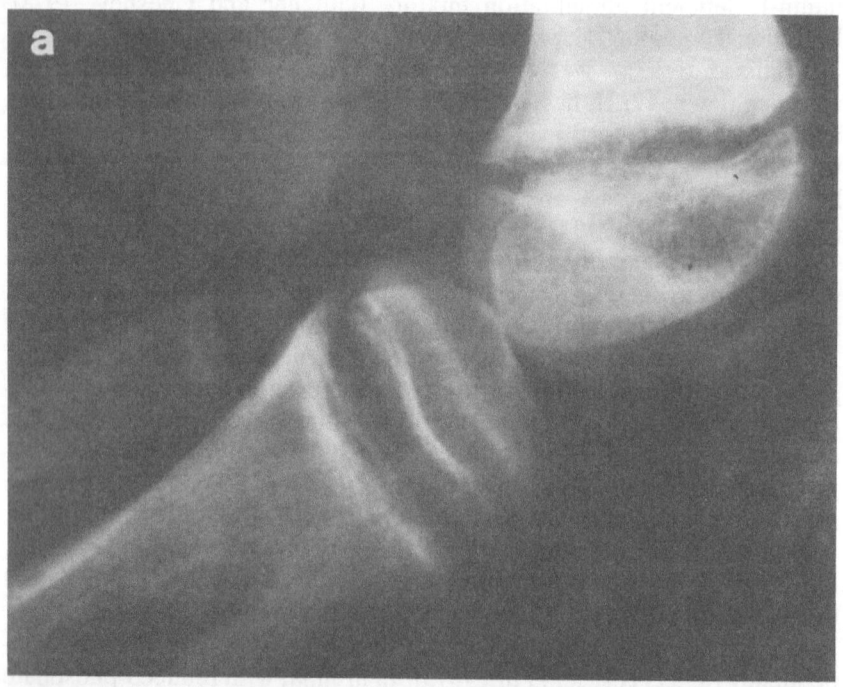

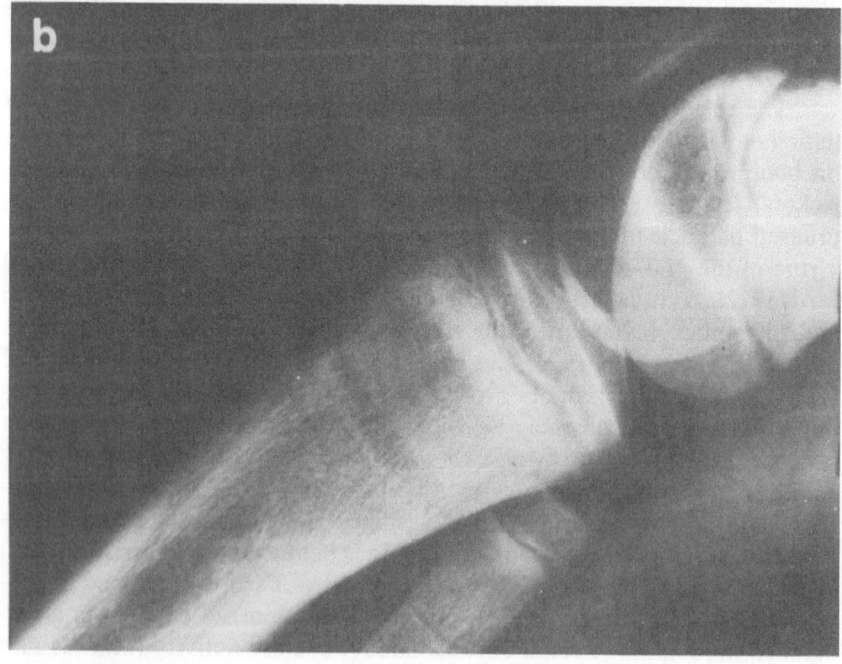

Aurbach, 1971). As reviewed in previous chapters of this volume, PTH acts on numerous sites along the nephron to produce nephrogenous cAMP (Broadus *et al.*, 1977). Since intraluminal cAMP may possibly induce phosphaturia, the accumulation of cyclic nucleotides derived from several locations may augment net phosphate excretion (Butlen and Jard, 1972). As suggested by others (Morris *et al.*, 1976), PTH may also play a role in the distribution of intrarenal blood flow, thereby augmenting phosphate excretion.

The therapy of D deficiency is directed by its cause: Simple D deficiency is reversed by 400 IU (10 µg) of D_2 daily; a dose of 7 µg of 25OHD$_3$ or 0.5–1.0 µg of 1,25(OH)$_2$D$_3$ will also be curative. Vitamin D dosage must be increased in those patients with malabsorption, hepatic disorders, or anticonvulsant-induced D deficiency (Avioli and Haddad, 1973). In the latter condition, a dose of 800 IU daily usually suffices (Hahn *et al.*, 1972). The role of ultraviolet light, once commonplace therapy in urban well-child clinics (Park, 1933), should not be forgotten in patients whose D deficiency is due to malabsorption. In all instances, once intestinal calcium absorption returns to normal, serum ionized calcium will rise, decreasing PTH secretion and reversing the phosphaturia. Thus, phosphate leak is primarily "calciopenic" (Scriver, 1974). In the rare instance where massive vitamin D doses are required to reverse stage III rickets, the genetic condition mentioned next should be considered.

2.2.2. Vitamin-D-Dependency Rickets

This autosomal recessive disorder is almost universally called vitamin D dependency, but the term "pseudodeficiency rickets" (pseudo-Mangel richitis) has been used since it resembles typical D deficiency in its clinical features. First described by Fraser and Salter (1958) and Prader *et al.* (1961), the striking similarity to D deficiency is evident from Table 3. D dependency may be clinically apparent by the age of 12 weeks. Muscle weakness, which is distinctly different from primary hypophosphatemic rickets, is another distinguishing feature. Other abnormalities include hypocalcemia, generalized hyperaminoaciduria, hypoplasia of dental enamel, and growth failure (Scriver, 1974). As the name suggests, this disorder is unaltered by physiologic doses of vitamin D_2 or D_3 (<400 IU/

Fig. 1. Serial knee radiographs from a patient with the idiopathic Fanconi syndrome before (a) and after (b) 23 months of therapy with 1,25(OH)$_2$D$_3$ (1.0 mg/day). During this time, serum 1,25(OH)$_2$D$_3$ levels rose from 2 to 59 pg/ml, serum immunoreactive PTH levels fell from 660 to 240 µEq/ml, and serum calcium rose from 8.3 to 10.0 mg/dl. Both healing of rickets and the filling in of a lesion of osteitis fibrosa cystica are evident in this patient described in Chesney *et al.* (1978) and Friedman *et al.* (1978).

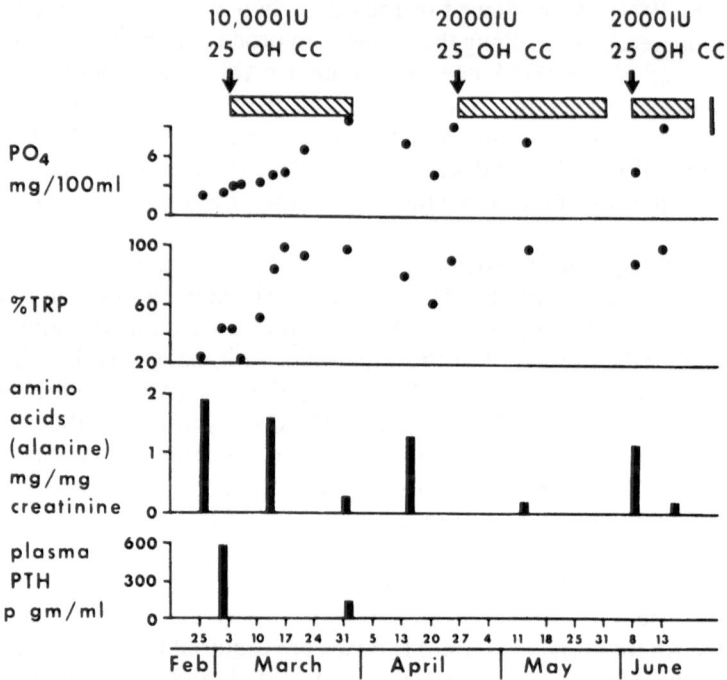

Fig. 2. The correction of the urinary abnormalities in a patient with the Fanconi syndrome secondary to bowel surgery, hepatitis, and vitamin D deficiency. Cross-hatched bars indicate the length and dose of 25OHD therapy. With treatment, serum phosphate rose, the percentage of TRP rose, and aminoaciduria disappeared. A fall in plasma immuno-reactive PTH levels is evident after vitamin D treatment. As vitamin D therapy was stopped, the findings of the Fanconi syndrome recurred. (From Chesney and Harrison, 1975. Reprinted with permission of the *Journal of Pediatrics*.)

day). Vitamin D is curative, but only at 100 times (25,000–100,000 IU/day) the physiologic dose, or approximately 1–2 mg daily. 1αOHD$_3$ and 1,25(OH)$_2$D$_3$ can completely reverse disease symptoms in the physiologic range (Fraser *et al.*, 1973; Reade *et al.*, 1975). The term "dependency" denotes that vitamin D will completely reverse all clinical and biochemical abnormalities, albeit in the pharmacologic range.

The major defect in the pathogenesis of this disorder is reduced calcium absorption (Hamilton *et al.*, 1970), which leads to the exact pathogenic sequence found in D-deficiency rickets (Scriver, 1974). Three patients with this disorder have been shown to have clear-cut hyperparathyroidism (Arnaud *et al.*, 1970), and malabsorption of vitamin D was excluded by elevated circulating 25OHD$_3$ levels in patients from whom oral vitamin D was withheld until recurrence of symptoms (Fraser *et al.*, 1973; Reade *et al.*, 1975). The study of Fraser *et al.* of providing $1,25(OH)_2D_3$ in physiologic amounts (1 μg daily) indirectly implies an inherited deficiency of 25OHD 1α-hydroxylase enzyme activity in renal cortical cells, particularly since the hypophosphatemia and hyperparathyroidism that prevail in these patients should actually enhance 1α-hydroxylase activity (DeLuca, 1976). However, to date, circulating $1,25(OH)_2D_3$ concentrations have not been reported. Should the thesis of Fraser *et al.* (1973) be correct, undetectable levels of this active D metabolite and elevated 25OHD levels should be found.

2.3. Phosphate Loss as Part of a Complex Tubulopathy

The excessive urinary loss of amino acids, phosphate, glucose, bicarbonate, uric acid, and tubular proteins (<50,000 mol. wt.) in conjunction with renal tubular acidosis and vasopressin-resistant polyuria defines the complex tubulopathy commonly termed the Fanconi syndrome (Harrison, 1958; Schneider and Seegmiller, 1972). Other features are rickets or osteomalacia, short stature, and, in children, delayed bone age for chronologic age. Other electrolytes, including calcium, magnesium, sodium, lithium, and potassium, may be lost. Low-molecular-weight proteins lost include many β-globulins, insulin, $β_2$-microglobulin, λ-L-chains, and lysozyme (Heinemann *et al.*, 1974). The fraction of radiolabeled λ-L-chains metabolized in patients with the Fanconi syndrome is reduced as an indication of tubular dysfunction (Waldmann *et al.*, 1972). The increased fractional excretion of all of these solutes is probably related to reduction of net tubular reabsorption, but net secretion of such compounds as *para*-aminohippurate may also be impaired (Houston *et al.*, 1968).

Leaf (1966) has written an excellent historical resume, making the point that "the recognition of the Fanconi syndrome has been confused by uncertainty as to just which features it encompasses and which eponyms should be applied to it. Not all the features recognized today as part of the syndrome were appreciated by earlier workers." Abderhalden, in 1903, is generally credited with the first description of cystinosis that showed it to be familial. (The reader is referred to Leaf, 1966, for these early references.) The separation of the cystinotic form from the other forms of this disorder, sometimes called the DeToni–Debré–Fanconi syndrome, was first made by McCune *et al.* (1943). McCune also was the first to show that the organic aciduria reported by Fanconi (1936) was largely due to excessive excretion of amino acids, later confirmed by Dent

(1947) using the paper chromatographic technique. Nonetheless, since the late 1930's the term encompassing all of the features of this complex tubulopathy is the Fanconi syndrome.

The numerous causes of the Fanconi syndrome and their accepted modes of inheritance are listed in Table 4. Many secondary disorders leading to the syndrome are genetically transmitted. An autosomal recessive mode of inheritance is evident in cystinosis, Wilson's disease, tyrosinemia, hereditary fructose intolerance, vitamin-D-dependent rickets, and glycogen storage disease (Garty et al., 1974; Morris et al., 1976). Lowe's syndrome is an X-linked recessive disorder (Scriver et al., 1976). Primary or idiopathic Fanconi syndrome, in which no obvious cause is found, may be sporadic or genetically transmitted (Figs. 3 and 4). Dominant inheritance has been noted in the reports of Hunt et al., (1966), Smith et al. (1976), Ben Ishay et al. (1961), and Friedman et al. (1978). In the latter case, renal failure at an early age was seen in two generations. Autosomal recessive inheritance has also been found (Doolan et al., 1962; Illig and Prader, 1961), as well as one possible instance of X-linked recessive inheritance (Neimann et al., 1968). Genetic factors are unimportant in the syndrome induced by exogenous toxins. Many of the causes listed in Table 4 have been reported only once or, at most, twice. Fanconi syndrome caused by outdated tetracycline is of interest, since it was a disease of physicians' and nurses' families using expired professional samples (Gross, 1963).

Little is known about the pathogenesis of the phosphate leak in the Fanconi syndrome other than in the form of the syndrome secondary to vitamin D deficiency in which excessive PTH secretion leads to phosphaturia (Chesney and Harrison, 1975; Fraser et al., 1967). The pathogenic mechanisms are best understood for hereditary fructose intolerance, where Morris and his co-workers (1971, 1976) have demonstrated the role of intracellular phosphate depletion and presumed insufficiency of high-energy phosphate compounds, leading to excessive solute excretion; unfortunately, excessive phosphaturia does not complicate hereditary fructose intolerance. The finding of "negative reabsorption" in some patients with the syndrome suggest more than decreased levels or loss of the phosphate or amino acid carrier(s) (Scriver et al., 1976). In any form of the syndrome, the defect could involve excessive backflux of solute from the luminal pole into the tubular fluid, either in the proximal tubule or in more distal sites in the nephron. Alternatively, phosphaturia could involve the presence of more leaky tubular membranes, particularly at the tight junctions between cells. Abnormalities of renal tubular cell intermediary metabolism may alter the integrity of tubular membranes or permit excessive exodus of solutes at the tubular apical pole.

Table 4. Causes and Genetics of the Fanconi Syndrome[a]

Disease	Mode of transmission
I. Disorders with a Demonstrable Inheritance Pattern	
A. Cystinosis	
1. Infantile (nephropathic)	Autosomal recessive
2. Adolescent	Autosomal recessive
3. Adult[b]	Autosomal recessive
B. Lowe's oculocerebrorenal syndrome	X-linked recessive
C. Tyrosinemia	Autosomal recessive
D. Galactosemia	Autosomal recessive
E. Glycogen storage disease	Sporadic or autosomal recessive
F. Hereditary fructose intolerance	Autosomal recessive
G. Wilson's disease	Autosomal recessive
H. Familial nephrotic syndrome	Autosomal recessive
II. Disorders in Which the Fanconi Syndrome Has Been Infrequently Reported	
A. Renal allografts	None
B. Myeloma of the kidney	None
C. Amyloidosis with Bence Jones proteinuria	Sometimes autosomal recessive
D. Nephrotic syndrome	None
E. Sjögren's syndrome	None
F. Pancreatic carcinoma	None
G. Hyperparathyroidism	None
H. Vitamin deficiency (B_{12}, C, D)	None
I. Potassium depletion	None
J. Interstitial nephritis with anit-tubular-basement-membrane antibodies	None
K. Infantile renal vein thrombosis	None
III. Chemical or Physical Toxins	
A. Heavy metals	None
1. Cadmium	
2. Mercury	
3. Organomercurials	
4. Leads	
5. Uranium	
B. Other chemicals	None
1. Lysol	
2. Salicylate	
3. Nitrobenzene	
4. Maleic acid	
5. Methyl-3-chrome	
6. Out-of-date tetracycline	

[a] Adapted from Scriver *et al.* (1976); Scriver and Bergeron (1974); Morris *et al.* (1976); Schneider and Seegmiller (1972); and Scriver and Rosenberg (1973a,b).
[b] Not associated with the Fanconi syndrome.

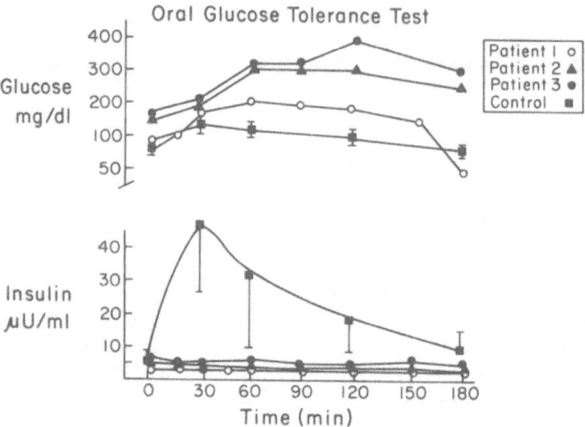

Fig. 3. Glucose intolerance and insulin hyposecretion in three patients with the idiopathic Fanconi syndrome. Each patient was given glucose by mouth (1.5 g/kg) after an 18-hr fast. The normal values for glucose concentrations and insulin concentrations for 44 control patients are shown. Ketonuria was also present in the patients with the Fanconi syndrome. (From Chesney et al., 1979.)

2.3.1. Miscellaneous Complex Tubulopathies Involving Phosphate Leaks

Luder–Sheldon Syndrome. This term is used to describe a family with generalized aminoaciduria and glucosuria in three successive generations inherited in an autosomal dominant fashion (Luder and Sheldon, 1955; Sheldon et al., 1960). The twin girls of the youngest generation developed renal phosphaturia and renal tubular acidosis, with rickets, hypophosphatemia, and genu valgum at least five years later. Phosphate supplementation was not curative, but it was administered only every 8 hr, and serum phosphate levels were not corrected. Vitamin D and phosphate therapy healed rickets. The separation in time of the features of this disorder makes it of interest, but the reasons for this finding are unclear.

Hypophosphatemia with Glycinuria, Glucosuria, and Glycylprolinuria. Rickets, bone pain, and growth failure developed between the ages of seven and nine years in a boy described in 1964 with this group of findings (Scriver et al., 1964). Continuous hypophosphatemia was related to excessive urinary excretion and glucosuria to a reduction in Tm for glucose. L-Proline infusion produced greater phosphaturia, and calcium infusion did not improve the percentage of TRP. Glycinuria was increased by proline infusion. Muscle weakness and biopsy-proven osteomalacia were cured at age 17 by oral phosphate. Glycylproline and bound hy-

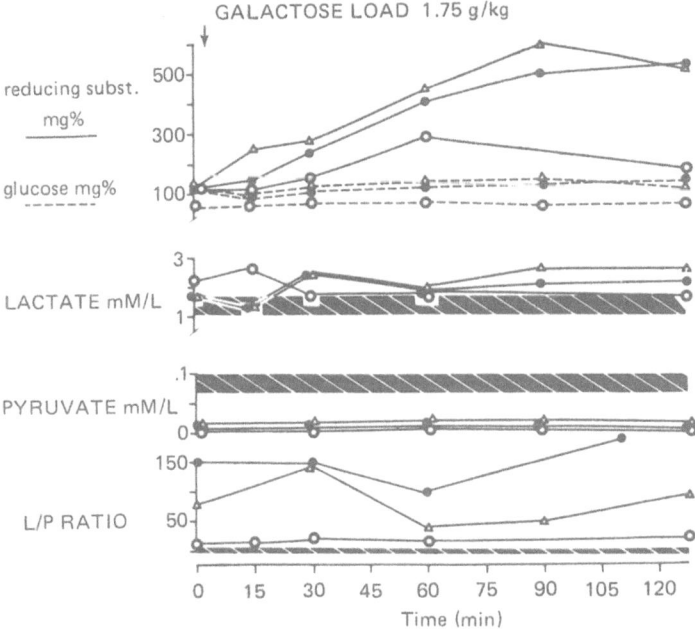

Fig. 4. Failure of galactose conversion to glucose with lactic acidosis in the same three patients with the idiopathic Fanconi syndrome. The upper portion of the curve shows the values for aldo sugars measured by the o-toluidine method and for glucose measured by the glucose oxidase method. The cross-hatched area represents normal values in healthy children. The lactate/pyruvate (L/P) ratios in these patients were altered, possibly because of an altered redox state (O, 1; △, 2; ●, 3). (From Chesney et al., 1979.)

droxyproline excretion disappeared after therapy, implying loss from bone. This patient also had intestinal calcium malabsorption and resembled in many ways those patients with adult-onset hypophosphatemic osteomalacia (Dent and Stamp, 1971; Segar et al., 1956).

3. CONDITIONS ASSOCIATED WITH INCREASED RENAL TUBULAR RETENTION OF PHOSPHATE

3.1. Pseudohypoparathyroidism (PHP)

Decreased urinary excretion of phosphate due to the absence of PTH action on the renal tubule is seen after surgical PTX; in idiopathic hypoparathyroidism (Schneider and Sherwood, 1975), familial hypoparathyroidism (Root and Harrison, 1976), Turner's syndrome, the Candida endocrinopathy syndrome (Chesney et al., 1977; Kirkpatrick et al., 1971), and the DiGeorge syndrome (absence of third and fourth pharyngeal pouches) (Harvey *et al.*, 1970); and after hypomagnesemic hypoparathyroidism, wherein PTH is not normally secreted by the parathyroids in response to hypocalcemia (Anast *et al.*, 1972). The mechanisms of this augmented retention of phosphate in the absence of PTH are amply covered in earlier portions of this book.

Originally, the term "pseudohypoparathyroidism" (PHP) was used by Albright and his colleagues (1942) to designate a disorder characterized by round facies, short stature, short fourth and fifth metacarpal and metatarsal bones, strabismus, cataracts, metastatic calcification of subcutaneous and basal ganglia, mental retardation, and hypocalcemic tetany (Potts, 1972). These patients have the laboratory and clinical features of hypoparathyroidism but do not have a phosphaturic response to exogenously administered PTH. Albright (Albright *et al.*, 1942), therefore, postulated that PHP was due to end-organ resistance to the phosphaturic action of PTH and likened this condition to the Seabright bantam rooster. Ten years later, Albright and his colleagues (1952) further described patients with similar developmental anomalies, but normal serum calcium and phosphorus levels, and termed this variant "pseudopseudohypoparathyroidism" (PPHP). PHP and PPHP can occur within the same kindred (Mann *et al.*, 1962), and hypocalcemia may be evident only after maturation with stresses such as pregnancy (Spranger, 1968). Today, however, PHP is the term used to designate a group of disorders in which resistance to the action of PTH is found (Chase *et al.*, 1969; Potts, 1972), and many of these patients have none of the somatic features mentioned above.

The genetic transmission of PHP is controversial. In most kindreds, an X-linked dominant or sex-influenced autosomal transmission seems most likely for the type known as Albright's hereditary osteodystrophy, or PHP type I (Gellis *et al.*, 1977; Mann *et al.*, 1962; Potts, 1972). Autosomal recessive transmission is possible in rare instances. The pattern for those forms without the typical somatic features of PHP type I is generally sporadic.

PTH-induced phosphaturia occurs after the steps of binding to a receptor in the basolateral membrane of the tubule and activation of adenyl cyclase to generate cAMP (Chase *et al.*, 1969; Marx *et al.*, 1972; Potts, 1972). Administration of PTH to normal individuals strikingly increases the plasma levels and urinary excretion of cAMP (Kaminsky *et al.*, 1970; Tomlinson *et al.*, 1976), and a brisk rise in cAMP excretion follows PTH infusion into hypoparathyroid and PPHP subjects (Chase *et al.*, 1969). As predicted by Albright *et al.* (1942), PHP patients do not show the rise in urinary excretion (Chase *et al.*, 1969) or in blood levels (Tomlinson *et al.*, 1976) of cAMP after exogenous PTH. Indeed, PHP patients have elevated levels of endogenous immunoreactive PTH, as expected from hypocalcemia, and these levels fall normally in response to calcium infusion (Potts, 1972). Fragments of PTH that are capable of promoting phosphaturia in normal subjects, hypoparathyroid subjects, and patients with PPHP, do not lead to cAMP excretion in PHP patients, indicating that a defect in metabolism and generation of the 1–34 fragment of PTH is unlikely (Neer *et al.*, 1977). These data seem to indicate that PTH nonresponsiveness represents the absence of or an abnormal form of the adenyl cyclase system in kidney and, by inference, in bone. Further evidence for this thesis is provided by the finding that cAMP, in this instance, dibutyryl cAMP, infused into PHP patients causes calcium retention and phosphaturia, identical to the situation in normal or hypoparathyroid subjects (Bell *et al.*, 1972). However, kidney cortex homogenates from a woman with PHP type I who died of pulmonary emboli demonstrate normal generation of cAMP following PTH stimulation (Marcus *et al.*, 1971). The authors speculated that any abnormal spatial relationship between membrane receptor binding and cyclase enzyme might have been distorted by preparation and freezing of her cortex, or, alternatively, the basic defect in PHP resides at a site beyond generation of this "second messenger."

Further investigations make the latter hypothesis seem plausible. Drezner *et al.* (1973) have described a patient without the physical stigmata of PHP type I but with hypocalcemia and PTH-resistant hyperphosphatemia who demonstrated normal urinary cAMP responses to PTH infusion. The authors termed this "PHP type II" (Drezner *et al.*, 1973). Rodriguez *et al.* (1974) have reported a patient who had the typical somatic features of Albright's hereditary osteodystrophy but a PHP type II renal response: increases in cAMP excretion following PTH infusion but no phosphaturia. In addition, the renal phosphaturic response to PTH was restored by calcium infusion; correction of the renal defect by vitamin D administration and normalization of serum calcium have also been shown (Suh *et al.*, 1970). Calcium may be responsible for the activation of physiologic or enzymatic reactions distal to the cAMP generation step in these patients, accounting for the phosphaturia.

To further confuse the pathophysiologic sequence that seemed likely after the studies of Chase *et al.* (1969), patients have been described with normal calcium levels and the physical and laboratory findings of PHP type I: absent phosphaturia and no rise in urinary cAMP after PTH (Balachander *et al.*, 1975). Another patient with PHP type I somatic features demonstrated PTH-induced phosphaturia but no rise in cAMP after normalization of calcium by vitamin D (Stögman and Fischer, 1975). Whether these patients reside at the vague borderlands between PHP and PPHP or have the absence of hypocalcemia and hyperphosphatemia often found in the first years of life is unclear (Monn *et al.*, 1976), but the term "PPHP" should probably be reserved for patients with persistent normocalcemia and normal urinary responses to PTH (Nusynowitz *et al.*, 1976). It is highly likely that other variants will be differentiated as the steps between the generation of cAMP and the final tubular responses of PTH are more clearly defined. Indeed, marked variability within a single family in terms of PTH levels and cAMP excretion has been described (Williams *et al.*, 1977).

Another class of patient demonstrates PHP and osteitis fibrosa cystica (Costello and Dent, 1963), wherein renal resistance to PTH is found but skeletal responsiveness is evident. These patients may have a normal phenotype or typical PHP type I somatic features (Frame *et al.*, 1972). These data suggest that hypocalcemia in this disorder, and indeed in all forms of PHP, could be the result of impaired formation of $1,25(OH)_2D_3$, leading to decreased, impaired gut calcium absorption and hyperparathyroidism (Bell *et al.*, 1964). $1,25(OH)_2D_3$ therapy has led to decreased fecal calcium excretion, reduction of immunoreactive PTH levels, and elevation of serum calcium concentrations (Kooh *et al.*, 1975; Sinha *et al.*, 1977). Furthermore, after PTH infusion into PHP subjects, impaired urinary calcium reabsorption is present, indicating additional tubular defects (Moses *et al.*, 1976). Where measured, serum $1,25(OH)_2D_3$ levels have been reduced (Drezner *et al.*, 1976; Metz *et al.*, 1977), and the hypocalcemia in this disorder appears to be related to a defect in the production of $1,25(OH)_2D_3$ (H. F. DeLuca and C. R. Scriver, personal communication). The provision of this active form of vitamin D corrects hypocalcemia and heals osteomalacia but, in general, does not alter the impaired cAMP or hypophosphaturic response. Long-term $1,25(OH)_2D_3$ therapy seems to ultimately reduce serum phosphate levels, possibly by the influence of prolonged normocalcemia (Werder *et al*, 1976). The reasons for the failure of $1,25(OH)_2D_3$ production in normal quantities by renal tubular cells are not known but could involve the inhibition of intracellular hyperphosphatemia (DeLuca, 1976), a blunted response to PTH which normally increases $1,25(OH)_2D_3$ production (Wright, 1975), or other factors. Therapy with 1α analogues of vitamin D seems indicated by these studies.

Other evidence suggests that PHP is a heterogeneous hormonal disorder, and deficiencies of prolactin (Carlson *et al.*, 1977) and thyrotropin secretion (Zisman *et al.*, 1969) and excessive thyrotropin response to thyrotropin-releasing factor with hypothyroidism have been described (Marx *et al.*, 1971; Werder *et al.*, 1975). The significance of these other deficiencies is unclear.

The major clinical forms of PHP are listed in Table 5.

A peculiar form of PHP has been described in a patient without somatic features of PHP type I. This patient had normal to high levels of

Table 5. Clinical Variation within Pseudohypoparathyroidism

1. Pseudohypoparathyroidism type I
   Skeletal and renal resistance to PTH; phenotypic somatic features (Albright *et al.*, 1942; Chase *et al.*, 1969; Potts, 1972)
2. Pseudopseudohypoparathyroidism
   Skeletal and renal responsiveness to PTH; phenotypic somatic features (Albright *et al.*, 1952; Chase *et al.*, 1969; Mann *et al.*, 1962; Potts, 1972)
3. Hypohyperparathyroidism
   Renal resistance to PTH with skeletal responsiveness (osteitis fibrosa cystica); normal features (Bell *et al.*, 1972)
4. Pseudohypoparathyroidism
   Renal resistance to PTH with skeletal responsiveness (osteitis fibrosa cystica); phenotypic somatic features (Bell *et al.*, 1964; Frame *et al.*, 1972)
5. Pseudohypoparathyroidism
   Skeletal resistance to PTH with renal responsiveness; phenotypic somatic features (Nusynowitz *et al.*, 1976)
6. Skeletal resistance to PTH with renal responsiveness with $1,25(OH)_2D_3$ deficiency; normal features (Metz *et al.*, 1977)
7. Pseudohypoparathyroidism type II
   Abnormal renal tubular response to cAMP with correction of responsiveness with normalization of serum calcium; phenotypic somatic features (Rodriguez *et al.*, 1974; Suh *et al.*, 1970)
8. Pseudohypoparathyroidism type II
   Abnormal renal tubular response to cAMP; normal features (Drezner *et al.*, 1973)
9. Pseudohypoparathyroidism
   Renal and skeletal resistance to PTH; phenotypic somatic features with normocalcemia (Balachandar *et al.*, 1975)
10. Pseudoidiopathic hypoparathyroidism
    High biologically inactive levels of PTH; normal features (Nusynowitz and Klein, 1973)

immunoreactive PTH to which his renal tubules and bone were unresponsive, but exogenous PTH led to normal urinary responses (Nusynowitz and Klein, 1973). These findings suggest abnormal metabolism of PTH or production of defective hormone in this patient.

3.2. Other Conditions of Phosphate Retention

Hyperphosphatemia of renal failure is discussed extensively in Chapter 12. Hyperphosphatemia from an increase in Tm for phosphate is commonly found in states of excessive growth hormone secretion (Cattaneo *et al.*, 1964). Administration of this hormone to humans causes phosphate retention within a day, independent of changes in glomerular filtration rate and serum phosphate levels (Corvilain *et al.*, 1962; Ikkos *et al.*, 1959). Thyroparathyroidectomy of experimental animals does not influence growth-hormone-induced decreases in phosphate excretion; PTH administration to these animals results in brisk phosphaturia (Lambert and Corvilain, 1963). Elevated Tm for phosphate and phosphate retention are seen in acromegaly (Cattaneo *et al.*, 1964) and in children in the growth phase (Harrison, 1977). Serum phosphate values from 4.6 to 8.1 mg/dl may be normal at various ages during childhood. The effects of these various hormones on urinary and serum phosphate are discussed in detail in Chapter 6. The mechanisms for increased phosphate retention in phosphate deprivation are discussed in Chapter 9.

ACKNOWLEDGMENTS. It became apparent in the writing of this chapter that proper recognition of the contributions of individual laboratories in the generation of data on the tubular disorders of phosphate transport would expand the number of references beyond a reasonable number, and, hence, many secondary references are cited. I hope that no investigator will interpret a lack of primary citation as a lack of appreciation of his or her efforts. I am grateful for the opportunity to collaborate with Drs. Harold E. Harrison, Charles R. Scriver, and Hector F. DeLuca over the past decade. Discussions with L. V. Avioli, E. McSherry, R. R. McInnes, H. Tenenhouse, S. F. Wen, and T. H. Steele were particularly helpful in the preparation of this chapter. The secretarial assistance of Kathy Chenoweth-Corby is gratefully appreciated. The writing of this chapter was supported, in part, by NIH grant AM19489.

4. REFERENCES

Albright, F., Butler, A. M., and Bloomberg, E., 1937, Rickets resistant to vitamin D therapy, *Am. J. Dis. Child.* **54**:529.

Albright, F., Burnett, C. H., Smith, P. H., and Parson, W., 1942, Pseudohypoparathyroidism—an example of the "Seabright–Bantam" syndrome, *Endocrinology* **30**:922.

Albright, F., Forbes, A. P., and Henneman, P. H., 1952, Pseudopseudohypoparathyroidism, *Trans. Assoc. Am. Physicians* **65**:337.

Albright, F., Henneman, P., Benedict, P. H., and Forbes, A. P., 1953, Idiopathic hypercalciuria, *Proc. R. Soc. Med.* **46**:1077.

Anast, C. S., Mohs, J. M., Kaplan, S. L., and Burns, T. W., 1972, Evidence for parathyroid failure in magnesium deficiency, *Science* **177**:606.

Arnaud, C., Maijer, R., Reade, T., Scriver, C. R., and Whelan, D. T., 1970, Vitamin D dependency: An inherited postnatal syndrome with secondary hyperparathyroidism, *Pediatrics* **46**:871.

Arnaud, C., Glorieux, F., and Scriver, C. R., 1971, Serum parathyroid hormone in X-linked hypophosphatemia, *Science* **173**:845.

Arnstein, A. R., and Hansen, C. A., 1969, Nature of renal phosphate leak, *N. Engl. J. Med.* **281**:1427.

Aschinberg, L. C., Solomon, L. M., Zeis, P. M., Justine, P., and Rosenthal, I. M., 1977, Vitamin D-resistant rickets associated with epidermal nevus syndrome: Demonstration of a phosphaturic substance in the dermal lesions, *J. Pediatr.* **91**:56.

Avioli, L. V., and Haddad, J. G., 1973, Vitamin D: Current concepts, *Metabolism* **22**:507.

Avioli, L. V., Williams, T. F., Lund, J., and DeLuca, H. F., 1967, Metabolism of vitamin D$_3$-^{3}H in vitamin D-resistant rickets and familial hypophosphatemia, J. Clin. Invest. 46:1907.

Balachandar, V., Pahuja, J., Maddaiah, V. T., and Collipp, P. J., 1975, Pseudohypoparathyroidism with normal serum calcium levels, Am. J. Dis. Child. 129:1092.

Balsan, S., and Garabedian, M., 1972, 25-Hydroxycholecalciferol. A comparative study in deficiency rickets and different types of resistant rickets, J. Clin. Invest. 51:749.

Beck, N., Singh, H., Reeds, S. W., and Davis, B. B., 1974, Direct inhibitory effect of hypercalcemia on renal action of parathyroid hormone, J. Clin. Invest. 53:717.

Bell, N. H., Gerard, E. S., and Bartter, F. C., 1964, Pseudohypoparathyroidism with osteitis fibrosa cystica and impaired absorption of calcium, J. Clin. Endocrinol. Metab. 23:759.

Bell, N. H., Avery, S., Sinha, T., Clark, C. M., Jr., Allen, D. O., and Johnson, C., Jr., 1972, Effects of dibutyryl cyclic adenosine 3',5'-monophosphate and parathyroid extract on calcium and phosphorus metabolism in hypoparathyroidism and pseudohypoparathyroidism, J. Clin. Invest. 51:816.

Ben-Ishay, D., Dreyfuss, F., and Ullman, T. D., 1961, Fanconi syndrome with hypouricemia in an adult, Am. J. Med. 31:793.

Bianchine, J. W., Stambler, A. A., and Harrison, H. E., 1971, Familial hypophosphatemic rickets showing autosomal dominant inheritance. The clinical delineation of birth defects. X. The endocrine system, Birth Defects Orig. Artic. Ser. 7(6):287.

Blackard, W. G., Robinson, R. R., and White, J. E., 1962, Familial hypophosphatemia: Report of a case with observations regarding pathogenesis, N. Engl. J. Med. 266:899.

Bordier, P., Ryckewart, A., Gueris, J., and Rasmussen, H., 1977, On the pathogenesis of so-called idiopathic hypercalciuria, Am. J. Med. 63:398.

Brickman, A. S., Coburn, J. W., Kurokawa, K., Bethune, J. E., Harrison, H. E., and Norman, A. W., 1973, Actions of 1,25-dihydroxycholecalciferol in patients with hypophosphatemic, vitamin D-resistant rickets, N. Engl. J. Med. 289:495.

Broadus, A. E., Mahaffey, J. E., Bartter, F. C., and Neer, R. M., 1977, Nephrogenous cyclic adenosine monophosphate as a parathyroid function test, J. Clin. Invest. 60:771.

Brunette, M. G., Chabardès, D., Imbert-Teboul, M., Clique, A., Montegut, M., and Morel, F., 1977, Hormone sensitive adenylate cyclase activity along the nephron of genetic hypophosphatemic mice, Kidney Int. 12:454.

Butlen, D., and Jard, S., 1972, Renal handling of 3'5'-cyclic AMP in the rat. The possible role of luminal 3',5'-cyclic AMP in the tubular reabsorption of phosphate, Pflügers Arch. 331:172.

Carlson, H. E., Brickman, A. S., and Bottazzo, G. F., 1977, Prolactin deficiency in pseudohypoparathyroidism, N. Engl. J. Med. 296:140.

Cartier, P., Leroux, J. P., Balsan, S., and Royer, P., 1970, Etude de la glycolyse et de la perméabilité des erythrocytes aux ions orthophosphates dans le rachitisime vitamerésistant hypophosphatémique héréditaire, Clin. Chim. Acta. 29:261.

Cattaneo, C., Martini, P. F., and Modica, A., 1964, The maximum tubular reabsorption of phosphate in acromegaly, Acta Endocrinol. 45:203.

Chabardès, D., Imbert, M., Clique, A., Montegut, M., and Morel, F., 1975, PTH-sensitive adenyl cyclase activity in different segments of the rabbit nephron, Pflügers Arch. 354:229.

Chase, L. R., Melson, G. L., and Aurbach, G. D., 1969, Pseudohypoparathyroidism: Defective excretion of 3'5'-AMP in response to parathyroid hormone, J. Clin. Invest. 48:1832.

Chesney, R. W., and Harrison, H. E., 1975, Fanconi syndrome following bowel surgery and hepatitis reversed by 25-hydroxycholecalciferol, J. Pediatr. 86:857.

Chesney, R. W., Horowitz, S. D., Kream, B. E., Eisman, J. A., Hong, R., and DeLuca,

H. F., 1977, Failure of conventional doses of 1α,25-dihydroxycholecalciferol to correct hypocalcemia in idiopathic hypoparathyroidism, *N. Engl. J. Med.* **297**:1272.

Chesney, R. W., Moorthy, A. V., Jax, D. K., Eisman, J. A., Mazess, R. B., and DeLuca, H. F., 1978, Increased linear growth after long term oral 1,25(OH)₂ vitamin D therapy in childhood renal osteodystrophy, *N. Engl. J. Med.* **298**:238.

Chesney, R. W., Colle, E., Scriver, C. R., McInnes, R. R., Kaplan, B. S., Dupont, C. H., Mohyuddin, F., Goldman, H., and Drummond, K. N., 1979, Glucose intolerance and altered lactate/pyruvate ratio in idiopathic Fanconi syndrome, *Pediatr. Res.* (in press).

Clarkson, T. W., and Kench, J. E., 1962, Urinary excretion of amino acids by men absorbing heavy metals, *Biochem. J.* **62**:361.

Condon, J. R., Nassim, J. R., and Rutter, A., 1971, Pathogenesis of rickets and osteomalacia in familial hypophosphatemia, *Arch. Dis. Child.* **46**:269.

Corvilain, J., Abramow, M., and Bergans, M., 1962, Some effects of human growth hormone on renal hemodynamics on tubular phosphate transport in man, *J. Clin. Invest.* **41**:1230.

Costello, J. M., and Dent, C. E., 1963, Hypo–hyperparathyroidism, *Arch. Dis. Child.* **38**:397.

Cowgill, L., Goldfarb, S., Goldberg, M., Slatopolsky, E., and Agus, Z. S., 1977, Nature of the renal defect in familial hypophosphatemic rickets, *Clin. Res.* **25**:505A.

Daum, F., Rosen, J. F., Roginsky, M., Cohen, M. I., and Finberg, L., 1975, 25-Hydroxy-vitamin D₃ (25-OHD₃) metabolism in children with biliary atresia, *Pediatr. Res.* **9**:302.

DeLuca, H. F., 1976, Recent advances in our understanding of the vitamin D endocrine system, *J. Lab. Clin. Med.* **87**:7.

DeLuca, H. F., Lund, J., Rosenbloom, A. R., and Lobeck, C. C., 1967, Metabolism of tritiated vitamin D₃ in familial vitamin D-resistant rickets with hypophosphatemia, *J. Pediatr.* **70**:828.

Dent, C. E., 1947, The amino aciduria in Fanconi syndrome: A study making extensive use of techniques based on paper partition chromatography, *Biochem. J.* **41**:240.

Dent, C. E., and Friedman, M., 1964, Hypophosphatemic osteomalacia with complete recovery, *Br. Med. J.* **1**:1676.

Dent, C. E., and Gertner, J. M., 1976, Hypophosphatemic osteomalacia in fibrous dysplasia, *Q. J. Med.* **45**:411.

Dent, C. E., and Stamp, T. C. B., 1971, Hypophosphatemic osteomalacia presenting in adults, *Q. J. Med.* **40**:303.

Doolan, P. D., Morris, M. D., and Harper, H. A., 1962, Amino-aciduria in an elderly man with the nephrotic syndrome and in a young man with a variant of the Fanconi syndrome, *Ann. Intern. Med.* **56**:448.

Drezner, M. K., and Feinglos, M. N., 1977, Osteomalacia due to 1α,25-dihydroxychole-calciferol deficiency, *J. Clin. Invest.* **60**:1046.

Drezner, M. K., Neelon, F. A., and Lebovitz, H. E., 1973, Pseudohypoparathyroidism type II: A possible defect in the reception of the cyclic AMP signal, *N. Engl. J. Med.* **289**:1056.

Drezner, M. K., Neelon, F. A., Haussler, M., McPherson, H. T., and Lebovitz, H. E., 1976, 1,25-Dihydroxycholecalciferol deficiency: The probable cause of hypocalcemia and metabolic bone disease in pseudohypoparathyroidism, *J. Clin. Endocrinol. Metab.* **42**:621.

Earp, H. S., Ney, R. L., Gitelman, H. J., Richman, R., and DeLuca, H. F., 1970, Effects of 25-hydroxycholecalciferol in patients with familial hypophosphatemia and vitamin D-resistant rickets, *N. Engl. J. Med.* **283**:627.

Eicher, E. M., Southard, J. L., Scriver, C. R., and Glorieux, F. H., 1976, Hypophospha-temia: Mouse model for human familial hypophosphatemic (vitamin D-resistant) rickets, *Proc. Natl. Acad. Sci. U.S.A.* **73**:4667.

Falkson, G., and Frame, B., 1958, Phosphate diabetes, a review, *Henry Ford Hosp. Med. Bull.* **6:**244.

Falls, W. F., Jr., Carter, N. W., Rector, F. W., and Seldin, D. W., 1968, Familial vitamin D-resistant rickets: Study of six cases with evaluation of the pathogenic role of secondary hyperparathyroidism, *Ann. Intern. Med.* **68:**553.

Fanconi, G., 1936, Der fruhinfantile nephrotische-glykosurische Zwergwuchs mit hypophosphatämischer Rachitis, *Jahrb. Kinderheilkd.* **147:**299.

Fanconi, G., 1956, Variations in sensitivity to vitamin D, in: *Ciba Foundation Symposium on Bone Structure and Metabolism* (G. E. W. Wolstenholme and G. M. O'Connor, eds.), pp. 187–205, J. and A. Churchill, London.

Fanconi, A., and Fischer, J. A., 1976, Parathyroid hormone in hereditary diseases of mineral metabolism, in: *Inborn Errors of Calcium and Bone Metabolism* (H. Bickel and J. Stern, eds.), pp. 52–62, University Park Press, Baltimore.

Fanconi, G., and Girardot, P., 1952, Familiarer pessistierender Phosphatdiabetes mit D-Vitamin-resistenter Rachitis, *Helv. Paediatr. Acta* **7:**14.

Fanconi, A., Fischer, J. A., and Prader, A., 1974, Serum parathyroid hormone concentration in hypophosphatemic vitamin D resistant rickets, *Helv. Paediatr. Acta* **29:**187.

Field, M. J., and Reiss, E., 1960, Vitamin D-resistant rickets: The effect of calcium infusion on phosphate reabsorption, *J. Clin. Invest.* **39:**1807.

Frame, B., Smith, R. W., Jr., Fleming, J. L., and Hanson, G., 1963, Oral phosphates in vitamin D-refractory rickets and osteomalacia, *Am. J. Dis. Child.* **106:**147.

Frame, B., Hanson, C. A., Frost, H. M., Block, M., and Arnstein, A. R., 1972, Renal resistance to parathyroid hormone with osteitis fibrosa "pseudohypohyperparathyroidism," *Am. J. Med.* **52:**311.

Fraser, D., and Salter, R. B., 1958, The diagnosis and management of the various types of rickets, *Pediatr. Clin. North Am.* **26:**417.

Fraser, D., and Scriver, C. R., 1976, Familial forms of vitamin D-resistant rickets revisited. X-linked hypophosphatemia and autosomal recessive vitamin D dependency, *Am. J. Clin. Nutr.* **29:**1315.

Fraser, D., Kooh, S. W., and Scriver, C. R., 1967, Hyperparathyroidism as the cause of hyperaminoaciduria and phosphaturia in human vitamin D deficiency, *Pediatr. Res.* **1:**425.

Fraser, D., Kooh, S. W., Kind, H. P., Holick, M. F., Tanaka, Y., and DeLuca, H. F., 1973, Pathogenesis of hereditary vitamin D-dependent rickets. An inborn error of vitamin D metabolism involving defective conversion of 25-hydroxyvitamin D to 1α,25-dihydroxyvitamin D, *N. Engl. J. Med.* **289:**817.

Friedman, A. L., Chesney, R. W., and Trygstad, C., 1978, Autosomal dominant idiopathic Fanconi syndrome with early renal failure, *Am. J. Med. Genet.* **2:**225.

Fritzell, S., Jagenburg, R., and Schnürer, L. B., 1964, Familial occurrence of coarse nodular cirrhosis, renal tubular defects and vitamin D resistant rickets associated with impaired tyrosine metabolism, *Acta Paediatr. Scand.* **53:**18.

Frymoyer, J. W., and Hodgkin, W., 1977, Adult-onset vitamin D-resistant hypophosphatemic osteomalacia, *J. Bone Jt. Surg.* **59A:**101.

Garty, R., Cooper, M., and Tabaelinek, E., 1974, The Fanconi syndrome associated with hepatic glycogenosis and abnormal metabolism of galactose, *J. Pediatr.* **85:**821.

Gellis, S. S., Feingold, M., Farriaux, J. P., and Fontaine, G., 1977, Pseudohypoparathyroidism, *Am. J. Dis. Child.* **131:**807.

Gerbaux-Balsan, S., 1965, L'absorption intestinale du phosphore dans le rachitisme vitamine-résistant hypophosphatémique héréditaire. Effets de fortes surcharges de phosphore et des régimes très pauvres en calcium, *Rev. Fr. Etud. Clin. Biol.* **10:**65.

Glanville, H. J., and Bloom, R., 1965, Case of renal tubular osteomalacia (Dent type 2) with later development of autonomous parathyroid tumors, *Br. Med. J.* **2**:26.

Glorieux, F., and Scriver, C. R., 1972, Loss of a parathyroid hormone-sensitive component of phosphate transport in X-linked hypophosphatemia, *Science* **175**:997.

Glorieux, F. H., and Scriver, C. R., 1973, Transport, metabolism and clinical use of inorganic phosphate in X-linked hypophosphatemia, in: *The Clinical Aspects of Metabolic Bone Disease* (B. Frame, A. M. Parfitt, and H. Duncan, eds.), pp. 421–426, Excerpta Medica ICS, Amsterdam.

Glorieux, F. H., and Scriver, C. R., 1974, Parathyroid hormone secretion in X-linked hypophosphatemia, *N. Engl. J. Med.* **290**:1329.

Glorieux, F. H., Scriver, C. R., Reade, T. M., Goldman, H., and Roseborough, A., 1972, Use of phosphate and vitamin D to prevent dwarfism and rickets in X-linked hypophosphatemia, *N. Engl. J. Med.* **287**:481.

Glorieux, F. H., Scriver, C. R., Holick, M. F., and DeLuca, H. F., 1973, X-linked hypophosphatemic rickets: Inadequate therapeutic response to 1,25-dihydroxycholecalciferol, *Lancet* **2**:287.

Glorieux, F. H., Morin, C. L., Travers, R., Delvin, E. E., and Porier, R., 1976, Intestinal phosphate transport in familial hypophosphatemia, *Pediatr. Res.* **10**:691.

Gray, R. W., Wilz, D. R., Caldas, A. E., and Lemann, J., Jr., 1977, The importance of phosphate in regulating plasma 1,25-(OH)$_2$-vitamin D levels in humans: Studies in healthy subjects, in calcium stone formers and in patients with primary hyperparathyroidism, *J. Clin. Endocrinol. Metab.* **45**:299.

Grose, J. H., and Scriver, C. R., 1968, Parathyroid-dependent phosphaturia and aminoaciduria in the vitamin D-deficient rat, *Am. J. Physiol.* **214**:370.

Gross, J. M., 1963, Fanconi syndrome (adult type) developing secondary to the ingestion of outdated tetracycline, *Ann. Intern. Med.* **58**:523.

Gutcher, G., and Chesney, R. W., 1978, Hyperalimentation rickets: The failure to provide calcium and vitamin D in alimentation therapy, *Clin. Pediatr.* **17**:817.

Haddad, J. G., Jr., Chyu, K. J., Hahn, T. J., and Stamp, T. C. B., 1973, Serum concentrations of 25-hydroxyvitamin D in sex-linked hypophosphatemic vitamin D-resistant rickets, *J. Lab. Clin. Med.* **81**:22.

Hahn, T. J., Hendin, B. A., Scharp, C. R., and Haddad, J. G., Jr., 1972, Effect of chronic anticonvulsant therapy on serum 25-hydroxycholecalciferol levels in adults, *N. Engl. J. Med.* **287**:900.

Hahn, T. J., Scharp, C. R., Halstead, L. R., Haddad, J. G., Karl, D. M., and Avioli, L. V., 1975, Parathyroid hormone status and renal responsiveness in familial hypophosphatemic rickets, *J. Clin. Endocrinol. Metab.* **41**:926.

Hamilton, J. R., Harrison, J., Fraser, D., Radde, I., Morecki, R., and Paunier, L., 1970, The small intestine in vitamin D dependent rickets, *Pediatrics* **45**:364.

Harrison, H. E., 1958, The Fanconi syndrome, *J. Chronic Dis.* **7**:346.

Harrison, H. E., 1959, Discussion after paper by Fraser *et al.*, *Helv. Paediatr. Acta* **14**:504.

Harrison, H. E., 1973, Oncogenous rickets: Possible elaboration by a tumor of a humoral substance inhibiting tubular reabsorption of phosphate, *Pediatrics* **52**:432.

Harrison, H. E., 1977, Vitamin D and the metabolism of calcium, phosphate and bone, in: *Pediatrics* (A. M. Rudolph, ed.), pp. 235–237, Appleton-Century-Crofts, New York.

Harrison, H. E., and Harrison, H. C., 1975, Rickets then and now, *J. Pediatr.* **87**:1144.

Harrison, H. E., Harrison, H. C., Lifshitz, F., and Johnson, A. D., 1966, Growth disturbance in hereditary hypophosphatemia, *Am. J. Dis. Child.* **112**:290.

Harrison, J. E., Cumming, W. A., Fornasier, V., Fraser, D., Kooh, S. W., and McNeill, K. G., 1976, Increased bone mineral content in young adults with familial hypophosphatemic vitamin D refractory rickets, *Metabolism* **25**:33.

Harvey, J. C., Dungan, W. T., Elders, M. J., and Hugher, E. R., 1970, Third and fourth pharyngeal pouch syndrome associated with vascular anomalies and hypocalcemic seizures, *Clin. Pediatr.* **9**:496.

Haussler, M. R., and McCain, T. A., 1977, Basic and clinical concepts related to vitamin D metabolism and action, *N. Engl. J. Med.* **297**:974.

Haussler, M. R., Baylink, D. J., Hughes, M. R., Brumbach, P. F. Wergedal, J. E., Shen, F. H., Nielsen, R. S., Counts, S. S., Bursac, K. M., and McCain, T. A., 1976, The assay of 1α,25-dihydroxyvitamin D_3: Physiologic and pathologic modulation of circulating hormone levels, *Clin. Endocrinol.* **5**:151s.

Heinemann, H. O., Maack, T. M., and Sherman, R. L., 1974, Proteinuria, *Am. J. Med.* **56**:71.

Henneman, P. H., Dempsey, E. F., Carroll, E. L., and Henneman, D. H., 1962, Acquired vitamin D-resistant osteomalacia: A new variety characterized by hypercalcemia, low serum bicarbonate and hyperglycinuria, *Metabolism* **11**:103.

Houston, I. B., Boichis, M., and Edelman, C. M., 1968, Fanconi syndrome with renal sodium wasting and metabolic alkalosis, *Am. J. Med.* **44**:638.

Hunt, D. D., Stearns, G., McKinley, J. B., Froning, E., Hicks, P., and Bonfiglio, M., 1966, Long-term study of family with Fanconi syndrome without cystinosis (DeToni–Debré–Fanconi syndrome), *Am. J. Med.* **40**:492.

Ikkos, D., Luft, R., and Gemzell, C. A., 1959, The effect of human growth hormone in man, *Acta Endocrinol.* **32**:341.

Illig, V. R., and Prader, A., 1961, Primaire tubulopathien. II. Ein fall von idiopathischem gluko-amino-phosphat-diabetes (DeToni–Debré–Fanconi syndrome), *Helv. Paediatr. Acta* **16**:622.

Jowsey, J., 1972, Calcium release from the skeletons of rachitic puppies, *J. Clin. Invest.* **51**:9.

Kaminsky, N. I., Broadus, A. E., Hardman, D., Jones, J., Jr., Ball, J. H., Sutherland, E. W., and Liddle, G. W., 1970, Effects of parathyroid hormone on plasma and urinary adenosine 3′5′-monophosphate in man, *J. Clin. Invest.* **49**:2387.

Kirkpatrick, C. H., Rich, R. R., and Bennett, J. E., 1971, Chronic mucocutaneous candidiasis: Model building in cellular immunity, *Ann. Intern. Med.* **74**:955.

Kistler, H. J., Bonetti, A., Frey, P., and Fischer, J. A., 1976, Sporadische hypophosphatämische vitamin-D-resistente Osteomalazie (Phosphatdiabetes) im Erwachsenenalter and Hyperparathyreoidismus, *Schweiz. Med. Wochenschr.* **106**:1855.

Kleerekoper, M., Coffey, R., Greco, T., Nichols, S., Cooke, N., Murphy, W., and Avioli, L. V., 1977, Hypercalcemic hyperparathyroidism in hypophosphatemic rickets, *J. Clin. Endocrinol. Metab.* **45**:86.

Knox, F. G., Osswald, H., Marchand, G. R., Spielman, W. S., Haas, J. A., Berndt, T., and Youngberg, S. P., 1977, Phosphate transport along the nephron, *Am. J. Physiol.* **233**:F261.

Kooh, S. W., Fraser, D., DeLuca, H. F., Holick, M. F., Belsey, R. E., Clark, M. B., and Murray, T. M., 1975, Treatment of hypoparathyroidism and pseudohypoparathyroidism with metabolites of vitamin D: Evidence for impaired conversion of 25-hydroxyvitamin D to 1α,25-dihydroxyvitamin D, *N. Engl. J. Med.* **293**:840.

Kooh, S. W., Fraser, D., Reilly, B. J., Hamilton, J. R., Gall, D. G., and Bell, L., 1977, Rickets due to calcium deficiency, *N. Engl. J. Med.* **297**:1264.

Kranhold, J. F., Loh, D., and Morris, R. C., Jr., 1969, Renal fructose-metabolizing enzymes: Significance in hereditary fructose intolerance, *Science* **165**:402.

Lambert, P. P., and Corvilain, J., 1963, Site of action of parathyroid hormone and role of growth hormone in phosphate excretion, in: *Hormones and the Kidney* (P. C. Williams, ed.), pp. 139–147, Academic Press, London.

Lavender, A. R., and Pullman, T. N., 1963, Changes in inorganic phosphate excretion induced by the renal arterial infusion of calcium, *Am. J. Physiol.* **205:**1025.

Leaf, A., 1966, The syndrome of osteomalacia, renal glycosuria, aminoaciduria and increased phosphate clearance (the Fanconi syndrome), in: *Metabolic Basis of Inherited Disease* (J. B. Stanbury, J. B. Wyngaarden, and D. S. Fredrickson, eds.), pp. 1205–1220, McGraw-Hill, New York.

Lewy, J. E., Cabana, E. C., Repetto, H. A., Canterbury, J. M., and Reiss, E., 1972, Serum parathyroid hormone in hypophosphatemic vitamin D-resistant rickets, *J. Pediatr.* **81:**294.

Lotz, M., Zisman, E., and Bartter, F. C., 1968, Evidence for a phosphorus-depletion syndrome in man, *N. Engl. J. Med.* **278:**409.

Luder, J., and Sheldon, W., 1955, A familial tubular absorption defect of glucose and amino acids, *Arch. Dis. Child.* **30:**160.

Maltz, H. E., Fish, M. B., and Holliday, M. A., 1970, Calcium deficiency rickets and the renal response to calcium infusion, *Pediatrics* **46:**865.

Mann, J. B., Alterman, S., and Hills, A. G., 1962, Albright's hereditary osteodystrophy comprising pseudohypoparathyroidism and pseudo-pseudohypoparathyroidism, *Ann. Intern. Med.* **56:**315.

Marcus, R., and Aurbach, G. D., 1971, Adenyl cyclase from renal cortex, *Biochim. Biophys. Acta* **242:**410.

Marcus, R., Wilber, J. F., and Aurbach, G. D., 1971, Parathyroid hormone-sensitive adenyl cyclase from the renal cortex of a patient with pseudohypoparathyroidism, *J. Clin. Endocrinol. Metab.* **33:**537.

Marx, S. J., Hershman, J. M., and Aurbach, G. D., 1971, Thyroid dysfunction in pseudohypoparathyroidism, *J. Clin. Endocrinol. Metab.* **33:**822.

Marx, S. J., Fedak, S. A., and Aurbach, G. D., 1972, Preparation of characterization of a hormone-responsive renal plasma membrane fraction, *J. Biol. Chem.* **247:**6913.

Massry, S. G., Friedler, R. M., and Coburn, J. W., 1973, Excretion of phosphate and calcium. Physiology of their renal handling and relation to clinical medicine. *Arch. Intern. Med.* **131:**828.

McCune, D. J., Mason, H. H., and Clarke, H. T., 1943, Intractable hypophosphatemic rickets with renal glycosuria and acidosis (the Fanconi syndrome), *Am. J. Dis. Child.* **65:**81.

McEnery, P. T., Silverman, F. N., and West, C. D., 1972, Acceleration of growth with combined vitamin D-phosphate therapy of hypophosphatemic resistant rickets, *J. Pediatr.* **80:**763.

Metz, S. A., Baylink, D. J., Hughes, M. R., Haussler, M. R., and Robertson, R. P., 1977, Selective deficiency of 1,25-dihydroxycholecalciferol. A cause of isolated skeletal resistance to parathyroid hormone, *N. Engl. J. Med.* **297:**1084.

Moncrieff, M., and Fadahunsi, T. O., 1974, Congenital rickets due to maternal vitamin D deficiency, *Arch. Dis. Child.* **49:**810.

Monn, E., Osnes, J. B., Øye, I., and Wefring, K. W., 1976, Pseudohypoparathyroidism, a difficult diagnosis in early childhood, *Acta Paediatr. Scand.* **65:**487.

Morgan, J. M., Hawley, W. L., Chenoweth, A. I., Retan, W. J., and Diethelm, A. G., 1973, Renal transplantation in hypophosphatemia with vitamin D-resistant rickets, *Arch. Intern. Med.* **134:**549.

Morris, R. C., McSherry, E., and Sebastian, A., 1971, Modulation of experimental renal dysfunction of hereditary fructose intolerance by circulating parathyroid hormone, *Proc. Natl. Acad. Sci. U.S.A.* **68:**132.

Morris, R. C., Jr., McInnes, R. R., Epstein, C. J., Sebastian, A., and Scriver, C. R., 1976,

Genetic and metabolic injury of the kidney, in: *The Kidney* (B. M. Brenner and F. C. Rector, eds.), pp. 1193–1256, W. B. Saunders, Philadelphia.

Moser, C. R., and Fessel, W. J., 1974, Rheumatic manifestations of hypophosphatemia, *Arch. Intern. Med.* **134:**674.

Moses, A. M., Breslau, N., and Coulson, R., 1976, Renal responses to PTH in patients with hormone-resistant (pseudo) hypoparathyroidism, *Am. J. Med.* **61:**184.

Neer, R. M., Tregear, G. W., and Potts, J. T., Jr., 1977, Renal effects of native parathyroid hormone and synthetic biologically active fragments in pseudohypoparathyroidism and hypoparathyroidism, *J. Clin. Endocrinol. Metab.* **38:**420.

Neimann, N., Pierson, M., Marchal, C., Ranker, G., and Gregnou, G., 1968, Néphropathie familiale glomérulo-tubulaire et un syndrome de DeToni–Debré–Fanconi, *Arch. Fr. Pédiatr.* **25:**43.

Nigrin, G., Cochrane, W. A., Jannigan, D., and Ernst, A., 1962, Results of calcium infusion and renal biopsy studies in refractory rickets, *Am. J. Dis. Child.* **104:**478 (Abstract).

Nordin, B. E., Peacock, M., and Wilkinson, R., 1972, Hypercalciuria and calcium stone disease, *Clin. Endocrinol. Metab.* **1:**169.

Nusynowitz, M. L., and Klein, M. H., 1973, Pseudoidiopathic hypoparathyroidism. Hypoparathyroidism with ineffective parathyroid hormone, *Am. J. Med.* **55:**677.

Nusynowitz, M. L., Frame, B., and Kolb, F. O., 1976, The spectrum of hypoparathyroid states: A classification based on physiologic principles, *Medicine* **55:**105.

O'Doherty, P. J. A., DeLuca, H. F., and Eicher, E. M., 1976, Intestinal calcium and phosphate transport in genetic hypophosphatemic mice, *Biochem. Biophys. Res. Commun.* **71:**617.

Offerman, G., von Herrath, D., and Delling, G., 1976, Idiopathische hypophosphatämische Osteomalagie, *Dtsch. Med. Wochenschr.* **101:**1684.

O'Regan, S., Carson, S. W., Chesney, R. W., and Drummond, K. N., 1977, Electrolyte and acid-base abnormalities in leukemia, *Blood* **49:**345.

Osman, A. A., 1924, Hereditary renal diseases, in: *The Chances of Morbid Inheritance* (C. P. Blacher, ed.), p. 280, William Wood, Baltimore.

Pak, C. Y., DeLuca, H. F., Bartter, F. C., Henneman, D. H., Frame, B., Simopoulos, A., and Delea, C. S., 1972, Treatment of vitamin D-resistant rickets with 25-hydroxycholecalciferol, *Arch. Intern. Med.* **129:**894.

Parfitt, A. M., 1972, Hypophosphatemic vitamin D refractory rickets and osteomalacia, *Orthop. Clin. North Am.* **3:**653.

Park, E. A., 1923, The etiology of rickets, *Physiol. Rev.* **3:**106.

Park, E. A., 1933, Rickets, in: *Diseases of Infancy and Childhood* (L. Parsons and S. Barling, eds.), pp. 318–341, Oxford Press, London.

Peacock, M., Heyburn, P. J., and Aaron, J. E., 1977, Treatment of vitamin D resistant hypophosphatemic osteomalacia with 1α-hydroxyvitamin D₃, *Calcif. Tissue Res.* **22:**55.

Pollack, J. A., Schiller, A. L., and Crawford, J. D., 1973, Rickets and myopathy cured by removal of a nonossifying fibroma of bone, *Pediatrics* **52:**364.

Potts, J. T., Jr., 1972, Pseudohypoparathyroidism, in: *The Metabolic Basis of Inherited Disease* (J. B. Stanbury, J. B. Wyngaarden, and D. S. Fredrickson, eds.), pp. 1305–1319, McGraw-Hill, New York.

Poujeol, P., Chabardès, D., Roinel, N., and de Rouffignac, C., 1976, Influence of extracellular volume expansion on magnesium, calcium and phosphate handling along the rat nephron, *Pflügers Arch.* **365:**203.

Prader, A., Illig, R., Uelinger, E., and Studler, G., 1959, Rachitis ufolge knocheintumors, *Helv. Paediatr. Acta* **14:**554.

Prader, V. A., Illig, R., and Heierli, E., 1961, Eine besondere form der primären vitamin

D resistenten rachitis mit hypocalcämie und autosomaldominanten erbgang die hereditäre pseudo-mangelrachitis, *Helv. Paediatr. Acta* **16**:452.

Rasmussen, H., and Anast, C., 1978, Familial hypophosphatemic (vitamin D-resistant) rickets and vitamin D-dependent rickets, in: *The Metabolic Basis of Inherited Disease* (J. B. Stanbury, J. B. Wyngaarden, and D. S. Fredrickson, eds.), pp. 1537–1562, McGraw Hill, New York.

Rasmussen, H., and Bordier, P., 1974, *The Physiologic and Cellular Basis of Metabolic Bone Disease*, Williams and Wilkins, Baltimore.

Rasmussen, H., Anast, C., Parks, J., Haussler, M., Lane, J., and Pechet, M., 1976, $1\alpha(OH)D_3$ in the treatment of hypophosphatemic rickets, *Clin. Res.* **24**:486 (Abstract).

Reade, T. M., Scriver, C. R., Glorieux, F. H., Nogrady, B., Delvin, E., Poirier, R., Holick, M.F., and DeLuca, H. F., 1975, Response to crystalline 1α-hydroxyvitamin D_3 in vitamin D dependency, *Pediatr. Res.* **9**:593.

Reitz, R. E., and Weinstein, R. L., 1973, Parathyroid hormone secretion in familial vitamin D-resistant rickets, *N. Engl. J. Med.* **289**:941.

Rizzoli, R., Fleisch, H., and Bonjour, J.-P., 1977, Role of 1,25-dihydroxyvitamin D_3 on intestinal phosphate absorption in rats with a normal vitamin D supply, *J. Clin. Invest.* **60**:639.

Robertson, B. R., Harris, R. C., and McCune, D. J., 1942, Refractory rickets: Mechanism of therapeutic action of calciferol, *Am. J. Dis. Child.* **64**:948.

Rodriguez, H. J., Villarreal, H., Jr., Klahr, S., and Slatopsky, E., 1974, Pseudohypoparathyroidism type II: Restoration of normal renal responsiveness to parathyroid hormone by calcium administration, *J. Clin. Endocrinol. Metab.* **39**:693.

Roof, B. S., Piel, C. F., and Gordan, G. S., 1972, Nature of defect responsible for familial vitamin D-resistant rickets (VDRR) based on radioimmunoassay for parathyroid hormone (PTH), *Trans. Assoc. Am. Physicians* **85**:172.

Root, A. W., and Harrison, H. E., 1976, Recent advances in calcium metabolism. II. Disorders of calcium homeostasis, *J. Pediatr.* **88**:177.

Rosen, J. F., and Finberg, L., 1972, Vitamin D-dependent rickets: Actions of parathyroid hormone and 25-hydroxycholecalciferol, *Pediatr. Res.* **6**:552.

Rosenberg, L. E., 1969, Hereditary diseases with membrane defects, in: *Biological Membranes* (R. M. Dowben, ed.), pp. 255–295, Little, Brown, Boston.

Royer, P., Habib, R., Mathieu, H., Broyer, M., and Walsh, A., 1974, Familial hypophosphatemia, in: *Pediatric Nephrology*, pp. 62–64, W. B. Saunders Co., Philadelphia.

Russell, R. G. G., Smith, R., Preston, C., Walton, R. J., Woods, G. G., Henderson, R. G., and Norman, A. W., 1975, The effect of 1,25-dihydroxycholecalciferol on renal tubular reabsorption of phosphate, intestinal absorption of calcium and bone histology in hypophosphatemic renal tubular rickets, *Clin. Sci. Mol. Med.* **48**:177.

Schneider, A. B., and Sherwood, L. M., 1975, Pathogenesis and management of hypoparathyroidism and other hypocalcemic disorders, *Metabolism* **24**:871.

Schneider, J. A., and Seegmiller, J. E., 1972, Cystinosis and the Fanconi syndrome, in: *The Metabolic Basis of Inherited Disease* (J. B. Stanbury, J. B. Wyngaarden, and D. S. Fredrickson, eds.), pp. 1581–1604, McGraw-Hill, New York.

Scriver, C. R., 1974, Rickets and the pathogenesis of impaired tubular transport of phosphate and other solutes, *Am. J. Med.* **57**:43.

Scriver, C. R., 1976, Hereditary hypophosphatemic bone disease, *N. Engl. J. Med.* **294**:1012.

Scriver, C. R., and Bergeron, M., 1974, Amino acid transport in kidney: The use of mutation to dissect membrane and transepithelial transport, in: *Heritable Disorders of Amino Acid Metabolism* (W. L. Nyhan, ed.), pp. 515–592, Wiley, New York.

Scriver, C. R., and Rosenberg, L. E., 1973a, Tyrosine, in: *Amino Acid Metabolism and Its Disorders*, pp. 338–369, W. B. Saunders, Philadelphia.

Scriver, C. R., and Rosenberg, L. E., 1973b, Generalized disorders of amino acid transport, in: *Amino Acid Metabolism and Its Disorders*, pp. 197–206, W. B. Saunders, Philadelphia.

Scriver, C. R., Goldbloom, R. B., and Roy, C. C., 1964, Hypophosphatemic rickets with renal hyperglycinuria, renal glycosuria and glycylprolinuria. A syndrome with evidence for renal tubular secretion of phosphorus, *Pediatrics* **34**:357.

Scriver, C. R., McInnes, R. R., Tenenhouse, H., Reade, T., and Glorieux, F. H., 1974, The further delineation of acquired vitamin D deficiency, autosomal recessive vitamin D dependency and X-linked hypophosphatemia, in: *Calcium Regulating Hormones* (R. V. Talmage, M. Owen, and J. A. Parsons, eds.), pp. 421–430, Excerpta Medica, Amsterdam.

Scriver, C. R., Chesney, R. W., and McInnes, R. R., 1976, Genetic aspects of renal tubular transport: Diversity and topology of carriers, *Kidney Int.* **9**:149.

Scriver, C. R., MacDonald, W., Reade, T., Glorieux, F. H., and Nogrady, B., 1977, Hypophosphatemic nonrachitic bone disease: An entity distinct from X-linked hypophosphatemia in the renal defect, bone involvement and inheritance, *Am. J. Med. Genet.* **1**:101.

Segal, S., 1972, Disorders of galactose metabolism, in: *The Metabolic Basis of Inherited Disease* (J. B. Stanbury, J. B. Wyngaarden, and D. S. Fredrickson, eds.), pp. 174–195, McGraw-Hill, New York.

Segar, W. E., Iber, F. L., and Kyle, L. H., 1956, Osteomalacia of unknown etiology, *N. Engl. J. Med.* **254**:1011.

Sheldon, W., Luder, J., and Webb, B., 1960, A familial tubular absorption defect of glucose and amino acids, *Arch. Dis. Child.* **35**:90.

Short, E. M., Binder, H. J., and Rosenberg, L. E., 1973, Familial hypophosphatemic rickets: Defective transport of inorganic phosphate by intestinal mucosa, *Science* **179**:700.

Short, E., Morris, R. C., Jr., and Spencer, M., 1976, Exaggerated phosphaturic response to circulating parathyroid hormone in patients with familial X-linked hypophosphatemic rickets, *J. Clin. Invest.* **58**:152.

Silver, J., Davies, T. J., Kupersmitt, E., Otme, M., Petrie, A., and Vajda, F., 1974, Prevalence and treatment of vitamin D deficiency in children on anticonvulsant drugs, *Arch. Dis. Child.* **49**:344.

Singer, F. R., Powell, D., Minkin, C., Bethune, J. E., Brideman, A., and Coburn, J. W., 1973, Hypercalcemia in reticulum cell sarcoma without hyperparathyroidism or skeletal masses, *Ann. Intern. Med.* **78**:365.

Sinha, T. K., DeLuca, H. F., and Bell, N. H., 1977, Evidence for a defect in the formation of $1\alpha,25$-dihydroxyvitamin D in pseudohypoparathyroidism, *Metabolism* **26**:731.

Smith, R., Lindenbaum, R. H., and Walton, R. J., 1976, Hypophosphataemic osteomalacia and Fanconi syndrome of adult onset and dominant inheritance, *Q. J. Med.* **179**:387.

Spranger, J., 1968, Skeletal dysplasia: Albright's hereditary osteodystrophy, in: *Birth Defects: The First Conference* (D. Bergsma, ed.), pp. 122–128, National Foundation, White Plains, N.Y.

Stamp, T. C. B., 1971, The hypocalcemic effect of intravenous phosphate administration, *Clin. Sci.* **40**:55.

Stamp, T. C. B., and Baker, L. R. I., 1976, Recessive hypophosphatemic rickets, and possible aetiology of the "vitamin D-resistant" syndrome, *Arch. Dis. Child.* **51**:360.

Steele, T. H., 1976, Renal resistance to parathyroid hormone during phosphorus deprivation, *J. Clin. Invest.* **58**:1461.

Steendijk, R., 1960, The renal tubular reabsorption of inorganic phosphate in primary refractory rickets, *Acta Paediatr.* **49**:609.

Stickler, G. B., Hayles, A. B., and Roserear, J. W., 1965, Familial hypophosphatemic vitamin D-resistant rickets, *Am. J. Dis. Child.* **110**:664.

Stickler, G. B., Jowsey, J., and Bianco, A. J., Jr., 1971, Possible detrimental effect of large doses of vitamin D in familial hypophosphatemic vitamin D-resistant rickets, *J. Pediatr.* **79**:68.

Stögman, W., and Fischer, J. A., 1975, Pseudohypoparathyroidism. Disappearance of the resistance to parathyroid extract during treatment with vitamin D, *Am. J. Med.* **59**:140.

Suh, S. M., Fraser, D., and Kooh, S. W., 1970, Pseudohypoparathyroidism: Responsiveness to parathyroid extract induced by vitamin D_2 therapy, *J. Clin. Endocrinol. Metab.* **30**:609.

Tarwalkar, Y. B., Musgrave, J. E., Buist, N. R. M., Campbell, R. A., and Campbell, J. R., 1974, Vitamin D-resistant rickets and parathyroid adenomas. Renal transport of phosphate, *Am. J. Dis. Child.* **128**:704.

Tashjian, A. H., Jr., Levine, L., and Munson, P. L., 1964, Immunochemical identification of parathyroid hormone in non-parathyroid neoplasma associated with hypercalcemia, *J. Exp. Med.* **119**:467.

Teitelbaum, S. L., Rosenberg, E. M., Bates, M., and Avioli, L. V., 1976, The effects of phosphate and vitamin D therapy on osteopenic, hypophosphatemic osteomalacia of childhood, *Clin. Orthop. Relat. Res.* **116**:38.

Tenenhouse, H. S., and Scriver, C. R., 1975, Orthophosphate transport in erythrocyte of normal subjects and of patients with X-linked hypophosphatemia, *J. Clin. Invest.* **55**:644.

Tenenhouse, H. S., Scriver, C. R., and McInnes, R. R., 1977, The apparent defect in phosphate transport in kidney of *Hyp* mice: A likely model of X-linked hypophosphatemia in man, *Clin. Res.* **25**:692A.

Thomas, W. C., Jr., and Fry, R. M., 1970, Parathyroid adenomas in chronic rickets, *Am. J. Med.* **49**:404.

Tomlinson, S., Hendy, G. N., and O'Riordan, J. L. H., 1976, A simplified assessment of response to parathyroid hormone in hypoparathyroid patients, *Lancet* **1**:62.

Waldmann, T. A., Strober, W., and Mogrelnicki, R. P., 1972, The renal handling of low molecular weight proteins. II. Disorders of serum protein catabolism in patients with tubular proteinuria, the nephrotic syndrome, or uremia, *J. Clin. Invest.* **51**:2162.

Walshe, J. M., 1972, The biochemistry of copper in man and its role in the pathogenesis of Wilson's disease (hepatolenticular degeneration), in: *Biochemical Aspects of Nervous Diseases* (J. N. Cumings, ed.), pp. 111–150, Plenum Press, New York.

Walton, J., 1976, Familial hypophosphatemic rickets. A delineation of its subdivisions and pathogenesis, *Clin. Pediatr.* **15**:1007.

Walton, R. J., and Bijvoet, O. L. M., 1975, Nomogram for derivation of renal threshold phosphate concentration, *Lancet* **2**:309.

Werder, E. A., Illig, R., and Bernasconi, S., 1975, Excessive thyrotropin response to thyrotropin-releasing hormone in pseudohypoparathyroidism, *Pediatr. Res.* **9**:12.

Werder, E. A., Kind, H. P., Egert, F., Fischer, J. A., and Prader, A., 1976, Effective long-term treatment of pseudohypoparathyroidism with oral 1α-hydroxy and 1,25-dihyroxycholecalciferol, *J. Pediatr.* **89**:266.

West, C. D., Blanton, J. C., Silverman, F. N., and Holland, N. H., 1964, Use of phosphate salts as an adjunct to vitamin D in the treatment of hypophosphatemic vitamin D-refractory rickets, *J. Pediatr.* **64**:469.

Williams, A. J., Wilkinson, J. L., and Taylor, W. H., 1977, Pseudohypoparathyroidism, variable manifestations within a family, *Arch. Dis. Child.* **52**:798.

Williams, T. F., Winters, R. W., and Burnett, C. H., 1972, Familial (hereditary) vitamin D-resistant rickets with hypophosphatemia, in: *The Metabolic Basis of Inherited Dis-*

ease (J. B. Stanbury, J. B. Wyngaarden, and D. S. Fredrickson, eds.), pp. 1465–1485, McGraw-Hill, New York.

Willis, M. R., Pak, C. Y. C., Hammond, W. G., and Bartter, F. C., 1969, Normocalcemic primary hyperparathyroidism, *Am. J. Med.* **47**:384.

Wilson, D. R., York, S. E., Jaworski, Z. F., and Yendt, E. R., 1965, Studies in hypophosphatemic vitamin D-refractory osteomalacia in adults. Oral phosphate as an adjunct to therapy, *Medicine* **44**:99.

Winters, R. W., Graham, J. B., Williams, T. F., McFalls, V. W., and Burnett, C. H., 1958, A genetic study of familial hypophosphatemia and vitamin D-resistant rickets with a review of the literature, *Medicine* **37**:97.

Witmer, G., and Balsan, S., 1968, Biopsie osseuse dans quatre cas de rachitisme vitamine D-résistant idiopathique, *Pathol. Biol.* **16**:421.

Wright, D. R., 1975, The pieces of a vitamin D puzzle fall into place—almost, *N. Engl. J. Med.* **293**:872.

Wyman, A. L., Paradinas, F. J., and Daly, J. R., 1977, Hypophosphatemic osteomalacia associated with a malignant tumor of the tibia: Report of a case, *J. Clin. Pathol.* **30**:328.

Zisman, E., Lotz, M., Jenkins, M. E., and Bartter, F. C., 1969, Studies in pseudohypoparathyroidism: Two cases with a probable selective deficiency of thyrotropin, *Am. J. Med.* **46**:464.

Index

Acetazolamide
    and bicarbonate conductance of basolateral membrane, 236
    bicarbonate reabsorption and, 230
    as carbonic anhydrase inhibitor, 275–277
    intracellular pH and, 234
    mechanism of action of, 233–236
    phosphate absorption and, 234
    phosphate excretion and, 120, 210, 234
    phosphate loss following, 218–219
    proximal tubular pH and, 234
    urine alkalinization and, 93
Acid–base balance, in phosphate transport, 92–96
Acidification studies, phosphate in, 227–231
Acidosis, metabolic, 93
Adenyl cyclase
    calcitonin-activated, 155
    parathyroid hormone and, 97
Adenyl cyclase-cAMP system, in phosphaturia, 123–126, 130
ADH, see Antidiuretic hormone
Adult sporadic hypophosphatemic osteomalacia, 338–339
Alkaline phosphatase, molecular mechanism of, 86–87
Alkaline phosphate, preferential transport of, 94
Alligator mississippiensis, 64
    phosphate secretion by kidneys of, 64–65
para-Aminohippurate, 345
para-Aminohippuric acid, 62
Amphibians, phosphate secretion in, 62–63
Angiotensin II, tubular transport and, 177–178
Animal studies, calcium infusion in, 293–295
Anions, physicochemical properties of, 231–233
Antidiuretic hormone
    phosphate level and, 142
    phosphaturic action of, 143

Antidiuretic hormone (*cont.*)
    in renal handling of phosphate, 142–145
    and tubular reabsorption of phosphate, 143–144

Bartter's syndrome, 178
Benzothiadiazines, as diuretics, 277–280
Bicarbonate, mechanism of action of, 233–236
Bicarbonate buffer
    acidification of, 231
    proximal tubular pH and, 235
    titration curves for, 225
Bicarbonate diuresis, phosphate excretion and, 276
Bicarbonate infusion, proximal tubular phosphate reabsorption and, 214
Bicarbonate reabsorption
    and acidification of nonbicarbonate buffer systems, 228
    inhibition of, 230
Bicarbonate reabsorption rate, formula for, 228
Bicarbonaturic effect, of parathyroid hormone, 129, 233
Birds, phosphate secretion from kidneys, of, 65–67
Bone disease
    nonrachitic, 337–338
    phosphaturia and, 326–327
Bone metabolism, calcium and phosphate in, 296–298
Bowman's capsule, 265
Brisk phosphaturia, 353–354
Brush border, of luminal plasma membrane, 81–82
Brush-border membrane
    enzymes of, 84–87
    glucose-binding site in, 83
    phosphate transport by, 90–91

Brush-border vesicles, hyperpolarization of, 90
Bumetamide, 280

Calciopenic rickets, 340–341
Calcitonin
  calcium level and, 288–290
  glucagon in release of, 158
  in phosphate metabolism, 152
  phosphaturic response and, 153
  in proximal tubular reabsorption, 156
  renal effects of, 152–154
  in renal handling of phosphate, 154–157
  serum phosphate levels and, 151–152
Calcium
  animal studies in infusion of, 292–295
  in bone metabolism, 296–298
  glomerular filtration rate and, 290–291
  hypoparathyroidism and, 302–303
  in renal handling of phosphate, 287–303
  renal hemodynamics and, 290–291
  in renal tubule phosphate absorption, 291–292
  in tubular phosphate reabsorption, 301, 310
  in vitamin-D-resistant rickets, 300–302
Calcium excretion, growth hormone and, 141
Calcium infusion, in primary hyperparathyroidism, 298
Calcium metabolism
  pathologic studies in, 296–303
  phosphorus and, 1–2
Calcium reabsorption, parathyroid hormone and, 124
cAMP (adenosine 3′,5′-cyclic monophosphate), 123–126
  alkaline phosphatase and, 87
  calcitonin and, 154–155
  dibutyryl, 124–126
  inhibition of, 124
  parathyroid hormone and, 97–99
  phosphate reabsorptive capacity and, 121
  phosphaturic effect of, 145
  urinary excretion of, 99–100, 104
  in vitamin-D-resistant rickets, 330
cAMP-dependent phosphorylation, 103
cAMP-dependent protein kinase, 101
cAMP excretion
  EHDP and, 258–259
  in hyperthyroidism, 150

cAMP excretion (cont.)
  phosphaturia and, 27
  in pseudohypoparathyroidism, 351
cAMP generation, PTH-induced, 126
cAMP level
  and alkalinization of proximal tubular fluid, 123
  parathyroid hormone and, 123–124
cAMP production, sodium transport and (see also cAMP generation), 122
Carbonic anhydrase activity, parathyroid hormone and, 129
Carbonic anhydrase inhibitors, diuretics as, 274–277
Cardiac glucosides, in sodium and phosphate excretion, 89
Catecholamine receptors, in renal tissue, 165
Catecholamines
  phosphate level and, 163
  in renal handling of phosphate, 163–167
Cellular mechanisms, of phosphate transport (see also Phosphate transport), 79–104
cGMP levels, changes in, 102
Clearance studies, phosphate reabsorption and, 210–212
Clinical medicine, tubular deficits of phosphate reabsorption in, 321–354
Creatinine clearance (see also Glomerular filtration rate)
  measurement of, 14–15
  phosphate clearance and, 17–18
CT, see Calcitonin
Cyclic nucleotides, phosphate regulation by (see also cAMP; cGMP), 96–103
Cytosolic protein kinase, 100

DeToni–Debré–Fanconi syndrome, 345–347
Dibutyryl cAMP, 124–126
Dietary phosphate (see also Phosphate)
  EHDP and, 250–251
  segmental tubular transport and, 256–257
  tubular adaptation to supply of, 246–247, 257
1-25-Dihydrocholecalciferol, 199
1,25-Dihydroxyvitamin D$_3$, 179, 252–254
Diphosphonate disodium ethane-1-hydroxy-1, 1-diphosphonate, see EHDP
Distal tubular microperfusion (see also Microperfusion studies), 47–48
  evaluation by, 52–54

Diuretics
  benzathiadiazenes as, 277–280
  bicarbonate as, 276
  bumetamide as, 280
  carbonic anhydrase inhibitory activity of, 274
  loop, 279–280
  mercurial, 273–275
  osmotic agents as, 272–273
  phosphate excretion and, 271–280
  potassium-sparing, 280
Dog(s)
  calcium infusion in, 293–295
  extracellular fluid volume expansion in, 266–270

ECV, see Extracellular fluid composition and volume
ECVE, see Extracellular fluid volume expansion
EHDP (ethane-1-hydroxy-1,1-diphosphonate)
  cAMP excretion and, 250–253
  dietary phosphate and, 258
EHDP treatment, phosphate demand and, 257–258
Epinephrine, hypophosphaturic response to, 164
Escherichia coli, 85
Estrogens
  bone sensitivity and, 174
  phosphate level and, 173–174
  in phosphate metabolism, 174
  receptor affinity for, 176
  in renal handling of phosphate, 175–177
Ethacrynic acid, 279–280
Extracellular fluid composition and volume, constancy of, 265–266
Extracellular fluid volume expansion
  fluid backleak in, 265
  parathyroid hormone and, 271
  phosphaturia during, 270–271
  in rat and dog, 266–270
  in renal handling of phosphate, 265–280
  in renal phosphate transport, 312
  sodium reabsorption in, 265

Fanconi syndrome, 345–347
  causes and genetics of, 347
  glucose intolerance in, 348
Filtered load, reabsorbed fraction of, 20–22

Fishes, phosphate secretion by kidneys of, 61–62
Furosemide, 279–280

Galactose conversion, failure of, 348–349
GFR, see Glomerular filtration rate
GH, see Growth hormone
Glomerular filtrate
  composition of, 2–4
  PO_4 concentration in, 3
Glomerular filtration, 2–8
  limit or threshold in, 5–8
  maximum reabsorption and, 9–11
Glomerular filtration rate
  in amphibians, 62–63
  calcium and, 290–291
  nephron and, 16
  phosphate clearance and, 19
  phosphate filtration and, 4
  plasma inulin and, 6–7
  plasma phosphate concentration and, 3, 27–29
  following renal transplantation, 317
  tubular transport capacity and, 244–245
Glucagon
  in calcitonin release, 158
  in renal handling of phosphate, 157–159
  serum phosphate level and, 157
Glucorticoids
  circadian rhythm and, 172–173
  parathyroid hormone and, 171
  phosphate level and, 167–168
  in renal handling of phosphate, 167–172
Glucose, in phosphate transport, 91–92
Glucosuria, 348
Glycinuria, 348
Glycylprolinuria, 348
Growth hormone
  biphasic effect of, 138
  calcium excretion and, 141
  hyperphosphatemia and, 353–354
  phosphate level and, 138–139
  and renal handling of phosphate, 139–141
  and tubular transport of phosphate, 141–142

Henderson–Hasselbalch equation, 225
Henle's loop, see Loop of nephron
Hydropenia, peritubular-to-luminal flux in, 70–71
25-Hydroxycholecalciferol, 199

Hyperaminoaciduria
  rickets and, 336
  in vitamin-D-dependency rickets, 343
Hypercalcemia
  cAMP and, 125
  in primary hyperparathyroidism, 298
Hyperparathyroidism (see also Primary hyperparathyroidism)
  low renal phosphate threshold in, 24
  phosphaturia in, 115
  primary, see Primary hyperparathyroidism
  reabsorbed fraction of filtered load in, 23
Hyperphosphatemia
  growth hormone and, 353
  phosphate reabsorption and, 215
Hyperphosphaturia, defined, 24–25
Hyperthyroidism, phosphate levels in, 145–146
Hypocalcemia
  parathyroid hormone and, 273
  phosphate reabsorption in, 215
  phosphate transport in, 296
Hypokalemia, intracellular pH and, 96
Hypomagnesemia, cAMP, and, 125
Hypoparathyroidism
  calcium metabolism and, 302–303
  vitamin D therapy in, 197
Hypophosphatemia
  parathyroid hormone and, 115
  in primary hyperparathyroidism, 298
  vitamin-D-resistant rickets in, 300–302
Hypophosphatemic nonrachitic bone disease, 337–338
Hypophosphatemic osteomalacia, 178–179
Hypophosphaturia, defined, 24–25

Idiopathic hypercalciuria, phosphate leak in, 339–340
Insulin
  phosphate level and, 159–160
  in renal handling of phosphate, 160–163
Inulin, fractional recovery of, 70

Kidney(s) [see also Renal (adj.)]
  of alligator, 64
  of amphibians, 62–63
  of birds, 65–67
  calcitonin effect on, 153–154
  of fishes, 61–62
  of lower vertebrates, 61–67

Kidney(s) (cont.)
  mammalian, 67–71
  in phosphate metabolism, 59–76
  in phosphate regulation, 1–2
  phosphate secretion by, 59–76
  of reptiles, 63–65
  transepithelial phosphate transport in (see also Phosphate transport), 79–104

Late accessible proximal tubule, phosphate delivery in [see also Proximal tubular reabsorption; Tubular (adj.)], 41–42
Leak, in idiopathic hypercalciuria (see also Phosphate leak), 339–340
Levamisole, 86
Loop diuretics, 279–280
Loop of nephron (Henle's loop)
  characteristics of phosphate reabsorption in, 48–49
  in vivo and in vitro microperfusion of, 47–48
  pars recta transport in, 117–118
  phosphate transport in, 45–49
Lophius piscatorius, 61–62
Luder–Sheldon syndrome, 348
Lumen–bath fluxes, 220–221
Luminal buffer base concentrations, steady-state level of, 229
Luminal membrane vesicles, 223–224
Luminal plasma membrane, "brush-border" arrangement of (see also Brush border), 81–82

Magnesium reabsorption, parathyroid hormone and, 124
Mammalian kidney
  peritubular-to-luminal flux of phosphate in, 69–76
  phosphate secretion by, 67–76
  renal clearance techniques in assessment of phosphate secretion by, 67–69
Mannitol, 272–273
Membranes, composition and structure of, 80–83, 223–224
Metabolic acidosis, phosphate transport and, 93
Michaelis constant, splay and, 16–17
Microperfusion
  distal tubular, see Distal tubular microperfusion
  loop reabsorption evaluation by, 47–48

Microperfusion studies, phosphate reabsorption and, 216–222
Micropuncture, evaluation by, 45–47, 311
Micropuncture studies, in phosphate reabsorption, 213–216
Microtubules, structure of [see also Tubular (adj.)], 82–83
Microvillus membrane, of renal brush border, 81
Myxine glutinosa, 61

"Natriuretic hormone," phosphate level and, 178
Natrix genus, 63
Necturus genus, 3, 63
Nephron (see also Tubular phosphate reabsorption)
  distal segments as sites of peritubular-to-luminal flux in, 74–76
  late accessible proximal tubule of, 39–42
  "leakiness" of, 74
  loop of, see Loop of nephron
  peritubular-to-luminal flux in, 70
  phosphate reabsorption in, 39–55
  superficial, 39–42
  terminal, 50–54
Nephron segments, phosphate transport in, 118–120
Norepinephrine, phosphate excretion and, 164

25OHD₃, see 25-Hydroxycholecalciferol; 1,25-Dihydroxycholecalciferol
1,25(OH)₂D₃, see 1,25-Dihydroxyvitamin D₃
Oncogenous rickets, 335–337
Orthophosphoric acid, 1
Osteitis fibrosa cystica, 352
Osteomalacia
  hypophosphatemic, 338–339
  oncogenic, 178
  tubulopathy and, 345
  vitamin D and, 352

Papain, digestion of membranes with, 84
Parathyroid extract, 62–67, 308–309
Parathyroid hormone
  acute phosphaturic response to, 257–259
  adenylate cyclase stimulation by, 97
  bicarbonate and, 211
  bicarbonaturia and, 129, 233
  bone sensitivity to, 174

Parathyroid hormone (cont.)
  calcium and, 288–289
  carbonic anhydrase activity and, 129
  glucocorticoids and, 171
  hypocalcemia and, 273
  inhibitory effect of, 116
  mode of action of, 120–122
  in overall tubular transport capacity, 245–246
  phosphate clearance and, 20
  phosphate reabsorption in absence of, 42–43
  phosphate secretion and, 62–67
  phosphate reabsorption and, 216–217
  phosphaturia and, 122–123, 353–354
  in primary hypoparathyroidism, 299
  in pseudohypoparathyroidism, 349–350
  in renal failure, 314
  in renal handling of phosphate, 115–130, 216–217, 245–246, 308
  and renal phosphate excretion in reptiles, 65
  sodium reabsorption and, 126–128
  tubular phosphate reabsorption and, 216–217, 308
  in vitamin-D-resistant rickets, 329
  withdrawal of, 122
Parathyroid secretion, during volume expansion, 271
Pars recta PO₄ transport (see also Loop of nephron; Phosphate transport), 117–118
PEI, see Phosphate excretion index
Peritubular-to-luminal flux
  distal nephron as site of, 74–76
  in mammalian kidney, 69–76
  proximal tubule as site of, 72–74
pH
  acetazolamide effect and, 234
  phosphate buffer perfusion and, 230
  phosphate transport and, 223–227
  urinary, 209
Phentolamine, phosphaturia and, 166
Phosphate
  bath–lumen fluxes of, 220–222
  as buffer system, 224–227
  concentration of, see Phosphate concentration
  cyclic nucleotide regulation of, 96–103
  dietary, 245–249
  excretion rate for, see Phosphate excretion rate

Phosphate (*cont.*)
fasting level of, 138–139
hormonal regulation of at cellular level, 96–104
as inorganic radical, 1, 83
lumen–bath fluxes of, 220–221
peritubular-to-luminal flux of in mammalian kidney, 69–76
proximal tubule as site of peritubular-to-luminal flux in, 72–74
reabsorption of, *see* Phosphate reabsorption
in renal acidification studies, 227–231
renal handling of, *see* Renal handling of phosphate
renal tubular reabsorption of, *see* Phosphate reabsorption; Tubular phosphate reabsorption
renal tubular retention of, 349–353
splay for, 9–17
transmembrane movement of, 80–87
tubular adaptation to supply and requirement of, 243–261
tubular reabsorption of, *see* Tubular reabsorption of phosphate
urinary, *see* Urinary phosphate
Phosphate buffer system, titration curve for, 225
Phosphate clearance
creatinine clearance and, 17–18
defined, 19–20
Phosphate clearance rate, absolute, 20
Phosphate clearance studies, urinary phosphate excretion and, 210–212
Phosphate concentration
calcium effect on, 287–290
in glomerular filtrate, 2–4
limit or threshold in, 5–8
renal handling of phosphate and, 17–19
Phosphate demand, tubular adaptation to, 249–252
Phosphate excretion
acetazolamide and, 234
calcium and, 289–290
circadian rhythm of, 172–173
diet and, 24
diuretics and, 271–280
extracellular fluid volume expansion and, 266–270
vs. phosphate intake, 24–25

Phosphate excretion (*cont.*)
in rat and dog, 266–270
tubular cell secretory activity and, 59–60
Phosphate excretion index, 23
choice of, 29–32
Phosphate excretion rate, 24–25
plasma phosphate concentration and, 13–14
Phosphate homeostasis, abnormalities in, 296–302
Phosphate hyperexcretion, primary renal tubular, 323–340
Phosphate intake
vs. phosphate excretion, 24–25
plasma phosphate concentration and, 27–29
Phosphate ions, behavior of, 232
Phosphate leak
disorders involving, 324
in Fanconi syndrome, 346
Phosphate level
in adults, 139
calcitonin and, 151–152
catecholamines and, 163
estrogens and, 173–174
glucagon and, 157
glucocorticoids and, 167–168
hyperthyroidism and, 145–146
insulin and, 159–160
"natriuretic hormone" and, 178
Phosphate loss, in tubulopathy, 345–347
Phosphate–membrane interactions, 83–84
Phosphate metabolism
calcitonin and, 152
calcium and, 1–2
estrogens and, 174
glucocorticoids and, 168
growth hormone and, 139
kidney in control of, 59–76
thyroid hormone and, 146–147
Phosphate reabsorption, 20–24
in absence of parathyroid hormone, 42–43
acetazolamide and, 234
antidiuretic hormone and, 143–145
bicarbonate infusion and, 214
characteristics of in loop of nephron, 48–49
clearance studies and, 210–212
distal convoluted tubule and terminal nephron in, 118–120
extracellular volume expansion and, 210–211

Phosphate reabsorption (*cont.*)
  in intact animal, 39–42
  microperfusion studies in, 216–222
  micropuncture studies in, 213–216
  parathyroid hormone and, 216–217
  phosphate threshold concentration and, 5–8, 17
  in rat, 268–269
  renal tubular, *see* Tubular phosphate reabsorption
  tubular defects in, 321–354
  urinary alkalinization and, 209–237
  in vitamin-D-deficient rats, 247
  whole-kidney, 120–121
Phosphate reabsorptive capacity, 120–121
Phosphate secretion, by kidney [*see also* Kidney(s)], 59–76
Phosphate supply, tubular adaptation to, 254–257
Phosphate threshold concentration, 5–7
  equation for, 8
  plasma phosphate concentration and, 26–27
  and splay for phosphate, 9–17
Phosphate transport (*see also* Renal handling of phosphate)
  acetazolamide and, 218–219
  acid–base balance and, 92–96
  alkaline phosphatase in, 85–86
  angiotensin II and, 177–178
  brush-border alkaline phosphatase in, 85
  by brush-border membrane, 90–91
  cellular mechanisms in, 79–104
  characteristics of, 87–89
  in distal convoluted tubule and terminal nephron, 118–120
  between glomerulus and nephron, 39–45
  glucose and, 91–92
  in hypocalcemia, 296
  leak in, 324
  in loop of nephron, 45–49
  nonhormonal factors in, 89–96
  1,25(OH)$_2$D$_3$ role in, 252–254
  pH and, 223–227
  phosphate as buffer system in, 224–226
  sodium dependency of, 89–91
  sodium reabsorption and, 127
  in terminal nephron, 50–54
Phosphate turnover, in vertebrates, 4
Phosphate uptake, sodium-dependent, 90

Phosphaturia
  bone disorders related to, 326–327
  cAMP excretion and, 27
  parathyroid hormone and, 115, 353–354
  from urine alkalinization, 213
  during volume expansion, 270–271
Phospholipids, 102
Phosphorus, energy-harnessing ability of, 1
Phosphorus concentration
  in renal failure, 313–316
  renal insufficiency and, 308
Phosphorus excretion, calcium infusion and, 311
Phosphorylation, cAMP-dependent, 103
PHP, *see* Pseudohypoparathyroidism
Plasma concentration, constant (*see also* Phosphate concentration), 59
Plasma inulin, glomerular filtration rate and, 6–7
Plasma phosphate, splay and (*see also* Phospate), 7, 11
Plasma phosphate concentration (*see also* Phosphate concentration)
  factors affecting, 25–29
  glomerular filtration rate and, 27–29
  phosphate clearance and, 19
  phosphate excretion rate and, 13–14
  phosphate intake and, 27–29
  phosphate threshold concentration and, 26–27
  urinary phosphate excretion and, 13–15
Plasma phosphorus level, growth hormone and, 140
PO$_4$, *see* Phosphate
PPHP, *see* Pseudopseudohypoparathyroidism
Prednisolone maintenance therapy, 170
Pregnancy, reabsorption impairment in, 176
Primary hyperparathyroidism, defined, 298
Primary hypophosphatemic rickets (*see also* Vitamin-D-resistant rickets) 323–335
Primary renal tubular phosphate hyperexcretion, 323–340
Propranolol, phosphaturia and, 166
Prostaglandin secretion, phosphate level and, 178
Protein phosphorylation, 100–101
Proximal tubular micropuncture data, 144
Proximal tubular reabsorption
  bicarbonate infusion and, 214–215

Proximal tubular reabsorption (*cont.*)
    calcitonin in, 156
    luminal membrane of, 81
    phosphate secretion in, 43–45
Pseudohypoparathyroidism, 349–353
    cAMP excretion in, 351
    phosphaturic response to parathyroid hormone in, 197
    "Pseudohypoparathyroidism type II," 197–198
    vitamin D therapy and, 199
Pseudopseudohypoparathyroidism, 350

Raja erinacea, 61
Rat, extracellular fluid volume expansion in, 266–270
Reabsorped fraction of filtered load, 20–22
    equation for, 20
Renal acidification studies, phosphate in, 227–231
Renal clearance techniques, in assessment of phosphate secretion by mammalian kidney, 67–69
Renal disease, heredity in, 322
Renal failure
    parathyroid hormone levels in, 314
    phosphate excretion in, 315
    renal handling of phosphate in, 307–317
    serum phosphorus concentration in, 313–316
Renal handling of phosphate [*see also* Kidney(s); Phosphate]
    antidiuretic hormone and, 142–145
    calcitonin in, 154–157
    calcium and, 287–303
    catecholamines in, 163–167
    choice of indices in, 29–32
    diuretics in, 265–280
    estrogens in, 175–177
    extracellular fluid volume expansion and, 265–280
    growth hormone and, 139–141
    hormones other than growth or parathyroid, 137–179
    indices for measurement of, 1–32
    insulin and, 160–163
    parathyroid hormone in, 115–130, 308
    phosphate concentration threshold in, 5–8, 17–19
    in renal failure, 307–317

Renal handling of phosphate (*cont.*)
    following renal transplantation, 316–317
    thyroid hormones in, 147–151
    vitamin D and, 197–204
Renal hemodynamics, calcium effect on, 290–291
Renal phosphate handling, *see* Renal handling of phosphate; Phosphate
Renal phosphate reabsorption (*see also* Phosphate reabsorption), 209–231
Renal transplantation, 316–317
Renal tubular absorption, calcium infusion and, 291–292
Renal tubular reabsorption, *see* Tubular reabsorption; Phosphate
Renal tubular transport, *see* Tubular transport
Renal tubules
    hypersensitivity of, 328
    "pores" of, 231
Reptiles, phosphate secretion by kidneys of, 63–65
Respiratory acidosis and alkalosis, phosphate transport and, 92
Rickets
    calciopenic, 340–341
    oncogenous, 335–337
    primary hypophosphatemic, 323–335
    vitamin-D-resistant, 300–302

Secondary renal tubular phosphate hyperexcretion, 340
Serum inorganic phosphate, calcium effect on (*see also* Phosphate), 287–288
Serum phosphate, *see* Phosphate
Serum phosphorus concentration, in renal failure, (*see also* Phosphate; Phosphorus), 313–316
Sodium-dependent phosphate transport, 126–128
Sodium excretion, osmolar clearance and, 162
Sodium reabsorption, inhibition of, 126–128
Sodium transport, phosphate transport and, 127–128
Splay
    analysis of, 11–13
    cause of, 15–17
    defined, 11
    measurement of, 14–15

Splay (*cont.*)
  Michaelis constant and, 16
  phosphate threshold concentration and,
    9–16
Squalus acanthias, 61
Superficial nephron (*see also* Loop of nephron; Nephron)
  phosphate delivery in distal tubules of, 51
  phosphate reabsorption by loop of, 46

Terminal nephron (*see also* Nephron; Superficial nephron)
  phosphate transport in, 50–54
  possible sites of phosphate reabsorption
    in, 54
Thiazides, in phosphaturia, 278
Threshold concentration, in glomerular filtration, 5–11
Thyroid hormones
  phosphate levels and, 145–147
  phosphate metabolism and, 146–147
  and renal handling of phosphate, 147–151
Thyroparathyroidectomy, dietary phosphate response to, 248
Thyrotoxicosis, vitamin D metabolism in,
  148–149
Transmembrane channel, 83–84
Transmembrane movement, 80–87
TRP, *see* Tubular reabsorption of phosphate
Tubular adaptation
  mechanism of, 259–260
  to phosphate demand of organism, 249–252
  phosphate transport disorders and, 260
  role of $1,25(OH)_2D_3$ in, 252–254
Tubular cells, phosphate excretion and, 59–60
Tubular defects, in phosphate reabsorption,
  321–354
Tubular epithelium, permeability of to buffer
  system components, 226–227
Tubular fluid alkalinization
  cAMP level and, 123
  role of, 128–130
Tubular phosphate reabsorption, *see* Tubular reabsorption of phosphate
Tubular phosphate leak, 323–349
Tubular phosphate retention, disorders involving, 324
Tubular phosphate transport (*see also* Phosphate transport)
  controlled variables in, 243

Tubular phosphate transport (*cont.*)
  direction of, 4–5
  overall capacity of, 244–245
Tubular reabsorption of phosphate (*see also*
  Phosphate; Phosphate reabsorption),
  20–24, 31
  bicarbonate infusion and, 214
  calcium infusion and, 301, 310
  increased rate of, 16
  in pregnancy, 176
  sites of, 39–55
Tubule, proximal, *see* Proximal tubule
Tumoral hyperphosphaturia, phosphate level
  and, 178–179

Urinary acid excretion, phosphate excretion
  and, 161
Urinary pH, reduction of (*see also* pH), 209
Urinary phosphate excretion (*see also* Phosphaturia) 1
  plasma phosphate concentration and, 13–15
  in renal failure, 315
Urine alkalinization, 93–94
  phosphaturia form, 213

Vasopressin, phosphate level and (*see also*
  Antidiuretic hormone), 142
Vertebrates, phosphate turnover in, 4
Vitamin D (*see also* 1,25-Dihydroxyvitamin
  D_3)
  in osteomalacia, 352
  in renal handling of phosphate, 197–204
Vitamin D deficiency, phosphate reabsorption and, 340–343
Vitamin-D-dependency rickets (*see also* Vitamin-D-resistant rickets), 343–345
Vitamin D metabolism, in thyrotoxicosis,
  148–149
Vitamin-D-resistant rickets, 323–335
  cAMP levels in, 330
  clinical and laboratory features of, 325–328
  with hypophosphatemia, 300–302
  pathogenesis of, 328–334
  therapy in, 334
Vitamin D sterols, 137
Vitamin D therapy
  in animals, 200–202
  in hypoparathyroid subjects, 197

X-linked hypophosphatemic rickets (*see also*
  Vitamin-D-resistant rickets), 323–325